BLOOD CELLS IN NUCLEAR MEDICINE, PART II

DEVELOPMENTS IN NUCLEAR MEDICINE
Series editor Peter H. Cox

Cox, P.H. (ed.): Cholescintigraphy. 1981. ISBN 90-247-2524-0
Cox, P.H. (ed.): Progress in radiopharmacology 3. Selected Topics. 1982.
ISBN 90-247-2768-5
Jonckheer, M.H. and Deconinck, F. (eds.): X-ray fluorescent scanning of the
thyroid. 1983. ISBN 0-89838-561-X
Kristensen, K. and Nørbygaard, E. (eds.): Safety and efficacy of radiopharma-
ceuticals. 1984. ISBN 0-89838-609-8
Bossuyt, A. and Deconinck, F.: Amplitude/phase patterns in dynamic scinti-
graphic imaging. 1984. ISBN 0-89838-641-1
Hardeman, M.R. and Najean, Y. (eds.): Blood cells in nuclear medicine I. Cell
kinetics and bio-distribution. 1984. ISBN 0-89838-653-5
Fueger, G.F. (ed.): Blood cells in nuclear medicine II. Migratory blood cells.
1984. ISBN 0-89838-654-3

Blood cells in nuclear medicine, part II

Migratory blood cells

edited by

GERHARD F. FUEGER

Division of Nuclear Medicine
Department of Radiology
Karl Franzens University
Landeskrankenhaus
Graz, Austria

1984 **MARTINUS NIJHOFF PUBLISHERS**
a member of the KLUWER ACADEMIC PUBLISHERS GROUP
BOSTON / THE HAGUE / DORDRECHT / LANCASTER

Distributors

for the United States and Canada: Kluwer Boston, Inc., 190 Old Derby Street, Hingham, MA 02043, USA

for the UK and Ireland: Kluwer Academic Publishers, MTP Press Limited, Falcon House, Queen Square, Lancaster LA1 1RN, England

for all other countries: Kluwer Academic Publishers Group, Distribution Center, P.O.Box 322, 3300 AH Dordrecht, The Netherlands

Library of Congress Cataloging in Publication Data

```
Main entry under title:

Blood cells in nuclear medicine Part II, Migratory
   blood cells.

   (Developments in nuclear medicine)
   Based on a satellite symposium of the Third Congress
of thr World Federation of Nuclear Medicine and Biology,
held by the Austrian Society of Nuclear Medicine in
Graz, Sept. 4, 1982.
   Includes index.
   1. Radiolabeled leucocytes--Congresses. 2. Radio-
isotope scanning--Congresses. 3. Inflammation--
Research--Methodology--Congresses. 4. Nuclear medicine
--Technique--Congresses. I. Fueger, Gerhard F.
II. Österreichische Röntgengesellschaft--Gesellschaft
für Medizinische Radiologie und Nuklearmedizin.
III. World Federation of Nuclear Medicine and Biology.
World Congress (3rd : 1982 : Paris, France) IV. Series:
Developments in nuclear medicine (1984) [DNLM: 1. Cell
Movement--congresses. 2. Leukocytes--physiology--
congresses. 3. Nuclear Medicine--congresses. W1 DE998KF
/ WH 200 B6545 1982]
QP95.B56  1984        616.07        84-8055
ISBN 0-89838-654-3
```

ISBN 0-89838-654-3 (this volume)
ISBN 0-89838-660-8 (set)

Copyright

PRINTED IN THE NETHERLANDS

CONTENTS

VI

FOREWORD

G.F. FUEGER

Among the many processes in Physiology few appear more inviting to be studied by tracers and external imaging than the variety of the routes of migratory (blood) cells in health and disease. Much emphasis has been placed lately on the methods of labelling of the white blood cells. It is obviously quite important and necessary to refine the methods of leucocytic labelling, particularly to search for ways to label selectively a specific group of white blood cells, but there is also the need to review and keep abreast with the developing knowledge of the white blood cells themselves, especially their behaviour under pathological conditions, as seen by histology and scintigraphy, their biological properties, their immunological characteristics and the mechanisms of the control of leucocytic functions. Similarly, it appears desirable to analyze animal models of inflammation as well as to review the dosimetry and the biodistribution of labelled white blood cells in humans. This book is the result of a cooperative effort to review certain highlights of the physiology of leucocytes, labelled and unlabelled, as a corollary to the effort concerning the labelling of white blood cells.

In preparing this book we aim for a better understanding and definition of the goals to be achieved by the successful labelling of the migratory cells of the body.

CONTRIBUTORS

Becker, H.   Medizinische Universitaetsklinik der Uni-
                         versitaet Graz, Graz, Landeskrankenhaus,
                         haus, Austria

Bjurman, B.   Department of Radiation Physics, General
                         Hospital, Malmoe, Sweden

Chiles, C.   Radioisotope Service, VA Hospital, Palo
                         Alto, CA, USA

Colas-Linhart, N.   Universite Paris VII, Faculte de Medecine
                         Xavier Bichat, Laboratoire Biophysique,
                         Paris, France

Danpure, H.J.   MRC Cyclotron Unit, Hammersmith Hospital,
                         London, U.K.

Egger, G.   Institut fuer Funktionelle Pathologie,
                         Universitaet Graz, Graz, Austria

Fliedner, T.M.   Abteilung fuer Klinische Physiologie und
                         Arbeitsmedizin der Universitaet Ulm, Ulm/
                         Donau, FRG

Fueger, G.F.   Abteilung fuer Nuklearmedizin, Universi-
                         taetsklinik fuer Radiologie, Universitaet
                         Graz, Austria

Gainey, M.   Radioisotope Service, VA Hospital, Palo
                         Alto, CA, USA

Goodwin, D.A.   Radioisotope Service, VA Hospital, Palo
                         Alto, CA, USA

Haferkamp, O.   Abteilung fuer Pathologie, Universitaet
                         Ulm, Ulm/Donau, FRG

Hardeman, M.   Vaumont Laan 8, Heemstede, The Netherlands

Herbeck, R.   Max-Planck-Gesellschaft GI, Munich, FRG

Hofer, K.G.   Institute of Molecular Biophysics, Florida
                         State University, Tallahassee, USA

Johansson, L.   Research Institute of National Defence,
                         Umea, Sweden

Kirkpatrick, C.J.   Department of Pathology, University of
                         Ulm, Ulm/Donau, FRG

Krieves, D.   Radioisotope Service, VA Hospital, Palo
                         Alto, CA, USA

Lanzer, G.   Medizinische Universitaetsklinik der Uni-
                         versitaet Graz, Landeskrankenhaus, Graz,
                         Austria

Mc Dougall, I.R.   Department of Nuclear Medicine, Stanford
                         University Hospital, Stanford, CA, USA

Mattsson, S.   Radiophysics Department, General Hospital,
                         Malmoe, Sweden

Moisan, A.   Centre Eugene Marquis, Department des
                         Radio-isotopes C.H.R. de Pontchallou,
                         Rennes, France

Nicoletti, R.   Abteilung fuer Nuklearmedizin, Universi-
                         taetsklinik fuer Radiologie, Graz, Landes-
                         krankenhaus, Austria

Nosslin, B.   Department of Nuclear Medicine, General
                           Hospital, Malmoe, Sweden

Oberhausen, E.   Abteilung fuer Nuklearmedizin, Radiologi-
                           sche Universitaetsklinik, Homburg/S., FRG

Paldi, J.H.   Radioisotope Service, VA Hospital, Palo
                           Alto, CA, USA

Olsson, P.I.   Department of Radiation Physics, Univers-
                           ity Hospital, Lund, Sweden

Osman, S.   MRC Cyclotron Unit, Hammersmith Hospital,
                           London, U.K.

Persson, B.   Department of Radiation Physics, Univers-
                           ity Hospital, Lund, Sweden

Schroth, H.J.   Abteilung fuer Nuklearmedizin, Radiologi-
                           sche Universitaetsklinik, Homburg/S., FRG

Strand, S.E.   Radiophysics Department, University Hosp-
                           ital, Lund, Sweden

Thakur, M.L.   Division of Nuclear Medicine, Department
                           of Radiation Therapy and Nuclear Medicine,
                           Thomas Jefferson University Hospital,
                           Philadelphia PA, USA

Tilz, G.P.   Medizinische Universitaetsklinik der Uni-
                           versitaet Graz, Immunologielabor, Landes-
                           krankenhaus, Graz, Austria

Wissler, J.H.   Arbeitsgruppe Biochemie, Max-Planck-Insti-
                           tut fuer physikalische und klinische For-
                           schung, Bad Nauheim, FRG

ACKNOWLEDGEMENTS

Under the auspices of the Third Congress of the World Federation of Nuclear Medicine and Biology, the Austrian Society of Nuclear Medicine held a satellite symposium entitled "Labelled Migratory Blood Cells", in Graz, on September 4, 1982.

The meeting was organized by the Editor of this book and provided the opportunity for many distinguished scientists in this field to meet, and share their knowledge and experience. The review articles appearing in the present book are the result of this valuable scientific interaction.

The Dean of the Medical Faculty, Prof. Dr. M. Lechner, the head of the Universitaetsklinik fuer Radiologie, Prof. Dr. E. Vogler and the head of the Universitaetsklinik fuer Innere Medizin, Prof. Dr. S. Sailer, welcomed and supported the scientific effort.

My collegue contributors and I would like to express our appreciation to the Commissariat a l'Energie Atomique of France and Biomedica Radiopharmaceuticals, Vienna, whose generous support made the meeting possible.

Special thanks are due to Ms. C. Barowitsch who contributed so much to the organization of the meeting and the preparation of this book, to Ms. C. Dommayer who processed the manuscripts, and - last not least - to Ms. L. Ladurner who undertook the English language editing.

ABBREVIATIONS

10E12	= ten to the power of twelve (E = exponential)
10E-04	= ten to the negative power of four, i.e. 1/10000
cu.um	= cubic micrometre
deg.C	= degree Celsius (centigrade)
deg.F	= degree Fahrenheit
mCi	= millicurie
mSv	= millisievert
mGy	= milligray
SnCl(2)	= tin-II-chloride
u	= symbol used instead of greek letter "my"
uCi	= microcurie
ug	= microgram
ul	= microlitre

1 INTRODUCTION

J. G. McAFEE

In recent years, techniques for labelling blood cellular elements with gamma-emitting agents have attracted much interest. Labelled platelets have not become widely used clinically because their localization in thrombi more than one day old, and in atheromatous plaques, has not been completely satisfactory. Labelled platelets, however, have proved useful for research studies of platelet kinetics, vascular prostheses and drugs modifying platelet deposition. In contrast, many medical centres have established routine clinical techniques for leucocyte labelling, because the efficacy in localizing inflammatory foci has been better than with other agents. Nonetheless, many other centres have not adopted this approach, but rely on other modalities such as ultrasound, computed tomography and 67-Gallium imaging for abscess localization.

This book summarizes the current knowledge of the Physiology, Pathophysiology and some biochemical aspects of the various leucocyte populations. Different techniques of harvesting and labelling leucocytes are discussed in detail. Newer techniques of cell labelling are continually emerging in the literature, claiming efficacy for abscess localization. In our laboratory, however, we have found that many of these methods do not irreversibly label leucocytes. It is important to bear in mind that many radionuclides and their compounds will accumulate to some degree in abscesses merely as part of the humoral exudation from increased capillary permeability. Long ago, Pathologists studied abscesses by in-vivo injections of non-specific dyes and even inert colloidal carbon. The most important tests of any leucocyte-labelling method are: 1) measurement of the in-vivo recovery, survival in whole blood, circulating leucocyte pool, and plasma, and, 2) in-vivo tissue localization. Poor in-vivo distribution may not be reflected by in-vitro tests of cell function, as pointed out in this book.

The lipophilic chelates of 111-In still remain the best agents for non-discriminant labelling of leucocytes, judging by the inferior recovery, survival and organ distribution of their competitors. Even the 111-In labelled leucocytes do not closely mimic the behaviour of cells labelled with 32-DFP. The technique of labelling cells in small volumes of plasma with 111-In-tropolone is very appealing, but the in-vivo distribution is probably similar to that obtained with 111-In-oxinate, except for the lesser transient lung sequestration with tropolone. Labelling by phagocytosis of 99m-Tc colloids has not produced as high a recovery of leucocytes in the circulating pool as the 111-In chelates, apparently due to rapid hepatic sequestration. The profound metabolic changes triggered by phagocytosis may inevitably lead to their extraction from the circulation. Nevertheless, irreversible labelling with 99m-Tc, with good cell survival and recovery would have several advantages over the 111-In chelates.

The radiation dose calculations for 111-In leucocytes provided in Chapter 15 indicate higher levels, particularly for the spleen, than those encountered in other Nuclear Medical procedures. However, the biologically critical organ is probably the bone marrow - the site of radiosensitive undifferentiated blood cell precursors. In the USA, it is now common practice to administer 6 mCi of 67-Ga-citrate to adults to detect inflammatory lesions, as opposed to only 0.5 mCi of 111-In leucocytes. The resultant marrow radiation dose is estimated to be 3.5 rad (35 mGy) for the former, and 1.0 rad (10 mGy) for the 111-In leucocytes. The question of oncogenicity induced by chromosomal aberrations in radiation-sensitive labelled lymphocytes is again raised in this publication. The evidence from animal experiments, however, indicates that lymphocytes will not survive beyond 24 hours when 10E08 cells are labelled with more than 100 uCi of 111-In.

The authors of this book have pointed out the limitations and disadvantages of the "state of the art" techniques of leucocyte

3

harvesting and labelling. The current agents label many cell types indiscriminantly. Lymphocyte behaviour is markedly altered by the radiation effects from 111-In or other radionuclides accumulating in the nucleus. The most likely means of overcoming these limitations is the development of new ligands for specific cell-surface receptor proteins, for selective labelling of leucocyte types and subsets. Labelled monoclonal antibodies against cell surface antigens of human leucocytes, already developed for in-vitro cell sorting, should be explored for in-vivo applications.

The reader interested in leucocyte labelling and its application for in-vivo studies will find this book a valuable source of information.

2 HISTOPATHOLOGICAL INFILTRATIONS OF MIGRATORY BLOOD CELLS

C.J. KIRKPATRICK AND O. HAFERKAMP

2.1 INTRODUCTION

"Wenn man aber ... den Namen der "Eiterkoerperchen" fuer
die ein- oder mehrkernigen, farblosen, mit Contractili-
taet und dem Vermoegen amoeboider Formveraenderungen
begabten Zellen reservirt, so glaube ich in der
vorliegenden Arbeit neue Beweise dafuer beigebracht zu
haben, dass alle diese Koerperchen aus den Gefaessen
stammen, ganz sicher alle diejenigen, welche in den
ersten Zeiten einer acuten Entzuendung auftreten."

(If one reserves the term "pus body" for the mono- or
multinuclear colourless cells capable of contracting and
changing shape in an amoeboid way, then I think I have
contributed new evidence in the present article that all
these bodies originate in the blood vessels, and
certainly all those bodies which appear in the early
phases of acute inflammation.)

Julius Cohnheim (1869) (1)

The foundation of our knowledge of the histopathological appearances of inflammation goes back to the 1860's, to the studies
of Julius Cohnheim (1861) (2). His work included descriptions of
the microscopic appearances of inflamed tissues with the accumulation of inflammatory cells. Since then, our understanding of
the inflammatory process has deepened considerably, although many
questions remain unanswered. The function of the Pathologist's
rewiew paper in this book is to set the "morbid anatomical scene"
to remind us of the disease processes which we are trying to localize and study with the help of labelled migratory blood cells.

Inflammation is characterized by the infiltration of involved tissues by inflammatory cells. Histologically, the infiltrate can be composed of three basic cell types: neutrophils, lymphocytes and macrophages in various forms. We would like to take each of these three cellular components and briefly delineate some of the disease processes in which a particular inflammatory cell type tends to predominate. However, it should be stated at this point that this classification is somewhat artificial, as inflammatory infiltrates containing all three cell types in varying proportions may be present in an inflamed tissue. Nevertheless, it is possible to delineate certain disease processes in which one cell type is particularly conspicuous.

There are certain diseases in which the macrophage has one of the leading roles. The majority of macrophages are derived from blood monocytes. This was shown by various labelling experiments carried out in the 1960's, using, for example, tritiated thymidine (3,4) or carbon labelling (5). Paz and Spector (6) reported that a significant monocyte migration occurred within 6 hrs after an appropriate stimulus, with predominance of these cells in the lesion after 24 hrs. More recently, Issekutz et al. (1981) in Canada (7), using 51-Cr labelled autologous monocytes in rabbits, have shown that the accumulation of these cells in response to the intradermal injection of E. coli is substantial even one hour after inducing the lesion, although the maximum rate was observed at 3-4 hrs. They stressed that monocytes migrate out of the circulation simultaneously with neutrophils. In acute inflammation, the numbers of neutrophils that emigrate are large, but their short life-span means that their numbers decrease with time. Macrophages, on the other hand, have a life-span which can be measured in months (8).

2.2 MONOCYTES

Four disease processes can be presented as illustrative of inflammatory diseases with a tendency towards predominance of monocytes: interstitial pneumonitis, desquamative pneumonitis, Crohn's disease and chronic granulomatous disease of childhood.

The term "interstitial pneumonitis" describes a large group of disease entities often of unknown aetiology and affecting the interstitial tissues of the lung. In certain cases the agent responsible is a virus. Early changes include a mononuclear cell infiltration in the peribronchiolar and interstitial alveolar planes. In Figure 1a, blood monocytes can be seen marginating in the pulmonary capillaries and emigrating into the interstitial tissues. Other forms of interstitial pneumonitis include sarcoidosis of the lung (9) and so-called desquamative interstitial pneumonia (DIP) (10). The latter disease is now considered to be a response of the lung to injury and has been described in association with exposure to various forms of dust (11). Affected areas of lung are firm and greyish-yellow in colour. Histologically, in advanced cases, the alveoli are filled with alveolar macrophages (Figure 1b), and (from electron microscopic studies) type II pneumocytes (12).

Crohn's disease can affect the entire digestive tract from mouth to anus. The pathological changes are well known: skip lesions, cobblestone appearance of the mucosa, thickening of the bowel wall and formation of fissures and fistulas (13,14). Figure 1c shows the typical macroscopic appearance. Whilst lymphocytic, plasma cellular and neutrophilic infiltrations are present, in many cases granulomatous tubercles predominate. The granulomas formed are conspicuous by the paucity of neutrophils in many cases. Typically, epitheloid cells with Langhans-type giant cells are found (Figure 1d). Studies carried out during the last decade have shed light on the reason for the relative absence of neutrophils in certain cases (15,16). It has been observed that the leucocyte migration rate in patients with Crohn's disease shows a late phase in response to a chemotactic stimulus and is reduced compared with normal controls (15).

Chronic granulomatous disease of childhood is a syndrome consisting of chronic suppurative lymphadenitis, hepato-splenomegaly, eczematoid dermatitis and pulmonary infiltrations (17). The basic anomaly is an enzymatic neutrophil deficiency, the failure of the patient's neutrophils to kill bacteria after ingesting them. This appears to be due to the inability of the neutrophils to generate hydrogen peroxide (18). On histological examination, the skin shows extensive areas of necrosis with massive cellular infiltration. Interestingly, in advanced lesions, the predominant cell type is the monocyte with the formation of epitheloid cells and multinucleated giant cells (Figure 1e). Lymphocytes are also present. Figure 1f shows a monocytic infiltration around malignant cells from a colonic adenocarcinoma. However, it should be stressed that malignant infiltrations can be accompanied by practically the entire spectrum of migratory blood cells!

Fig. 1 a-f

a. Marginating (single arrow) and emigrated (double arrow) monocytes in and around a pulmomary venule in a case of interstitial pneumonitis.   Giemsa x 500

b. Pulmonary tissue from a case of desquamative interstitial pneumonia (DIP), showing the alveolar spaces filled with monocytes (arrow).   H + E x 35

c. Macroscopic picture of a segment of ileum affected by Crohn's disease. The bowel wall is thickened and the mucosa shows segmental areas of destruction (central portion of picture).

d. Microscopic appearance of the colon in Crohn's disease. Some lymphocytes and plasma cells can be seen. However, the histological feature is the granuloma formation (arrow) with monocyte-derived epitheloid cells and giant cells.   H + E x 350

8

e. Dermis taken from a case of chronic granulomatous disease
of childhood.   Infiltration by monocyte-derived epitheloid cells
(arrow), with giant cell formation.
Semi-thin section, toluidine blue   x 420

f. Monocyte   infiltration   (arrow)   surrounding   a   nest   of
malignant cells from a colon adenocarcinoma.   H + E x 350

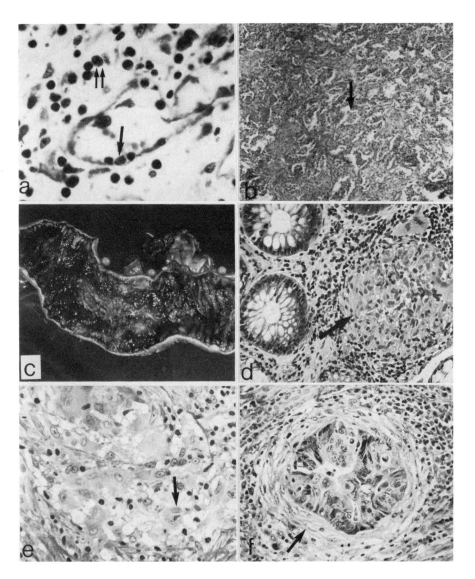

2.3 LYMPHOCYTES

T and B lymphocytes perculate through lymphatic tissues and mucosal barriers. The thymus-derived lymphocytes (T cells) are found in blood, in the thoracic duct, lymph, perifollicular and paracortical areas of lymph nodes, periarteriolar areas of the spleen and virtually all tissues to which lymphocytes have access. Lymphocytes are known to undergo a recirculation (19,20). T lymphocytes leave the bloodstream and enter lymph nodes via postcapillary venules in the paracortical regions, leave the lymph nodes via efferent lymphatics to the thoracic duct, and thence re-enter the bloodstream (21). Because of their long life and recirculation, these small lymphocytes are logical candidates for antigen recognition and immunological memory retention. The T cell plays the predominant role in cellular immunity. Immunity in this case is mediated by sensitized T lymphocytes. Delayed hypersensitivity, allograft rejection, graft-versus-host disease, immunity to intracellular parasites and contact allergy are examples of T lymphocyte involvement.

The essential pathological findings of two examples of T lymphocyte activity will now be briefly discussed: allograft rejection and graft-versus-host disease. Figure 2a shows the macroscopic appearance of a kidney which has undergone rejection. The outstanding feature is the widening of the renal cortex. The histopathological correlate is characteristic: marked tubular dilatation and extensive lymphocytic infiltration (Figure 2b). The acute graft-versus-host reaction, in which it is presumed that immunologically competent donor cells mount an immunological reaction against the host (22), is characterized by a triad of pathological changes: lesions in the skin, gastrointestinal tract and in the liver (23). Some histopathological findings taken from an autopsy case following severe graft-versus-host disease after bone marrow transplantation will be presented. In Figure 2c, the skin shows, among other changes, histiolymphocytic infiltration in the subepidermal region of the dermis with degeneration of individual keratinocytes (24). Various grades (I to IV) of skin involvement have been described (25). Chronic skin changes have also been reported. Thus, lichen planus-like lesions in the mouth and tongue and lichen planopilaris lesions on the trunk and limbs associated with a lymphocytic infiltrate can be present (26). In the liver the lymphocytic activity is focussed on the portal regions and can lead to a form of biliary cirrhosis (Figure 2d). A problem with the labelling of sensitized T lymphocytes is the fact that we are dealing in a particular situation with single clones of cells.

B lymphocytes tend to have a shorter life-span (days to weeks). They are located in the germinal centres of lymph nodes and spleen and in the subcapsular and medullary areas of lymph nodes. Stimulation of B lymphocytes to produce antibody and to become plasma cells is a complex process often requiring interactions between macrophages, T cells and B cells. The resulting sensitized B cell and plasma cell do not infiltrate through the tissues. They tend to stay at the site of stimulation (lymphatic tissue, mucosa) producing and excreting antibody immunoglobulin.

2.4 NEUTROPHILS

2.4.1 Tissue infiltration

Turning to the last of the cell types to be discussed here, it is obvious that labelling of this cell type holds much promise for the early diagnosis of acute inflammatory lesions. The disease processes in which the neutrophil predominates are legion. Disease processes of interest to those involved in the clinical application of blood cell labelling include pulmonary abscess, subphrenic abscess, ulcerative colitis, suppurative infection of orthopaedic implants and myocardial infarction.

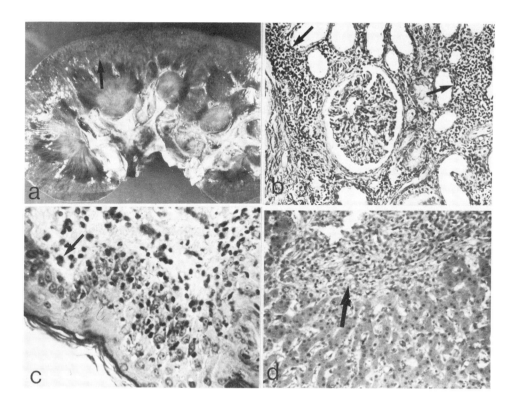

Fig. 2 a-d

    a. Macroscopic appearance of a renal allograft following
rejection. Note the marked widening of the renal cortex (arrow).

    b. Histological correlate of Figure 1a, showing marked
lymphocytic infiltration (arrow) of the renal cortex and
flattening of the tubular system.   H + E x 220

    c. Graft-versus-host disease in the skin, with
histiolymphocytic infiltration (arrow) of the subepidermal region
of the dermis. Signs of keratinocyte degeneration.   H + E x 350

    d. Liver tissue from a case of graft-versus-host disease,
showing a portal area (arrow) with three important pathological
changes: fibrosis, bile-duct proliferation and lymphocyte
infiltration.   H + E x 220

12

The authors wish to thank Professor Berno Heymer, Department of Pathology, University of Ulm, for kindly permitting us to publish the pictures comprising this figure.

2.4.1.1 The pulmonary abscess –

can assume various appearances, which are macroscopically apparent. Thus, the cut surface can be dry, as in the case of a fungal abscess (Figure 3a). The bacterial abscess lacks this dry appearance, although both forms show histologically a predominance of neutrophils. In the periphery of the abscess, in the so-called abscess membrane, necrotic lung tissue as well as numerous neutrophils are visible (Figure 3b). Many of these polymorphonuclear leucocytes are no longer viable.

2.4.1.2 Ulcerative colitis –

has been placed in the neutrophil group. As can be seen above, Crohn's disease was classified under the monocyte group. This was, of course, an oversimplification, because in both diseases practically all types of inflammatory cells can be found. However the histological hallmark of the early lesion of ulcerative colitis is the crypt abscess with accumulation of neutrophils in the crypts of Lieberkuehn and subsequent breakdown of the crypt wall. The extent of the mucosal destruction is evident in an advanced case, as illustrated in Figure 3c. Microscopically, a massive infiltration of the colonic mucosa with neutrophils was the predominant feature (Figure 3d).

2.4.1.3 Ischaemic disease of the bowel —

is often difficult to diagnose and is interesting because the histopathological picture is sometimes surprising. The material in Figure 3e originated from a 33-year-old man who suffered prolonged severe shock after polytrauma. The colonic mucosa displays segments that are necrotic and histologically characterized principally by neutrophils. The blood vessels were free from occlusion.

2.4.1.4 Occlusive ischaemic bowel disease —

In the case presented in Figure 3f, the patient suffered from atrial fibrillation and subsequent arterial embolisation with occlusion of the superior mesenteric artery. The result was acute haemorrhagic necrosis of the jejunum, ileum and part of the proximal colon. The microscopic alterations of the acute phase of ischaemic bowel disease are dominated by vascular congestion, oedema, haemorrhage and necrosis (27). The low-power histological view shows the typical mucosal and submucosal haemorrhage and necrosis (Figure 3g). However, on high-power examination (Figure 3h), we see mucosal necrosis, but a lack of neutrophilic infiltration. It is important in this disease to remember that at the optimal time for surgical intervention, the neutrophilic emigration has not yet occurred.

14

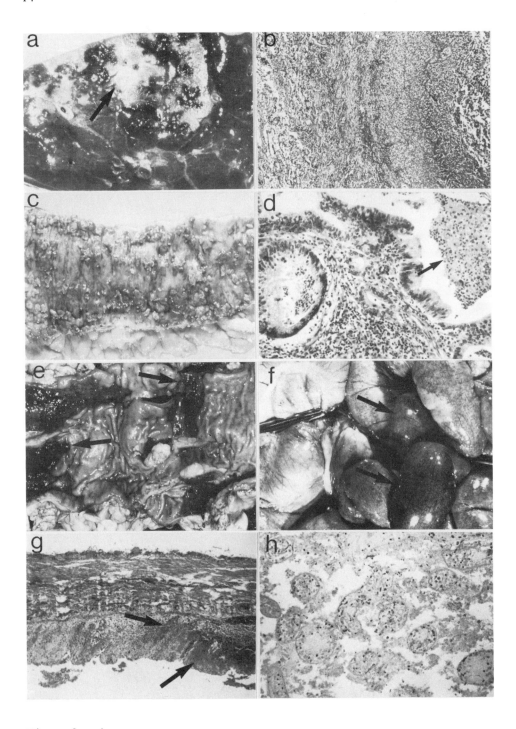

Fig. 3 a-h

Fig. 3 a-h

    a. Cut surface of a lung showing the dry lesion (arrow) of a fungal abscess.

    b. Histological appearance of the peripheral region of a bacterial abscess of the lung, showing necrotic pulmonary tissue containing numerous polymorphonuclear granulocytes.   H + E x 35

    c. Luminal aspect of a segment of colon affected by ulcerative colitis. Note the extensive mucosal destruction.

    d. Microscopic appearance of a crypt abscess, containing destruction of colonic epithelium and large numbers of neutrophils (arrow).   H + E x 280

    e. Luminal aspect of a colonic segment from a case of prolonged shock with ischaemia of the bowel. Discrete areas of mucosal necrosis are evident (arrows).

    f. Macroscopic appearance of the ileum in ischaemic bowel disease caused by occlusion of the superior mesenteric artery. Areas of haemorrhagic necrosis are marked (arrows).

    g. Histological picture of acute haemorrhagic necrosis of the small bowel with widespread destruction of the mucosa as well as focal areas of mucosal and submucosal haemorrhage. H + E x 35

    h. Higher-power view of acute haemorrhagic necrosis of the small bowel showing mucosal necrosis in the absence of a granulocyte infiltration. The dark precipitate is a processing artefact-formalin pigment.   H + E x 280

2.4.2 Intravascular margination

Next, we would like to turn our attention to a crucial aspect of the neutrophil, namely to its heterogeneity. This is of considerable importance in the labelling of migratory blood cells. Since the early 1960's, it has been known that intravascular neutrophils are distributed approximately equally between a circulating and a marginated pool (28). There are certain states in which a redistribution of the two neutrophil pools occurs, for example:
1) hydrocortisone-induced release of granulocytes from the bone marrow (29),
2) demargination induced by epinephrine (28), and
3) hypermargination caused during haemodialysis (30,31).

Fehr and Grossmann (32) regarded the circulating and marginated pools as functionally heterogenous. This conclusion was based on experiments using the above-mentioned methods of causing a shift in granulocyte pools. Thus, the activity of granulocyte alkaline phosphatase, a marker of cell maturity, as well as the ratio of segmented to non-segmented neutrophils, increased during epinephrine-induced demargination. This observation contradicted the concept of a qualitative equivalence of circulating and marginated pools of neutrophils.

This margination of neutrophils, which of course precedes emigration, can be seen histologically, for example, in myocardial infarction. In Figure 4a the typical macroscopic appearance of recent myocardial infarction can be seen with hyperaemic demarcation of the necrotic areas. Figure 4b illustrates what the older Pathologists used to term "leucocytic hyperaemia". The microscopic picture reveals that very many neutrophils are intravascular and aggregated, possibly as a result of intravascular activation of complement. The involvement of prostaglandins is also a possibility.

2.4.3 Pulmonary hypersequestration

Neutrophils are, of course, also implicated in the pathogenesis of pulmonary injury. Intra-alveolar generation of chemotactic activity causes the intra-alveolar accumulation of neutrophils - a familiar picture in bronchopneumonia (Figure 4c). By contrast, the intravascular generation of chemotactic activity (for example, complement activation during haemodialysis) causes shifting of neutrophils from the circulating to the marginated pool with increased cellular adherence to capillary and venular endothelium. The increased adherence is associated with sequestration of leucocytes in pulmonary microvessels. The neutrophils fail to migrate through the vessel wall because they are structurally, and possibly also functionally, altered. Furthermore, microvascular pressure is elevated.

In the past two years we have seen two such cases of pulmonary leucocyte hypersequestration in lung biopsies. The light microscopic picture revealed some areas of atelectasis and a definite widening of the alveolar septa caused by a hypercellularity (Figure 4e). Closer examination revealed that these granulocytes had been partially degranulated (Figure 4f).

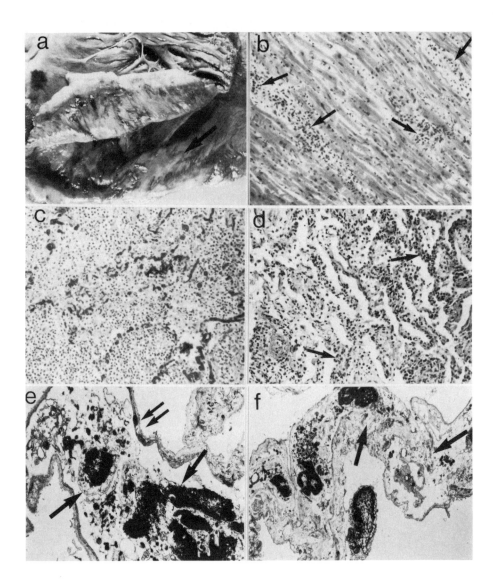

Fig. 4 a-f

Fig. 4 a-f

a. Typical appearance of a recent myocardial infarction with a hyperaemic and haemorrhagic zone (arrow) around the infarcted myocardial tissue.

b. Myocardial tissue adjacent to a myocardial infarct. Note the aggregation of neutrophils which are principally intravascular (arrows).   H + E x 220

c. Histological appearance of a bronchopneumonia, showing filling of the pulmonary alveoli with polymorphonuclear leucocytes.   H + E x 220

d. Pulmonary leucocyte hypersequestration, with broadening of the alveolar septa (arrows) and a definite hypercellularity.
                                                  H + E x 220

e. Electron micrograph of the case illustrated in Figure 4d. Note the aggregation of granulocytes (single arrows) within a pulmonary alveolar capillary (double arrow).   x 3150

f. Case presented in Figure 4 d + e, showing the partial degranulation of neutrophils (arrows).   x 2000

This type of phenomenon poses a problem for the labelling method, because, even if one can establish a localization of neutrophils in the tissue, how is one going to differentiate between intravascular and perivascular or intra-alveolar neutrophil accumulation?

Finally, it is hoped that this brief excursion into the realm of Pathology will serve as an "orientating introduction". The techniques for studying the in-vivo kinetics of labelled migratory blood cells should assist the clinician in detecting inflammatory lesions and thus aid prompt and effective treatment.

SUMMARY

Knowledge of the histopathological patterns of inflammatory cell infiltration of tissues is a prerequisite for a meaningful application of labelled migratory blood cells for diagnostic purposes. Each type of inflammatory cell is discussed separately and disease processes in which a particular cell type tends to predominate are presented both macroscopically and histologically. Monocyte involvement is illustrated in the context of interstitial and desquamative pneumonitis, Crohn's disease and chronic granulomatous disease of childhood. T lymphocyte activity is discussed using the examples of allograft rejection and graft-versus-host disease. Attention is drawn to the problems (from a Pathologist's point of view) associated with tracer labelling of the B lymphocyte. Of the innumerable acute inflammatory disease processes involving the neutrophil, the fungal and bacterial pulmonary abscess, ulcerative colitis and ischaemic disease of the bowel are presented. The concept of the circulating and marginated pools of intravascular neutrophils and its implications for tracer labelling are discussed, with reference to situations in which demargination or hypermargination may occur. The latter phenomenon is well seen histologically in acute myocardial infarction. Finally, observations on pulmonary leucocyte hypersequestration are presented.

REFERENCES

1. Cohnheim J.: Ueber das Verhalten der fixen Binde-gewebskoerperchen bei der Entzuendung. Virchows Arch. Path. Anat. 45:333-350, 1869.
2. Cohnheim J.: Ueber die Entzuendung seroeser Haeute. Virchows Arch. Path. Anat. 22:516-526, 1861.
3. Volkman A. and J.L. Gowans: The production of macrophages in the rat. Br. J. Exp. Pathol. 46:50-61, 1965.
4. Spector W.G., M.N.-I. Walters and D.A. Willoughby: The origin of the mononuclear cells in inflammatory exudates induced by fibrinogen. J. Pathol. Bacteriol. 90:181-192, 1965.
5. Hurley J.V., G.B. Ryan and A. Friedman: The mononuclear response to intrapleural injection in the rat. J. Pathol. Bacteriol. 91:575-587, 1966.
6. Paz R.A. and W.G. Spector: The mononuclear-cell response to injury. J. Pathol. Bacteriol. 84:85-103, 1962.
7. Issekutz T.B., A.C. Issekutz and H.Z. Movat: The in vivo quantitation and kinetics of monocyte migration into acute inflammatory tissue. Am. J. Pathol. 103:47-55, 1981.
8. Spector W.G. and D.A. Willoughby: The cells of the in-flammatory response. Eur. J. Rheumatol. Inflamm. 3:3-6, 1979.
9. Hagerstand I. and F. Linell: The prevalence of sarcoidosis in the autopsy material from a Swedish town. Acta Med. Scand. 176 (Suppl. 425), 171-173, 1964.
10. Liebow A.A.: Desquamative interstitial pneumonia. 59th Scientific Proc. Amer. Assoc. Pathol. and Bacteriol. Montreal. Am. J. Pathol. 41:127, 1962.
11. Patchefsky A.S., H.L. Israel, W.S. Hoch and G. Gordon: Desquamative interstitial pneumonia: relationship to interstitial fibrosis. Thorax 28:680-693, 1973.
12. Spencer H.: Pathology of the lung, Vol.2, p.770. Pergamon Press, Oxford, 1977.
13. Price A.B. and B.C. Morson: Inflammatory bowel disease. The surgical pathology of Crohn's disease and ulcerative colitis. Human Pathol. 6:7-29, 1975.
14. Haferkamp O.: Morbus Crohn und Colitis ulcerosa - Stand-ortbestimmung: pathologisch-anatomische Aspekte. Chirurg 52:737-743, 1981.
15. Segal A.W. and G. Loewi: Neutrophil dysfunction in Crohn's disease. Lancet 2:219-221, 1976.
16. Wandall J.H. and V. Binder: Leucocyte function in Crohn's disease. Studies on mobilisation using a quantitative skin window technique and on the function of circulating polymorphonuclear leucocytes in vitro. Gut. 23:173-180, 1982.
17. Millard M.: Lung, pleura and mediastinum. In: Pathology, edited by W.A.D. Anderson and J.M. Kissane, 7th Edition, p.1106. CV Mosby Co., St.Louis, 1977.
18. Stossel Th.P.: Congenital and acquired defects of neutrophil granulocytes. Schweiz. med. Wschr. 108:1577-1579, 1978.
19. Everett N.B., R.W. Caffrey and W.O. Rieke: Recirculation of lymphocytes. Ann. N.Y. Acad. Sci. 113:887-897, 1964.

20. Schnuda N.D.: Circulation and migration of small blood lymphocytes in the rat. I. Kinetics of lymphocyte circulation in the lymphoid organs. Am. J. Pathol. 93:623-638, 1978.
21. Mann R.B., E.S. Jaffe and C.W. Berard: Malignant lymphoma – a conceptual understanding of morphologic diversity. A review. Am. J. Pathol. 94:103-192, 1979.
22. Sale G.E., K.G. Lerner, E.A. Barker, H.M. Shulman and E.D. Thomas: The skin biopsy in the diagnosis of acute graft-versus-host disease in man. Am. J. Pathol. 89:621-636, 1977.
23. Slavin R.E. and J.M. Woodruff: The pathology of bone marrow transplantation. Pathol. Annual 9:291-344, 1974.
24. De Dobbeleer G.D., M.H. Ledoux-Corbusier and G.A. Achten: Graft versus host reaction. An ultrastructural study. Arch. Dermatol. 111:1597-1602, 1975.
25. Lerner K.G., G.K. Kao, R. Storb, C.D. Buckner, R.A. Clift and E.D. Thomas: Histopathology of graft versus host reactions in human recipients of marrow from HLA matched sibling donors. Transplant Proc. 6:367-371, 1974.
26. Saurat J.H., E. Gluckman, A. Bussel, L. Didierjean and A. Puissant: Graft versus host reaction and lichen planus-like eruption in man. Br. J. Dermatol. 93:675-681, 1975.
27. Alschibaja T. and B.C. Morson: Ischaemic bowel disease. J. Clin. Path. 30: Suppl. (Roy. Coll. Path) 11:68-77, 1977.
28. Athens J.W., S.O. Raab, O.P. Haab, A.M. Mauer, H. Ashenbrucker, G.E. Cartwright and M.M. Wintrobe: Leukokinetic studies. III. The distribution of granulocytes in the blood of normal subjects. J. Clin. Invest. 40:159-164, 1961.
29. Dale D.C., A.S. Fauci, G. DuPont and S.M. Wolff: Comparison of agents producing a neutrophilic response in man. J. Clin. Invest. 56:808-813, 1975.
30. Jensen O.P., L.H. Brubaker, K.D. Nolph, C.A. Johnson and R.J. Nothum: Hemodialysis coil-induced transient neutropenia and overshoot neutrophilia in normal man. Blood 41:399-408, 1973.
31. Craddock P.R., J. Fehr, A.P. Dalmasso, K.L. Brigham and H.S. Jacob: Hemodialysis neutropenia: pulmonary vascular leucostasis resulting from complement activation by dialyzer cellophane membranes. J. Clin. Invest. 59:879-888, 1977.
32. Fehr J. and H.-C. Grossmann: Disparity between circulating and marginated neutrophils: evidence from studies on the granulocyte alkaline phosphatase, a marker of cell maturity. Am. J. Hematol. 7:369-379, 1979.

3 PHYSIOLOGY AND PATHOPHYSIOLOGY OF MIGRATORY BLOOD CELLS

T.M. FLIEDNER

3.1 INTRODUCTION

This contribution reviews the cellular kinetics of the migratory blood cells, i.e. those cells in the blood of human beings that are in transit from one part of the organism to another, usually from the site of production to the site of emigration or removal (as in the case of granulocytes), but also from the site of transitory residence to another site of transitory residence (as in the case of "recirculating" lymphocytes). In the first part of this review, the principal functional structure of cell renewal systems is outlined in order to show that each migratory blood cell originates from a particular cell system that is under continuous renewal and guarantees a dynamic equilibrium between cell production and cell removal under the conditions of the normal steady state. In the second part of this presentation, data will be summarized to indicate, that each type of migratory blood cell has its own particular characteristics considering origin, migratory properties and destination. From this it will become evident that the term "leucocyte" is at best a historical term that should clearly be replaced by more specific terms not only in the case of neutrophilic, eosinophilic or basophilic granulocytes and monocytes but also in the case of lymphocytes, which again is a term embracing many types of mononuclear cells with quite different functional characteristics. As more subclasses of "mononuclear leucocytes" or of "lymphocytes" are being detected and characterized, it becomes obvious that there are among "lymphocytes" cells endowed with pluripotent haematopoietic potential which also need to be mentioned - at least briefly - when migratory blood cells are considered. They may well represent that population of leucocytes responsible for the maintenance of haemopoietic activity in the various sites of blood cell production distributed throughout the organism.

3.2 DETERMINATION OF THE KINETICS OF MIGRATORY BLOOD CELLS

The knowledge of the cellular renewal kinetics of the migratory blood cells and in particular of granulocytes, monocytes and lymphocytes is based on the use of cellular labelling techniques developed about 25 years ago, roughly between 1954 and 1964. Major advances were made possible through the possibility of labelling the DNA or RNA of cells during the different phases of their life cycle and to follow them or their progeny throughout their life span until death. Thus, the Physiology of the kinetics of most of the migratory cells of the blood of man became amenable to analysis when radioactive nuclides such as 32-P or 3-H were used to label cellular DNA of RNA or to bind to cellular enzymes as with 32-P-Di-isopropyl-fluorophosphate (32-P-DFP), (Table 1).

Ottesen in 1954 and Hamilton in 1956 labelled human lymphocytes and first suggested the existence of at least two populations with different cellular kinetics: about 20% were found to have a life span of two to three days, the remainder of 200 to 300 days. It was at the Brookhaven National Laboratory in December 1957 under the leadership of Eugene P. Cronkite, that the first human beings received tritiated thymidine to label haemopoietic precursor cells and to follow them through the various stages of maturation and function. With this approach, the first calculations about cellular renewal of granulocytes and monocytes were made and evidence for the longevity of lymphocytes was confirmed. The latter were then extensively studied in man by in-vitro labelling methods using tritiated cytidine which predominantly labelled RNA. In Salt Lake City, the group of Athens and Mauer introduced DFP labelled with 32-P or 3-H to label granulocytes. In our group these early studies were extended to the monocyte system, together with Meuret and in addition - together first with Cuttner and later in collaboration with Bremer

- to the lymphatic renewal system (reviewed in 1-6).

Table 1.   Early Labelling Methods to Study Leucocyte
                  Production and Migration Streams in Man

32-P:	Lymphocytes
Ottesen	1954
Hamilton	1956
3-H-TdR:	Granulocytes, Monocytes, Lymphocytes
Cronkite, Fliedner,	
Bond et al.	1958 - 1964
32-P- or 3-H-DFP:	Granulocytes, Monocytes
Athens, Mauer et al.	1958 - 1960
Meuret and Fliedner	1965 - 1969
3-H-C:	Lymphocytes
Fliedner, Cuttner,	
Bremer	1964 - 1975

More recently, the principal knowledge developed during the years up to about 1970 has been utilized in Nuclear Medicine to approach very practical problems: methods were developed to trace leucocytes to sites of infection and to determine cell kinetic parameters in a variety of disorders (Review 7,8).

Leucocytes were labelled in-vitro with 51-Cr-chromate. Although this method was used to study neutrophil turnover, it was apparent that leucocytes other than granulocytes became labelled. Thus, in cases of chronic lymphocytic leukemia, the autotransfusion of 51-Cr-labelled lymphocytes provided a tool for the study of the cellular turnover kinetics in this disorder. An advantage was that 51-Cr is a gamma emitting isotope that could be traced by external counting techniques. Thus, sites of sequestration and destruction could be detected, although they could not be imaged. However, due to the fact that several different types of leucocytes were being labelled, a careful evaluation of the results was necessary to recognize the migration properties of specific cells.

A group of most promising compounds to label leucocytes in-vitro for practical purposes are the relatively new 111-In-chelates, e.g. oxinate or tropolonate, 99m-Tc-colloids and others (see Thakur, Danpure, Oberhausen, Moisan, in this book). These compounds label blood cells effectively better than 85% in 15 minutes, and exhibit only minimal dilution, but, as was the case for other compounds, the In-chelates also are non-specific labels and attach to many cell types. Therefore, cell separation and purification procedures are necessary before exposing the cells to the compound. It has been shown that the collection and purification of neutrophils or other selected blood cells is feasible. The subsequent labelling with an 111-In-chelate and the autotransfusion make clinical studies possible. This general method has been developed best for the localization of abscesses. After an initial trapping in the lung, the cells migrate to the liver and spleen but accumulate in abscesses or other infiltrations of migratory blood cells if present in the body (see Kirkpatrick and Haferkamp, Chapter 2).

3.3 MIGRATORY CELLS AND THEIR ORIGIN IN CELL RENEWAL SYSTEMS

Migratory (blood) cells represent cell populations characterized by a very complex functional structure and dynamic development. In the adult mammalian organism all haematopoietic tissue such as is localized in bone cavities, in spleen, lymphnodes or thymus appears to be the result of the seeding of a cellular matrix by migrating cells. These migratory haematopoietic stem cells originate from extra-embryonic sites, such as the yolk sac, and find a transitory home in the foetal liver before the seeding into the stroma of thymus, spleen, lymphnodes and bone marrow occurs using the blood as a suitable vehicle (9). Thus, the most important migratory leucocytes are the stem cells that establish during embryogenesis the various sites of haematopoietic activity. Once these sites become haematopoietically active then the newly produced cells differentiate and will be discharged eventually into the blood stream to migrate to their final or transitory destination. "Migratory blood cells" in the adult organism originate from tissues, the function of which was established and initiated by some of their own kind, i.e. migratory stem cells. Therefore, it may be justified to consider all cells whose function is to establish and maintain haemopoietic activity (i.e. stem cells) as "first order" migratory cells in contrast to "second order" cells that originate from established intra- or extramedullary cell renewal systems and migrate to sites of functional activity. Second order migratory cells are the various forms of granulocytic, monocytic or lymphatic cells.

In the adult mammalian organism, migratory blood cells circulate as stem cells, or end cells (such as granulocytes or monocytes) or as transitory resting cells (such as "lymphocytes") originating from cell renewal systems, localized in the various sites of haemopoietic activity, such as bone marrow, spleen, lymphnodes, thymus. Their function is closely controlled by local microenvironmental mechanisms, but also by humoral as well as neural factors.

The structure of the cell renewal systems, the products of which may enter the blood stream and then migrate to sites of function, emigration or removal, is very similar in spite of the extensive differences in the migratory cells (10).

In the last 30 years, it has become evident on the basis of experimental studies, that all migratory blood cells have a common origin (Figure 1).

There is evidence for an omnipotent haematopoietic stem cell from which the T and B lymphocytes originate. However, between the stem cell pool and the migratory lymphocytes are developmental phases such as the "progenitor cells" of a restricted potentiality and residing in special microenvironmental sites (such as the thymus or "bursa equivalents"). In addition, the omnipotent haematopoietic stem cell pool feeds into the pluripotent "myeloid" stem cell pool, at least under regeneratory conditions. This part

28

of the haematopoietic tissue is localized under normal
circumstances in the bone marrow. These "myeloid" stem cells give
rise to progenitor cells with restricted potentiality (i.e.
granulocytic/monocytic, erythrocytic and megakaryocytic progenitor
cells) which can be measured by appropriate cell culture
techniques at least in certain animal species. The migratory
blood cells - neutrophils, monocytes, eosinophils - are the
products of the function of cell line specific renewal systems
(Review 7).

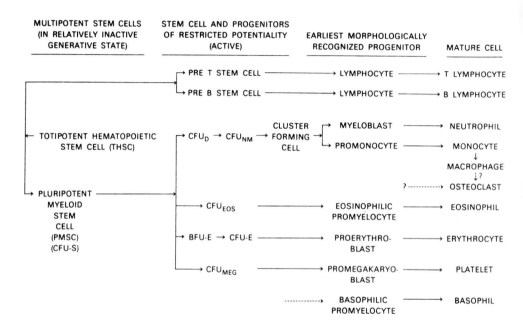

Fig. 1. Functional structure of blood cell forming
        systems as presented in Winthrobe 1981 (7)

In summary, the major "second order" migratory blood cells,
in particular the granulocytes, monocytes as well as T and
B lymphocytes, are products of cell renewal systems, each of which
possess their own functional structure, regulatory mechanisms and
turnover dynamics.

3.4   LIFE HISTORY OF MIGRATORY BLOOD CELLS

"Leucocytes" are so different in their characteristics that it is mandatory to study each cell type separately from the other. "Leucocyte studies" as such are relatively meaningless.

3.4.1   Neutrophilic granulocytes

It would be impossible to review the wealth of knowledge available today about the life history of the granulocyte (reviewed in 7). However, there is a consensus that the blood granulocyte pool consists normally of two subpools, the "circulating" (CGP) and the "marginal" (MGP) pool. It was found in 71 normal subjects (who were autotransfused with 32-P-DFP in-vitro labelled granulocytes) that these two pools are of about equal size [CGP = 31 x (95% limits 13-49) x 10E07 per kg body weight; MGP = 29 x (8-115) x 10E07 per kg body weight]. Under normal circumstances, the granulocytes disappear from the blood with a half life of 6.3 hours (95% limits 4-10 hours). According to 3-H-TdR autotransfusion studies, the time might be longer, such as 7.6 hours. - This means roughly that every day, the bulk of the blood granulocyte pool is turned over once. The blood granulocytes are released continuously from the sites of active blood cell formation. However, the mechanisms of the release are poorly understood. The "bone marrow-blood barrier" allows the retention of immature cells (such as metamyelocytes and myelocytes or promyelocytes). However, very immature cells, such as haematopoietic stem- or progenitor cells (which can be demonstrated by special cell culture methods (11) are able to enter the blood stream. The maturation time from the last division of granulocyte precursors to the release of their maturation products is about four days under normal conditions and may be shortened in infectious states to a minimum of two days (7). The transit time through the recognizable precursor compartments in which cell division occurs (myeloblasts,

promyelocytes, large and small myelocytes) is in the order of six
days as inferred from studies using tritiated thymidine as a cell
label. The fate of blood granulocytes is characterized by two
possibilities. A small fraction of cells remains in the
circulation and ages. Finally, these cells turn "pyknotic" and
are removed from the circulation. The time from release into the
blood until turning pyknotic has been found to be about 24 to
30 hours (12).

However, the great majority of cells emigrate from the blood
into the tissues. Labelled granulocytes have been traced normally
to the saliva. However, this may actually represent a response to
local inflammation in the oral cavity since the rate at which
granulocytes enter the oral cavity has been correlated with the
degree of gingivitis. Loss of granulocytes in the urine has also
been demonstrated in normal subjects. In addition, there are
losses into all relevant tissues such as lung, liver, spleen, and
gastro-intestinal tract. Whenever infection occurs as a local or
generalized phenomenon, there is a chain of events resulting in a
migration of granulocytes to the site of infection. This is
accompanied by marked undulations of the blood granulocyte
concentrations due to shifts between the circulating and marginal
blood granulocyte pools, to a shortening of granulocyte maturation
times, to an increase in granulocyte production in the marrow or a
sequential combination of all factors. The regulatory mechanisms
that are operative in the mobilization of granulocytes to
counteract the manifestation of bacterial infection or to act as
phagocytes have been reviewed extensively. It is enough to say
that many granulocyte changes relate to changing activities of the
adrenal cortex. The keyword "chemotaxis" should be mentioned (13)
since it is well known that granulocytes migrate to sites of
infection or digestion and that these unidirectional migratory
streams activate a variety of controlling factors (leucocytosis
inducing factor, "colony stimulating activity" etc.), (see
Wissler, Chapter 4). In cases of generalized bacterial infection,
the halflife of granulocytes in the blood may be shortened but
also prolonged (it varies between 4 and 14 hours). In cases of
neutropenia, the T 1/2 may vary from 2.2 to 7 hours.

3.4.2 Monocytes

The life history of blood monocytes has been studied extensively by Meuret et al. while working in our group (14). The model that is now generally accepted indicates very well that the blood monocyte is "in transit" from sites of production (bone marrow) to sites of activity (such as lung, spleen, liver, lymphnode, peritoneum, gastro-intestinal tract). The halflife of monocytes in the blood is about 8.4 hours with a blood compartment transit time of about 12 hours. The turnover rate of the blood monocyte pool was calculated to be about 7.0 x 10E06 cells per kg body weight per hour. The marginal monocyte blood pool is about 3.5 times the size of the circulating pool. The monocytes enter the blood at a rate of about 0.8 x 10E07 per kg per hour. They originate from a strong proliferating monocyte precursor pool that appears to be in equilibrium with a pool of non-proliferating, resting monocytes (in G(o)-cell cycle phase). There is evidence for at least two cell cycles between the stem cell level of cells and the non-dividing blood monocytes. The cell cycle time is comprised of a 10 hours DNA synthesis time, a 13 hours G 1- and 5 hours G 2-phase. After leaving the blood, monocytes transform into macrophages and become actively phagocytic. Traditionally one distinguishes between "fixed" and "wandering" forms. However, today there seems to be little if any reason for this subdivision and the differences noted may well be due to the different challenges that monocytes/macrophages have to face depending on the tissue site to which they have migrated. It is of interest to note that there are calculations to indicate that there are at least 50 times as many macrophages in the spleen, liver and bone marrow as there are monocytes in the blood. Of course, in cases of local or of generalized infection, there is a marked increase in the migratory stream of monocytes. The kinetics of these changes have to be carefully studied in individual patients. However, it has been found, that in septicemia, monocytopoiesis is enhanced in the marrow and the blood turnover rate is increased (see also Kirkpatrick and Haferkamp, Chapter 2, as well as Wissler, Chapter 4).

3.4.3 Lymphocytes

In contrast to neutrophilic granulocytes and to monocytes, the lymphocytes represent a very inhomogenous group of cells. Some years ago, Stutman and Good were able to distinguish 14 cell groups (that were all "lymphocytes" as far as light microscopical characteristics are concerned) with different functional potentialities (25). They appear to have one property in common: to recirculate (reviewed in 15). This property may be best characterized by a scheme as outlined in Figure 2.

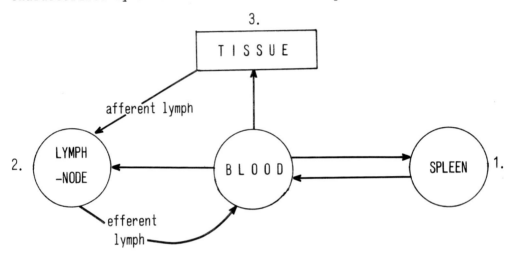

Fig. 2.   Lymphocyte migration streams as pre-
               sented in Theml and Begemann 1975 (15)

Small lymphocytes leave the blood stream on three routes and return on two. Every day, more than 10.0 x 10E09 lymphocytes enter the blood and leave it again. They all come from the lymphatic tissues and the bone marrow. Only a very small fraction of lymphocytes that enter the blood every day are newly formed. Most are "recirculating": they enter the blood, remain in it for a short period of time (about 30 minutes), and enter tissues where they remain for hours to days before they start the recirculation again. This recirculation may occur in three different ways: they may leave the blood, enter the white pulp of the spleen and return (Figure 2); they may leave the blood to enter lymphnodes and return to the blood via the efferent lymphatics (Figure 2), or they may go from the blood into the tissue, from there via the afferent lymphatics to the regional lymphnodes and from there via the efferent lymphatics to the blood (Figure 2).

The major part of the efferent lymph reaches the blood via the thoracic duct. Thus, lymphocyte kinetics can be studied effectively by thoracic duct drainage. The daily output of lymphocytes from the thoracic duct lymph is about equal to the total lymphocyte content of the blood (about 10.0 x 10E09 cells per day). The recirculating lymphocyte pool is about 25 times larger than the circulating lymphocyte pool. About 90% of blood lymphocytes circulate. The recirculating lymphocytes are mainly T cells. The portion of lymphocytes with "S"-characteristics in the thoracic duct lymph is (in the mouse) only 15%.

The life-span of lymphocytes is quite heterogenous. Short-lived lymphocytes (small, medium, large) have a life expectancy of 1-10 days; long-lived lymphocytes may reach a life-span of several hundred days. It may well be that there is no defined life span of lymphocytes and that they are eliminated from the blood at random. In the adult human only about 10% of the lymphocytes belong to the rapidly turning over cell population. The slowly turning over lymphocyte populations are mainly represented in the recirculating cell pool. These lymphocytes of slow turnover represent 90% of those present in the blood, 75% of those present in all of the tissues.

T lymphocytes are turning over slowly outside the thymus. In contrast, B lymphocytes outside the bone marrow consist of cells with slow as well as fast turnovers. Many of the plasma cells have a rapid turnover, their life span is in the order of 0.5-2 days. There are also "long-lived" plasma cells which are in the bone marrow but also in the blood.

It is of importance to finally point out the fate of lymphocytes. Three to five percent of lymphocytes are newly formed per day. Thus, an equal number has to disappear. The disappearance may occur in three ways. There is first the "transformation" of lymphocytes into other cells (for instance:

formation of immunoblasts that may form plasma cells). There is secondly the elimination of lymphocytes into the gastro-intestinal lumen; and there is finally cell death in all lymphatic tissues, primarily in thymus and lymphnodes (germinal centres) but also at sites of inflammation.

In diseases of the lymphocytic cell renewal, several aspects have been found to play a role in the clinical phenomenology (Figure 3).

PATHOPHYSIOLOGICAL FACTORS IN CLL

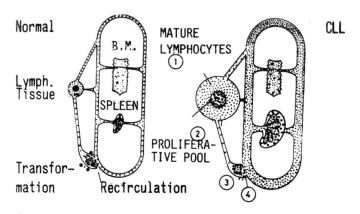

① Increased turnover times
② Increased production
③ Immunedefect
④ Perturbance of recirculation

Fig. 3. Model of lymphocyte migration streams under normal and diseased (CLL) conditions indicating the major sites of impairments

There is in chronic lymphocytic leukemia (CLL) an increased turnover time for lymphocytes and an increased production in the lymphopoietic tissue. In addition, there may well be cases with an immune defect and finally, there is evidence for a blockade of lymphocytes with respect to recirculation (Reviewed in 16,17,18).

3.4.4 Mixed versus selected populations of migratory blood cells

Thus, in summary, it is obvious that granulocytes, monocytes and lymphocytes have their very own characteristics of cell origin, cell developmental pattern, turnover and function. Therefore, any attempt to study "leucocytes" by radioactive labelling techniques can only be successful if the "leucocyte populations" are separated into classes of functional similarities. Whether the neutrophilic granulocytes are studied in health or disease, one has to purify and separate them from other cells (lymphocytes, monocytes). If the latter cells are to be studied, then granulocytes have to be removed and lymphocytes or monocytes can be studied separately. In autoradiographic labelling techniques, there is no need for cell separation since it is possible to distinguish the cells microscopically on the basis of their cytological characteristics in single cell autoradiography.

(Editor's note: For methods of cell separation see also round table discussion, Chapter 17)

3.5 CIRCULATING HAEMOPOIETIC STEM- AND PROGENITOR CELLS

Circulating haemopoietic stem- and progenitor cells were considered above as "first order migratory blood cells". The knowledge about this cell population has been reviewed extensively (15,19,20). It was A. Maximow in 1909 who published an article on "The Lymphocyte as a common stem cell of the different blood elements during embryogenesis and in the postfoetal life of mammals". Since then, the existence of a subpopulation of cells, morphologically indistinguishable from other mononuclear cells, termed "lymphocytes", has been first suspected and finally proven experimentally by haemopoietic reconstitution of lethally irradiated animals by mononuclear cells derived from blood (21). Since then, techniques became available to prove the existence of stem- or haemopoietic progenitor cells in suspensions of mononuclear blood leucocytes. These in-vitro techniques allowed, in mice, the demonstration in appropriate cell cultures of the existence of granulocytic, erythrocytic as well as megakaryocytic progenitor cells (11). The spleen colony forming assay by Till and McCullough (22) was used to show the presence of pluripotent stem cells in a cell suspension. In larger animals and in man, the essential findings of the murine system were confirmed. Therefore, the present "state of the art" with respect to circulating stem- and progenitor cells may be summarized as follows (23):

There is, in the blood, a small, but significant population of stem- and progenitor cells among blood mononuclear cells under physiological conditions. In dogs, the frequency is about one granulocytic progenitor cell measured as CFU-C (colony forming unit in culture) per 10 000 to 15 000 lymphocytes. There is a dynamic equilibrium between the intravascular and extravascular progenitor cells. In mice and in dogs, there is a mobilization of such progenitor cells from the bone marrow into the blood by certain chemicals (such as dextran sulfate) but also as a consequence of leucocytophoreses. These blood progenitor cells disappear from the blood at the same rate as they enter it but it is unknown what their fate is. It must be assumed that some cells simply "age" and die. But others may leave the circulation to seed in ecological niches suitable and prepared to accept them in order to produce haemopoietic "colonies". Such a "seeding" would be normal in the bone marrow but also in the lymphatic organs, in order to guarantee and maintain a continuous blood cell formation in the many different locations of haemopoietic activity throughout the skeleton. It is well known that extramedullary haemopoiesis occurs under pathological conditions. In this case, haemopoietic stem cells are probably activated by local microenvironmental factors to differentiate along granulo-, erythro- or megakaryocytic pathways. In the adult human or in larger animals, this cell production is restricted to the bone marrow sites. In pathological situations, such as myelofibrosis but also after total body irradiation and bone marrow transplantation, extramedullary haemopoiesis occurs in the spleen (24). It is evident that the origin of this abnormal haemopoiesis is the "migratory" stem cell. It would be desirable to be able to isolate and to radioactively label selectively the circulating haemopoietic stem cells in order to study the stem cell migration streams in the organism under steady state as well as under pathological conditions.

3.6 CONCLUSIONS

This review of selected physiological and patho-physiological characteristics of "migratory blood cells" has made evident that the term migratory blood cells encompasses a large variety of cells: First order migratory cells are circulating stem cells, which may establish haemopoietic activity. Second order migratory cells are end cells such as "granulocytes" and "monocytes", or "lymphocytes". The term "lymphocyte" denotes an unknown large number of cell types of different origin and functional destiny. Two of these "lymphocyte" types were found to have stem- or progenitor cell potentials. Therefore the enormous heterogeneity of "migratory blood cells" (both with respect to origin as well as to functional properties and destiny) requires very careful cell separation procedures before they can be labelled and traced by radionuclide techniques. Only if autoradiographic techniques are used, may one distinguish various cell types labelled by the same compound or nuclide (such as tritiated thymidine, - cytidine or tritiated DFP) in cell smears of histological sections and thus be able to draw conclusions on the dynamic behaviour of individual "migratory blood cells". If these precautions and reservations are observed, the modern tools of Nuclear Medicine may contribute significantly to the elucidation of cell line specific questions regarding the kinetics, function and fate of blood cells under physiological conditions. In addition, many important questions can be answered by these tools when the Pathology of events has to be evaluated, including the localization of inflammatory sites and abscesses as well as mechanisms of stem cell migration and seeding in the formation of extramedullary haemopoiesis.

SUMMARY

In the adult mammalian organism all haematopoietic or
lymphatic cell renewal tissues such as are localized in bone
cavities, in spleen, lymph nodes or thymus are the result of the
seeding of a cellular matrix by migrating omnipotent stem cells
which originate from extra-embryonic sites, such as the yolk sac,
and transiently reside in the foetal liver before seeding the
matrix in thymus, spleen, lymphnodes and bone marrow. Thus, the
"first order" migratory cells of the body are the omnipotent stem
cells. After having established haematopoietic or lymphatic cell
renewal tissues newly produced cells are differentiated and
released into the blood stream and migrate to their transient or
final destination. They are the "second order" migratory cells
comprising the various forms of granulocytes, monocytes,
lymphocytes etc. Very immature cells, such as haematopoietic
progenitor cells may leave the bone marrow, whereas the more
mature, but still immature cells such as metamyelocytes,
myelocytes or promyelocytes are retained in the bone marrow by
some kind of poorly understood structural or functional barrier.
Progenitor cells, normally present at low frequency in blood, may
leave the circulation to producer haematopoietic "colonies", if
need be, also in extramedullary locations under pathological
conditions.

REFERENCES

1. Stohlman F., Jr. (Ed.): The Kinetics of Cellular Proliferation. Grune and Stratton, New York, 1959.
2. Cronkite E.P., T.M. Fliedner, V.P. Bond, J.R. Rubini and W.L. Hughes: Dynamics of the proliferating cell systems of man studied with tritiated thymidine. J. Clin. Invest. 37:887, 1958.
3. Athens J.W. et al.: A method for labeling leukocytes with di iso propylfluorophosphate (32-P-DFP). Blood 14:303-333, 1959.
4. Cuttner J.W., E.P. Cronkite, M. Kesse and T.M. Fliedner: Behaviour of autotransfused in vitro 3-H-cytidine labeled lymphocytes in chronic lymphocytic leukemia. J. Clin. Invest. 43:1236, 1964.
5. Bremer K. and T.M. Fliedner: RNA metabolism of circulating lymphocytes studied in man after autotransfusion and in-vitro 3-H-cytidine labeling. Acta haematol. (Basel) 45:181, 1971.
6. Meuret G., G. Hoffmann, T.M. Fliedner, M. Rau, S. Oehl, R. Walz and Klein-Wisenberg, A. v.: Neutrophil kinetics in man. Studies using autotransfusion of 3-H-DFP labelled blood cells and autoradiography. Blut 25:97-109, 1973.
7. Winthrobe M.M. (Ed.): Clinical hematology. Lea and Febiger, Philadelphia, 1981.
8. Thakur M.L.: Cell Labeling: Achievements, Challenges, and Prospects. J. Nucl. Med. 22:1011-1014, 1982.
9. Kelemen E., W. Calvo and T.M. Fliedner (Eds.): Atlas of Human Hemopoietic Development. Springer Verlag Berlin, Heidelberg, New York, 1979.
10. Fliedner T.M., K.H. Steinbach and D. Hoelzer: Adaptation to environmental changes: The role of cell-renewal systems. In: The effects of environment on cells and tissues, edited by E.S. Finckh and E. Clayton-Jones. Excerpta Medica, Amsterdam-Oxford, pp. 20/38, 1976.
11. Metcalf D. (Ed.): Hemopoietic colonies. Springer Verlag Berlin, Heidelberg, New York (Recent Results in Cancer Research, Vol. 61), 1977.
12. Fliedner T.M., E.P. Cronkite, S.A. Killman and V.P. Bond: Granulocytopoiesis II. Emergence and Pattern of labeling of neutrophilic granulocytes in human beings. Blood 24:683-700, 1964.
13. Bessis M.: Living blood cells and their ultrastructure. Springer-Verlag Berlin, Heidelberg, New York, 1973.
14. Meuret G., J. Bammert and G. Hoffmann: Kinetics of human monocytopoiesis. Blood 44:801-816, 1974.
15. Theml H. and H. Begemann (Eds.): Lymphozyt und klinische Immunologie. Springer Verlag Berlin, Heidelberg, New York, 1975.
16. Schiffer L.M.: Kinetics of chronic lymphocytic leukemia. Ser. Hematol. 1:3, 1968.
17. Bremer K., P. Schick, O. Wack, H. Theml, B. Brass and H. Heimpel: Rezirkulation von Lymphozyten bei Patienten mit malignen lymphatischen Systemerkrankungen. Blut 24:215, 1972.

18. Queisser W. (Ed.): Das Knochenmark. Georg Thieme Verlag, Stuttgart, 1978.
19. Zwaan F.E.: Haemopoietic Progenitor Cells in Peripheral Blood. Blut 45:87-95, 1982.
20. Barr R.D. and J.A. McBride: Haemopoietic engraftment with peripheral blood cells in the treatment of malignant disease. Br. J. Haemat. 51:181-187, 1982.
21. Ford C.E., J.L. Hamerton, D.W.H. Barnes and J.F. Loutit: Cytological identification of radiation-chimaeras.
22. Till J.E. and E.A. McCulloch: A direct measurement of the radiation sensitivity of normal mouse bone marrow cells. Radiation Research 14:213-222, 1961.
23. Fliedner T.M., W. Calvo, M. Koerbling, W. Nothdurft, H. Pflieger and W. Ross: Collection, Storage and Transfusion of Blood Stem Cells for the Treatment of Haemopoietic Failure. Blood Cells 5:313-328, 1979.
24. Fliedner T.M., U.B. Wandl and W. Calvo: Medullaere und extramedullaere Haemopoiese im Hund nach Ganzkoerperbestrahlung und Transfusion von aus dem Blut gewonnenen Stammzellen. Schweiz. med. Wschr. 112:1423-1429, 1982.
25. Stutman O. and R.A. Good: Heterogeneity of lymphocyte populations. Rev. Europ. Etudes Clin. Biol. 17:11, 1972.

4 INFLAMMATORY EFFECTORS AND MECHANISMS OF INFORMATION PROCESSING
FOR CELLULAR REACTIONS AND COMMUNICATION IN REGENERATIVE TISSUE
MORPHOGENESIS BY LEUCOCYTES: CHEMICAL SIGNALLING IN POIESIS,
RECRUITMENT, KINESIS, TAXIS, TROPISM, AND STASIS OF CELLS

J. H. WISSLER

Dedicated to Prof. Dr. Joerg Jensen, University of Miami,
at His 65th Birthday

4.1   INTRODUCTION: MECHANISMS IN REGENERATIVE MORPHOGENESIS

For the renewal of supramolecular structures of tissue
patterns and functions, highly organized signalling devices in
cells are necessary for the reliable, discriminative and efficient
transmission of specific information and the display of selective
cellular responses. White blood cells and plasma, as major
components of the body's defense system in the inflammatory
process, provide chemical information in the form of effector
molecules, i.e. mediators of inflammation and wound hormones.
Mediators are substances transmitting information by autocrine or
paracrine mechanisms; hormones are substances transmitting
information by endocrine mechanisms; these distinctions are
detailed elsewhere (1). Effector molecules instruct tissue cells
to initiate the renewal of injured morphogenetic patterns. They
participate in the regulation of maintenance, regeneration,
replacement or loss of biological functions in tissues at their
impaired sites (1). There are four types of tissue patterns in
interactive cell systems which may be formed or maintained in
regenerative growth processes:
(a) The complete renewal of the original (conservative), life-experienced, physiological tissue pattern, as expressed in ontogeny;
(b) the regenerative formation of life-compatible, impaired
(conservative) tissue patterns; e.g. the formation of a locally
limited scar by filling a wound with structured connective tissue;

Fueger, G.F. (ed.), Blood Cells in Nuclear Medicine, Part II. ISBN 089838-654-3
©*1984 Martinus Nijhoff Publishers, Boston/The Hague/Dordrecht/Lancaster − Printed in the Netherlands*

42

(c) the (transient) formation of life-compatible, non-conservative tissue patterns; e.g. the formation of abnormal patterns of one cell type within interactive tissue systems, as shown for blood vessel systems in membranes, skin and muscle (1-3,156,157);
(d) the formation of life-incompatible tissue patterns; e.g. tumours and other degenerative tissue patterns.

Known until now are six basic categories with several sub-groups of chemical mechanisms which operate the interactive cellular reactions and communication systems that are intrinsic to these processes of regenerative formation of tissue patterns. Those chemical mechanisms with their definitions are compiled in Table 1: Chemopoiesis, chemorecruitment, chemokinesis, chemotaxis, chemotropism and chemostasis of cells, biological units and organisms are based and dependent on the ability of displacement and motion of subcellular and cellular units. In tissue regeneration by inflammation and healing processes, leucocytes and other participating cells follow (and are confined) in their organized behaviour (to) such chemical mechanisms. Figure 1 schematically illustrates some of the steps involved in the organized displacement and motion of leucocytes from their birth in the bone marrow (in the myeloid phase of haematopoiesis) (4) to their functional committment at (injured) tissue sites on formation of a "secretory leucocytic tissue" (1). It represents a functional expression of the haematopoietic and immune systems (effector network) (1).

This mobile secretory tissue can be organized and activated at various places, at different times and in alternative or identical cellular compositions in the body on request. It provides effector molecules of tissue morphogenesis (1) in the forms of wound mediators and hormones. Table 2 compiles their nature. They operate the organization of the inflammation and the healing processes as well as the whole life cycles of leucocytes themselves. From and to any of the reaction steps schematically shown in Figure 1, chemical feedback regulation is initiated and controlled by complex effector and enzyme networks. Their knowledge is yet only fragmentary. Chemical information residing in different structures (Table 2) is transmitted in both directions between the wound and target cells proximate and remote to the injury site by autocrine, paracrine and endocrine mechanisms (1, 5-7).

Some of the reactions of displacement and motion of leucocytes occurring in the organized function of the haematopoietic
and immune systems have been clearly recognized as based or
dependent on active cellular locomotion, e.g. chemokinesis and
chemotaxis (6, 8-20). For others, the participation of active
locomotion terms is still in question, e.g. in chemorecruitment
(6,8,19-27,156). Passive displacement and motion of leucocytes
without participation of active locomotion is obviously the major
mechanism of movement of leucocytes in the blood circulation, at
least within larger vessels. This passive displacement of
leucocytes is based on the ability of endothelial cells to form
tubes and closed circulatory loops (156,157) with active
haemodynamics (1-3,7,28-35). Endothelial cells are ontogenically
related to leucocytes in terms of their common origin from blood
islets in the early mesenchymal phase of haematopoiesis (4). The
relation of endothelial cells to leucocytes makes these cell types
appear similar in many aspects of their biological potencies, e.g.
their chemotactic, chemokinetic, metabolic or other properties
(36,158). Whether or not such reactions are specifically expressed
by cells in response to the chemical effector network of
leucocytes, and which possible recognition mechanisms are
intrinsic and distinct to them has not yet been clarified.

Cellular reactions and communication in reproductive cycles
(such as fertilization, embryogenesis and tissue regeneration by
wound healing, etc.) use displacement and motion of cellular
elements as mechanisms for the organization of supramolecular
structures. On one hand, they aim at the renewal and conservation
of biological patterns. On the other hand, they are in a
continuous trial of the survival value of new patterns for the
future. Pattern formation in interactive tissues is based on a
complex variety of involved cellular reactions and biological
signalling devices (1). This paper presents our present models of
mechanistic actions of cellular signalling devices for specific
cellular responses as evoked by chemical signals in the form of
endogenous polypeptide effectors of the regenerative process of
tissue morphogenesis in inflammation and healing.

44

Table 1. Basic Chemical Mechanisms Operating Cellular Reactions and Communication for the Reproduction, Regenerative Growth and Morphogenesis of Tissue Patterns
----
The compilation of the subgroups is incomplete, and yet limited by their relevance to the subject of this article

1. CHEMOPOIESIS OF CELLS AND ORGANISMS:
   Chemical control of growth in random directions, of cellular committment and storage.

   1.1. Hyperplastic and hypertrophic growth
   1.2. Differentiation (switching on/off of un-/expressed genes)
   1.3. Maturation (modulation of phenotype profile)
   1.4. Storage and compartmentation (of biologically quiescent cells)

   DEFINITION: Chemopoiesis is a reaction between cells and chemicals in their environment governing random growth, committment and storage of cells and organisms.

2. CHEMORECRUITMENT OF CELLS AND ORGANISMS:
   Chemical control of mobilization from storage pools

   2.1. Mobilization from primary (poietic) storage pools
   2.2. Mobilization from secondary (marginal) storage sites

   DEFINITION: Chemorecruitment is a reaction governing the mobilization of (biologically quiescent) cells and organisms from their storage pools into sites of functional readiness by chemicals in their environment.

3. CHEMOKINESIS OF CELLS AND ORGANISMS:
   Chemical control of random locomotion

   3.1. Orthokinesis (speed and frequency of locomotion)
   3.2. Klinokinesis (frequency of turning)
   3.3. Haptokinesis (adhesion and aggregation)
   3.4. Endocytosis
   3.5. Mechanokinesis

   DEFINITION: Chemokinesis is a reaction governing the motility of cells and organisms migrating at random by chemicals in their environment.

Table 1 (continued)

4. CHEMOTAXIS OF CELLS AND ORGANISMS:
   Chemical control of the direction of locomotion by recognition
   of dissipative (metastable) physical and chemical structures.

   4.1. Chemotaxis (locomotion along solute gradients of
        informative molecules)
   4.2. Haptotaxis (locomotion along surface gradients of
        informative molecules)
   4.3. Mechanotaxis

   DEFINITION: Chemotaxis is a reaction governing the direc-
               tion of locomotion of cells and organisms by
               chemicals in their environment.

5. CHEMOTROPISM OF CELLS AND ORGANISMS:
   Chemical control of the direction of (hyperplastic and
   hypertrophic) growth by recognition of dissipative
   (metastable) physical and chemical structures.

   5.1. Chemotropism (growth along solute gradients of
        informative molecules)
   5.2. Haptotropism (growth along surface gradients of
        informative molecules)
   5.3. Mechanotropism

   DEFINITION: Chemotropism is a reaction governing the direc-
               tion of growth of cells and organisms by chemi-
               cals in their environment.

6. CHEMOSTASIS OF CELLS AND ORGANISMS:
   Chemical control of homeostatic regulatory mechanisms for

   6.1. Maintenance and auto-repair of cells and organisms
   6.2. Maintenance of micro-environment of cells and organisms
   6.3. Maintenance of system of organization of cells and
        organisms

   DEFINITION: Chemostasis is a reaction governing homeostatic
               regulatory mechanisms of cells and organisms by
               chemicals in their environment.

Table 2.   Definitions of Humoral and Cellular Effector Substances

"Mediators"		are substances trans- mitting information by		autocrine and paracrine mechanisms
"Hormones"				endocrine mechanisms

(For details see references (1,5,156)

HUMORAL EFFECTORS

They are products of plasma protein degradation formed by limited, bond-specific proteolysis of biologically quiescent protein parent molecules.

Their formation may occur in cell-free plasma on its modification by contact reactions with intruded exogenous materials or with unmasked endogenous substances.

They are mainly activators and regulators of the inflammatory process.

CELLULAR EFFECTORS (CYTOKINES)

They consist of various structural groups, e.g. amines, fatty acid derivatives, steroids, amino acids, peptides and proteins.

They are formed by activated cells and brought into biological function by the secretion or exudation either of preformed or newly synthetized compounds.

They are mediators of inflammation and healing and comprise wound hormones.

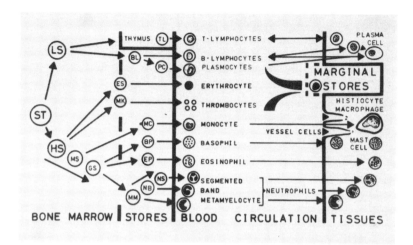

Fig. 1. Schematic representation of the course of life of white
cells from their production in the bone marrow (in the myeloid
phase of haematopoiesis) (4) to morphogenesis of a "SECRETORY
LEUCOCYTIC TISSUE", e.g. at injured tissue sites, as a functional
expression of the organization of the haematopoietic and immune
systems (1). It operates the various distinct types of chemical
mechanisms (Table 1) for cellular reactions and communication by
different (autocrine, paracrine and endocrine) transmission and
processing modes of the specific information intrinsic to chemical
signals of the effector network. Some of the reactions governing
the displacement and motion of leucocytes are clearly based on
active cellular locomotion (e.g. chemotaxis and chemokinesis). For
others, the participation of active locomotion is still in
question (e.g. chemorecruitment). Passive displacement and the
motion of leucocytes without participation of locomotion terms is
obviously the major mechanism of leucocyte movement within the
blood circulation, at least in larger vessels. For a further
description, see text and (1).

Abbreviations (alphabetically):

BL B-lymphocytes
BP basophil
EP eosinophil
ES erythroid stem cell
GS granulocyte stem cell
HS haematopoietic stem cell
LS lymphoid stem cell
MC monocyte

MK megakaryocyte
MM Metamyelocyte
MS myelopoietic stem cell
NB neutrophilic band
NS neutrophilic segmented WBC
PC plasma cell
ST pluripotent stem cell
TL T-lymphocyte

From (1).

4.2   ENDOGENOUS POLYPEPTIDES EFFECTING SPECIFIC CELLULAR RESPONSES

There are biologically specific effector polypeptides of humoral and cellular origin which regulate passive or active displacement, and motions of leucocytes and vascular (endothelial) cells. For their study, we have established methods for the isolation of polypeptide effector substances of humoral and cellular (leucocytic) origin. This is a little known group of signal molecules operating chemical mechanisms for cellular reactions and communication in regenerative morphogenetic pattern formation, as e.g. performed by inflammatory and healing processes. These signal peptides may be polypeptides of high biological specificity and they interact with the membranes of their target cells. As far as this process has been investigated, some conclusions could be drawn regarding the mechanisms of cellular recognition and transmembrane signal transmission.

As a result of these efforts, at least one representative of each group of specifically acting polypeptide effectors, either of humoral or of cellular origin (Table 2), have now been shown to exist for the selective operation of each of the basic categories of chemical mechanisms (Table 1). By the biotechnical methods devised (6,7,18,20,24,27, 33-35, 37-43,156), signal peptides can be isolated in a highly purified form and in physical (mg) amounts for further biological, chemical and clinical studies (1,2, 6-8, 10-19, 22-27, 33-47,157). In Table 3, a survey and summary of the work is given. The methods employed are reported in the references quoted.

Thus, earlier, humoral polypeptide mediators of inflammation specifically operating the chemotaxis of leucocytes (classical anaphylatoxin and cocytotaxin) have been described (6,8, 10-17, 19, 20, 44-46). Now additionally, in Figures 2 and 3, the cell- and reaction-specific actions of some of the recently isolated, biologically active polypeptide mediator preparations for cellular communication between adjacent cells in chemopoiesis (2A), chemotropism (2B), chemokinesis (3A) and chemotaxis (3B) are shown. They are cytokine representatives derived from leucocytes and represent chemical signals for short range intercellular com-

Table 3.   Summary of   Biotechnical Preparation and   Character-
            ization of Humoral and Cellular Polypeptide Effector
            Substances of the   Haematopoietic and Immune Systems
            (For details and references, see text)

1. Preparation of at   least 1 kilogram   (ca. 2.0 x 10E12) viable
   leucocytes of a physiologically composed population mixture
   from a minimum volume of ca. 200 litres of   aseptically   drawn,
   anticoagulated,   fresh blood, preferably porcine blood, per day
   and investigator by a new biotechnical process. Its first   step
   is   a   one-phase-batch   process   providing kilogram amounts of
   peripheral white blood cells in yields of (greater than or
   equal) 50% within a few hours. Concomitant preparation by the
   same process of all other blood components in their native
   state,   especially thrombocytes, erythrocytes, and blood plasma
   in kilogram amounts and at hectolitre scales, respectively, per
   day and per investigator.
2. Separation of the prepared kilogram amounts of mixed   leucocyte
   population into homogenous cell populations, especially neutrophil,   eosinophil and basophil granulocytes, monocytes and
   lymphocytes by a sequence of further (adsorption-desorption and
   flotation) steps of   the biotechnical process within a few
   hours.
3. Sterile culture of the kilogram quantities of   isolated   leucocytes   and   thrombocytes   in bioreactors of ten to fifty litre
   culture volumes in a new, fully synthetic,   serumfree,   chemically defined cell culture medium for production of cellular
   effectors (cytokines) operating basic chemical mechanisms of
   cellular   reactions and communication in regenerative tissue
   morphogenesis processes, with activities basic to functional
   expressions of the haematopoietic and immune system.
4. Twenty- to fifty-fold repetition of processes 1. to 3. provide
   from 10 000 litres of blood about fifty kilograms (one hundred
   trillion) of peripheral leucocytes of a physiological cell
   population mixture, or, correspondingly, about 29 kilograms
   (58%) neutrophil,   1.25 kilograms   (2.5%)   eosinophil   and
   0.25 kilograms (0.5%) basophil granulocytes, 3.5 kilograms (7%)
   monocytes (macrophages) and 16 kilograms (32%) lymphocytes.
5. Production, isolation, crystallization and characterization of
   biologically active,   humoral polypeptide effectors of
   inflammation from the isolated native blood plasma.
6. Production, physical isolation and characterization of
   biologically active polypeptide cytokine effectors for
   autocrine, paracrine (mediator) and endocrine (hormonal)
   information transmission in cellular communication systems: The
   kilogram amounts of isolated leucocytes and thrombocytes
   obtained from about 10 000 litres of blood result in ca.
   1 000 litres of culture supernatant solution. Then, on average,
   1-10 milligram quantities of highly purified, biologically
   active, reaction- and cell-specific inflammatory polypeptide
   mediators and wound hormones can be obtained with yields of
   about 10% by sequences of multiple purification steps. These
   polypeptide cytokine effectors display their reaction- and
   cell-specific biological activity above thresholds of picomolar
   concentrations or femtomol amounts.

50

7. For the first time, physical (milligram) quantities of at least one representative effector for the specific operation of each of the known basic categories of chemical mechanisms for cellular reactions and communication in regenerative tissue morphogenesis processes can be obtained separately by the biotechnical methods devised. These basic categories of chemical mechanisms are chemopoiesis, chemorecruitment, chemokinesis, chemotaxis, chemotropism and chemostasis of cells and biological units. Biological specificity of action of isolated leucocytic effector polypeptides implies specific mechanisms in signal reception, discrimination and transmission into cellular reactions within the cell and its membrane with which effectors interact.

8. "Wound hormones" as a new class of leucocytic effector polypeptides have been shown to exist for the first time. Hence, they substantiate this classical term by chemical objects and biological activities which were missing, so far. In contrast to leucocytic mediators, wound hormones specifically act by endocrine mechanisms of information transmission and conform to hormone definitions. Their existence proves leucocytes as truly unicellular, mobile endocrine glands ("secretory leucocytic tissue"). By their mediators, however, leucocytes may convey information also by autocrine and paracrine mechanisms of transmission for the operation of certain chemical mechanisms of cellular reactions and communication in regenerative tissue morphogenesis processes.

9. Wound hormones comprise novel cytokine entities for classical reactions in pathophysiology, e.g. the leucocytosis and, especially, "leftward shift reactions", i.e., the reactive increase in the number and the band/segmented ratio of circulating leucocyte phenotypes.

10. Molecular properties of mediators (angiotropins) for directional blood vessel sprouting (chemotropism of endothelial cells) suggest a novel mechanism operating the atherogenetic reaction: An endogenous "lesion" in the endothelium of the vessel ("intravascular leaky tip") is formed as a normal biological response in terms of a cellular reaction, i.e. impaired, intravascular sprouting, induced by angiotropins derived from intravascular monocytes. Such a "lesion" ("intravascular leaky tip") is not the response to intrinsic or extrinsic injury of endothelial cells itself, but a physiological, cellular reaction operated by wrong transmission mechanisms of information of the effector system to which cellular reactions and communication in the regenerative morphogenesis of tissues are subjected. Impaired (increased) permeability and perfusion disorders are brought about spot-wise in the asymmetrical endothelium of the vessel by this mechanism as a first step promoting the atherogenetic reaction. The directionally wrong hyperplastic growth of cells intrinsic to this mediator-disordered cellular reaction may be of monoclonal or of polyclonal origin.

11. Highly purified mediators of inflammation and wound hormones are potential models of natural pharmaceuticals whose specificity of action has been selected in evolution.

munication. They regulate displacement mechanisms of cells (Figure 1) within the haematopoietic and immune systems by active random and directional locomotion (Figures 2B,3A,3B) as well as displacement mechanisms for oriented movement of subcellular organelles (Figure 2A), e.g. in the mitotic cycle. Figures 4A and B show active polypeptide effector preparations for cellular communication between specific functional areas and distinct, remote biological units of the haematopoietic, immune and neural systems operating mechanisms of chemorecruitment and chemostasis. Thus, in chemorecruitment, displacement of cells from one biological unit (e.g. bone marrow storage pools of leucocytes) to another (e.g. blood circulation) occurs. At least for these endogenous chemorecruitment polypeptides isolated (6,7,23-27, 47,156), endocrine information transmission has been recognized as the underlying communication mechanism (1,6,7, 23-27, 47). Therefore, such polypeptides which are formed in wounds and which fulfil hormone definitions (5), are true "wound hormones". For the first time, they provide a chemical basis and biological function for this historic name (1,5,6). The cooperation of a number of such known, and probably some further still unknown, chemical mechanisms for the operation of cellular reactions and communication, make up tissue morphogenesis of life-compatible patterns in regenerative growth. As evidenced by the analysis of chemical factors involved, the regulation of of each of the basic categories of the operating chemical mechanisms (Table 1) is based on and composed of the interactive and cooperative actions of a diversity of chemical signals (1,2,5-8,12, 17-19, 24-27, 31-33, 36,38, 40-43, 48,49,156). The chemical effectors shown in this paper clearly represent only a few examples of the probably existing large diversity of factors. Most of them are still unknown today (1,2,6,7): The regenerative and interactive growth and turnover of blood vessel patterns in muscle and skin (2,157) can be initiated by one of the isolated chemotropism polypeptide effectors derived from monocytes ("monocyto-angiotropin", Figure 2B) (1,7,33-35). The self-regulation of their structure and (haemodynamic) functions, however, demonstrates this cooperative and interactive function of a multitude of chemical

52

signals (effector network) in the turnover of morphogenetic patterns of tissues (section 4.3.3.).

With highly purified, defined polypeptide effector substances, some new biological relationships between chemokinesis, chemotaxis and other mechanisms for cellular displacement, motion and locomotion reactions (with emphasis on chemorecruitment and chemotropism) could be elaborated so far. They are summarized below in the following topics (sections 4.2.1-4.2.4); namely, the biological cross-reactivity of endogenous polypeptide effectors in operating basic chemical mechanisms, the selectivity of mechanistic action of endogenous polypeptide leucotaxins, the regulation of random locomotion (chemokinesis) of leucocytes by endogenous polypeptide chemokinesins and the apparent existence of discriminating receptive units or reactions on cells for biologically specific cellular reactions and communication in tissue morphogenesis.

4.2.1 Biological cross-reactivity of polypeptide effector action

Basic groups of chemical mechanisms for cellular reactions and communication (Table 1) may be operated by the highly purified endogenous polypeptide effectors with high specificity, i.e. no cross-reactive cellular responses result from their action at their physiological concentrations. Thus, for example, leucotaxis and leucokinesis can be clearly distinguished from leucocyte recruitment as dissimilar chemical mechanisms. They are operated by effector polypeptides without cross-reactivity at physiologically relevant concentrations. This could be shown by the specificity of the action of all highly purified, and, in part, crystallized effector preparations obtained (6-8, 10-14, 18, 19, 24-27, 37, 40-47). Hence, mobilization of leucocytes from the bone marrow and their recruitment into the blood circulation is not operated by tactic or kinetic mechanisms which effect the infiltration of peripheral leucocyte types into tissue (formation of a "secretory leucocytic tissue"). Furthermore, chemotaxis and chemorecruitment of leucocytes may be elicited by polypeptide effectors with cell- and reaction-selectivity. Thus, these effectors have e.g. no febrile and (on endothelial cells) no chemotropic activity. The same lack in biological cross-reactivity can be shown for angiotropins, operating chemotropism of blood vessel (endothelial) cells (Figure 2B), in terms of chemotaxis, chemokinesis and chemorecruitment of leucocytes. All of them are also lacking leucocyte-proliferating activity at physiological relevant concentrations. Therefore, as far as we know at present, they do not operate major chemopoiesis mechanisms for leucocyte development (Figure 1), and are not directly involved in the homeostatic regulatory mechanisms of haematopoiesis (1,6,7,18,19,24-27, 33-35, 41-46, 47, 58,156) prior to storage reactions (47).

4.2.2 Selectivity in mechanistic action of leucotaxins

The high selectivity of mechanistic action and the lack of cross-reactivity of the highly purified endogenous polypeptide effectors (operating specific subgroups of a certain chemical mechanism of cellular reaction and communication) at present are best exemplified by leucotaxins, but similarly apply to others. Thus, the selectivity of the mechanistic action of chemotaxins for leucocytes does not appear to be constrained to the cell type chemo-attracted; or to the mechanisms of transmission operating local (paracrine) (1,5) or far range (endocrine or neural) signalling, (e.g. endocrine transmission mechanisms in leucocyte chemorecruitment) (Figure 4A): Chemotaxins also display high biological specificity not only in terms of chemotaxis and chemokinesis as defined major mechanistic categories, but also in terms of the subgroups (e.g. chemotaxis versus haptotaxis, etc.) of cellular reactions and communication (Table 1): In all cases, leucotaxins could be physically separated from leucokinesins, as is the case for leucorecruitment polypeptides and vice versa (Figures 3A, 3B and 4A).

1. Inhibitor of cell proliferation: Substance for braking distinct steps of the mitotic cycle (negative feed back mechanism)
2. Cell-specific action on (generative line of) secreting cell type family
3. Reversible, non-cytotoxic action
4. Local (short range) action

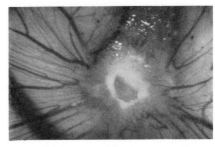

A.   B.

Fig. 2. Passive and active directional displacement and motion of subcellular organelles and cells regulated by leucocyte-derived effectors for the operation of cellular chemopoiesis and chemotropism mechanisms.

A.
Autocrine or paracrine cellular communication between mature, differentiated and immature, proliferating (generative) leucocytic phenotypes: Summary of a basic definition of a chalone (49,50). The reversibly acting, non-cytotoxic, cytostatic properties of some endogenous effector entities formed and exuded by leucocytes into supernatant solutions of biotechnical cultures conform to this definition (1,42,51,156). It applies to a purified granulocyte chalone preparation whose action is shown elsewhere [Figure 3 in reference (49)]. The effector reversibly inhibits the mitotic cycle and, thus, directed displacement of subcellular organelles in granulocyte proliferation and random colony formation in bone marrow leucocyte cultures. Together with a number of other identified, in part counteracting (mitogen) polypeptide effectors (41,43), it is one of the effector representatives for the (negative feedback) regulation of CHEMOPOIETIC mechanisms (randomly hyperplastic growth, Table 1).

B.
Paracrine cellular communication of leucocytes (monocytes) with vascular endothelial cells: Neovascularization of embryonic tissue (chorio-allantois membrane, CAM, of a chick embryo) by the biological action of a focally applied, monocyte-derived polypeptide effector ("monocyto-angiotropin", MAT) (1,156) for chemotropism (directional sprouting) of endothelial cells (1,7,33-35). MAT is one of the representatives of polypeptide mediators exuded by the different types of leucocytes on their biotechnical culture in-vitro or on their accumulation and activation in wounds in-vivo (e.g. in ischaemically injured, infarcted heart muscle sites), for the operation of CHEMOTROPIC mechanisms; i.e. active directional displacement and orientation of distinct cell types nascently formed by hyperplastic growth (Table 1). MAT (molecular weight given as hydrodynamic equivalent: 4 500) can be isolated in mg-amounts and in highly purified, biologically specific and active form after more than about 100 000-fold purification from about 1 000 liter supernatant solution of serum-free, mitogen-activated cultures of about 3.5 kg

55

(7 trillion) monocytes (macrophages). They can be processed by the
methods devised from about 10 000 kg porcine blood
(7,33-35,38-40,156). The figure shows an experimentally
vascularized CAM of an 8 day old embryo to which 5 fmol MAT has
been focally applied (on a filter paper) on the fifth day of its
life. The directional growth of blood vessels to the chemotropin
MAT is obvious. The resulting ("pathological") vessel pattern
shown deviates significantly from conservative ("normal")
reference patterns, as expressed without the addition of MAT in
the ontogeny of the embryo. Further details, reference patterns of
vascular structure, haemodynamic function, and turnover of
MAT-induced vascular patterns in other tissues are given elsewhere
(1,2,7,33-35,156,157). From (1).

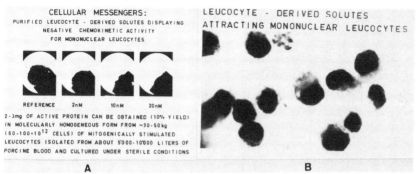

Fig. 3. Active random and directional displacement and locomotion
of cells regulated by leucocyte-derived effectors for operation of
cellular chemokinesis and chemotaxis mechanisms.

A.
Paracrine intercellular communication between the different
leucocyte types: Biological action of different concentrations (in
nmol/l) of a purified "lymphocyto-monoapokinesin" (LMAK)
polypeptide (molecular weight given as hydrodynamic equivalent
when derived from porcine lymphocytes: 14 000) in terms of
negative (apo-) chemokinesis (52) of porcine monocytes
(macrophages). Together with a number of other identified, in part
counteracting polypeptide mediators (17,18,156), this
lymphocyte-derived polypeptide is a representative for a
regulatory effector operating CHEMOKINETIC mechanisms in
leucocytes (monocytes): It reversibly inhibits (non-
cytotoxically) the displacement and motility of monocytes
migrating by active locomotion at random on surfaces. Its
preparation is achieved from activated, biotechnically cultured
porcine lymphocytes similarly to that, as quoted in Figure 2B for
MAT. The assay shown is performed according to the classical
method of Rich and Lewis (53) as inhibition of emigration of
monocytes from glass capillaries (Sahli type, 20 ul) in which the
cells had been densely packed. For reference assays, only the
reference medium comprising the components no. 1-93 of a
serum-free, fully synthetic, chemically defined cell culture
medium (7,39,156) is used. In the other assays the cytokine
polypeptide is added to this medium at the given concentration.

The migration areas of monocytes are measured after incubation of
the assembly at 37 deg.C [99% humidity, 3% CO(2)] for 20 hrs.
Polystyrol well-type incubation chambers (total volume: 500 ul) in
which the capillaries are mounted, are covered during the assay
with a gas-permeable membrane.

B.
Paracrine intercellular communication between different types of
leucocytes for chemotaxis of monocytes by granulocytes: Biological
action of a purified "granulocyto-monotaxin" (GMT) polypeptide
(molecular weight given as hydrodynamic equivalent when derived
from porcine granulocytes: 17 000) on porcine monocytes
(macrophages) in terms of their directional locomotion through a
filter membrane (8 um pore size). A modified Boyden assay system,
as described elsewhere, (19,46) was used for this purpose. The
figure shows monocytes which migrated through and adhered to the
lowermost surface of the filter after responding chemotactically
to 10 nmol/l GMT, and having been stained with Weigert's iron
haematoxylin by the described histological techniques (46).
Together with a number of other identified representatives (156)
of leucocyte-derived polypeptide mediators operating chemotactic
mechanisms in distinct leucocyte types, GMT is prepared from
biotechnically cultured porcine granulocytes similarly to the
other effector types presented (17,18,156).

The nomenclature used for the effectors is adapted from
agreed proposals (54,55). If not applicable, pre-syllables ("apo",
"pros-") are used according to Rothert (52) to specify "negative"
or "positive" chemokinesis. Three syllables are used for the main
name: The first is derived from the effector-producing cell; the
second from the target cell; the third specifies the reaction
operated by effectors.

Fig. 4. Displacement and conditioning of the microenvironment of
cells and biological units regulated by leucocyte-derived
effectors for operation of mechanisms of chemorecruitment and
chemostasis, respectively.

A.
Endocrine cellular communication between leucocytes and remote,
distinct biological units (leucocyte storage pools) of the bone
marrow in order to mobilize and recruit new leucocyte phenotypes
into blood circulation ("WOUND HORMONES"): Biological action of
"monocyto- leucorecruitin" (MLR) polypeptide in terms of an
endogenously induced transient, combined leucocytosis and leftward
shift reaction in a guinea pig by mobilization of immature and
mature leucocyte phenotypes from their bone marrow stores and
their recruitment into the blood circulation. The MLR polypeptide
(molecular weight given as hydrodynamic equivalent when derived
from porcine monocytes: 12 000) is one of several identified and
purified representatives of endogenous chemical signals for the
operation of CHEMORECRUITMENT mechanisms (1,6,7,156, 23-27). Its
preparation and purification is achieved from activated,
biotechnically cultured leucocytes (monocytes) similarly to that

quoted in Figure 2B for MAT. The figure shows the **blood** cell patterns and the kinetics of their changes prior, during (T = 0) and following the intravenous application (Vena saphena dextra) of 25 pmol MLR/kg guinea pig. These patterns and their kinetics were evaluated by periodical counting and differentiation of cell types in peripheral blood (Vena saphena sinistra) with classical haematological methods and given nomenclature (56-58). The reactive increase in the number (leucocytosis) combined with a reactive change of blood cell population differential in favour of immature cells (leftward shift) as long-lasting, transient response to MLR is obvious. For reasons of transparency, only granulocyte phenotypes are shown in the differential cell composition (upper panel). Endogenous substances for the induction of specific leftward shift reactions, as well as protein cytokines (chemorecruitins) for the induction of specific leucocytosis reactions combined with or without leftward shifts as classical phenomena in Pathology (6,57,58,156), were not at all known, so far. MLR and the other described chemorecruitin cytokines are the first evaluated polypeptides with these biological properties. They conform in their endocrine information transmission mechanism to the definition of hormone action (5).

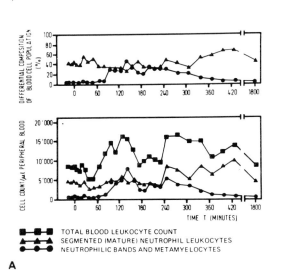

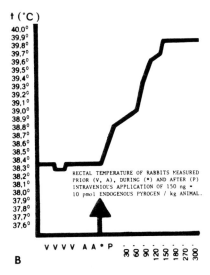

A

B

B.
The cellular communication of leucocytes (monocytes) with neural thermoregulatory centres (hypothalamus): The biological action of endogenous monocyto-pyrogen (MPY) polypeptide (molecular weight as hydrodynamic equivalent: 13 000) in terms of transiently and immediately induced febrile reaction of a rabbit (40). The assay is performed according to internationally standardized methods (59). MPY represents one of the signals operating chemostatic mechanisms (Table 1). However, whether it is a wound hormone, or a mediator, remains to be shown.

Thus, various biological and physico-chemical methods have shown (10-16, 60-63) that leucotaxins do not elicit any form of positive or negative leucokinesis. Furthermore, as far as evaluated for the humoral anaphylatoxin-associated leucotactic activity (6,8,19, 44-46), it was shown that by endogenous leucotaxins, neither the cellular speed in single steps of random locomotion is altered, as calculated from the distance travelled by the cell against time (12); nor do they change the total cellular velocity, i.e. the sum of cellular speeds and frequencies of locomotion and the magnitude and frequencies of cellular turning (change of direction), when calculated as displacement of the cell against time (12); e.g. from coordinates $(x,y,z) = (0,0,0)$ to $(x,y,z) = (a,b,c)$ as illustrated in Figure 5.

Therefore, the endogenous polypeptide chemotaxins investigated exert neither a positive, nor a negative effect, but they exert no chemokinetic activity on neutrophil leucocytes. Hence, they achieve accumulation of motile leucocytes specifically by chemo-attraction. The term "leucotaxin" (65) fully meets their properties. Chemotaxis by these highly purified leucotaxin preparations, thus, is a vector of cell migration constrained by the direction of an increasing concentration gradient of the leucotaxin. This vector of cell migration is superimposed on the normal, same locomotion scalar intrinsic to random cell migration which is subject to distinct regulation by endogenous polypeptide chemokinesins (e.g. Figure 3A).

Directional locomotion of leucocytes induced by the investigated endogenous polypeptide effectors is also not caused apparently by alteration of the intrinsic adhesion tendencies of cells to surfaces onto which they migrate. Therefore, in principle, chemotaxis of leucocytes by natural polypeptide effector substances in terms of direction finding (but not in terms of locomotion), is independent of the surface on which the leucocyte migrates by means of its intrinsic, surface-dependent motility: Contrary to the hypothesis of Carter (67) on surface-dependent cell taxis, Keller et al. (13,15,62) demonstrated that chemotaxis of leucocytes operated by endogenous polypeptide chemotaxins is no special case of cellular haptotaxis.

4.2.3 Regulation of random locomotion of leucocytes by effectors

The random locomotion, i.e. kinesis, of the leucocytes is regulated by endogenous polypeptide chemokinesins. Keller et al. (10-12,14) first defined a few humoral, positively acting chemokinetic substances (pros-chemokinesins) (52) for leucocytes. Their most prominent member was identified as serum albumin. Those workers clearly distinguished the pros-chemokinesins from the highly purified, humoral polypeptide mediators operating leucotaxis in terms of direction finding of a locomoting (positively chemokinetically activated) cell. The further search for defined endogenous substances regulating random cell locomotion has shown that chemokinesis of leucocytes is achieved by specific humoral AND cytokine polypeptide mediators distinctly different and physically separable from endogenous polypeptide leucotaxins of humoral or cellular origin (6,10-15, 17,18,51,62,63). Thus, endogenous positive and negative chemokinesins, i.e. pros- and apo-chemokinesins, respectively (52,55), for leucocytes exist. They can be isolated and separated from leucotaxins, leucorecruitins and other biologically active components present in plasma and supernatant solutions of biotechnically obtained, serum-free leucocyte cultures (6,17-19, 23-27, 33-35, 37, 40-46, 51,156). Figure 3A exemplifies the biological action (negative leucokinetic activity) of one of the isolated, lymphocyte-derived polypeptide mediators regulating the random locomotion of monocytes in terms of the inhibition of their migration (6,17,18). It substantiates the notion earlier made by Ward et al. (68) that lymphocytes may elaborate a factor inhibiting the migration of monocytes which is distinct from other cell-derived leucotactic activity. It also shows that in this case, migration inhibition of monocytes is due to a reversible, locomotion-regulative mechanism; namely by negative chemokinetic action, and not to cytotoxic effectors which are separable (156).

As far as mechanisms of action of reversibly acting, endogenous chemokinesins on cells have been investigated, the positive chemokinetic action of a polypeptide is most likely to be associated with lowering the average adhesion or aggregation tendencies of leucocytes to a given surface (6,13,15,16, 60-63). The negative chemokinetic activity of a polypeptide (e.g. as shown in Figure 3A) may be due to enforcing this average tendency. Therefore, the subtle equilibrium between reversible chemokinesin types, especially their capability to compete with the pros-chemokinetic action of the in-vivo ubiquitously present serum albumin, determines what average locomotion (in terms of displacement) prevails among the cells migrating at random; and what efficiencies the chemotaxins possess in terms of directional displacement (section 4.3.3). Clearly, the negative chemokinetic activity of a polypeptide can be distinguished from lowering of the efficiency of the average directional cellular displacement brought about by (diffusion non-equilibria of) chemotaxins in the form of solute-solvent boundaries (Figure 5B) by chemo-trapping of cells, as first shown by Wissler (8). It can be postulated that the positive chemokinetic action of serum albumin is possibly responsible for the low adhesion tendency of circulating leucocytes (Figure 5A). On one hand, positive chemokinesins are also necessary for efficient directional locomotion induced by chemotaxins (6,8,11-13, 15,19,62,66); since recognition of the direction of migration (vector, due to chemotaxins) can be shown not to account for the distances migrated by cells (scalar of locomotion, dependent on chemokinesins) (Figure 5) (6,8,10-12). However, serum albumin is always present in blood and extravascular, interstitial biological fluids. Hence, on the other hand, cytokine polypeptide effectors bearing negative leucokinetic activity (Figure 3A) may be of paramount importance in the accumulation of emigrated (pros-chemokinetically stimulated) leucocytes through the promotion of their cellular adhesion and aggregation tendencies at the reaction site of inflammation.

4.2.4 Specific cell responses by discriminating receptive units

Summarizing section 4.2, it becomes evident that the existence of discriminating receptive units or reactions on cells can be deduced from biologically specific, endogenous polypeptide effectors for cellular reactions and communication in tissue morphogenesis. The distinctive properties of the endogenous polypeptide effector substances are clearly superior (in molecular qualities) to the so far known, endogenous non-polypeptide mediators and to exogenous small peptides to which biological activity concerning the subject described could be attributed. Thus, for example, the biologically active, exogenous, synthetic small peptide leucotaxins (e.g. formyl-methionine derivatives), in contrast to the evaluated endogenous polypeptide effectors, display reaction- and cell-non-specificity: taxis, kinesis, adhesion, aggregation and also phagocytosis, etc., are biological reactions indiscriminately induced in leucocytes by them (69-75). Their properties suggested to postulate common receptors (69-74) at leucocyte membranes which indiscriminately convey information to the cell for concomitant display of such biological reactions. However, the existence of specifically acting polypeptide effectors clearly shows that cells are able to discriminate such signals: Discriminating receptive units or reactions for the different signals must exist at the cell surface; and cells are able to fulfil specific reactions dictated by a communication effector network of selective chemical signals. A direct comparison (in the same cellular reaction assay systems) of an exogenous small synthetic peptide with an endogenous polypeptide effector substance best exemplifies (62) that discriminating signal reception and transmission for specific cellular reactions are in existence.

Such molecular properties of effector substances or oligodisperse systems of them (effector network) can specifically operate distinct mechanisms for cellular communication in the regenerative growth of tissues. Their apparent intrinsic general principle is basic to any efficient and reliable information transfer in signalling devices: structure and specificity are information. The biological evolution is based on this principle of thermodynamics (76-78). This principle is also intrinsic to enzymology and immunology. It has been shown already to apply to mechanisms of chemo-attraction of phylogenetically primitive organisms (79). This work shows that in their fundamental behaviour, leucocytes are also confined to these laws of information theory: Active and passive displacement and motions of cells are basic expressions of life, and direction of motion makes expressions of life efficient.

4.3   MOLECULAR MECHANISMS OF CELLULAR RECOGNITION AND RESPONSE

4.3.1   Discriminative recognition mechanisms: Basic considerations

Discriminative mechanisms in effector-operated cellular reactions and communication can be visualized by means of models of molecular mechanisms of cellular recognition and responses. As demonstrated, the transmission of biological signals in the inflammatory and healing processes (Figure 1) are effected by mediators and hormones of different structural features to proximal and remote target cells and biological units. Targeting of biological units remote to the reaction site of inflammation and healing by specific chemical (polypeptide) signals emitted by secretory leucocytes and the wound plasma, has been exemplified in the chemorecruitment reactions, such as leucocytosis and leftward shift reactions (Figure 4A) (1,6,7, 23-27, 40). The direction finding of leucocytes and endothelial cells in chemotaxis and chemotropism (Figures 2B and 3B), and promotion or inhibition of motility and motions of cells and subcellular organelles in leucokinesis and leucopoiesis (Figures 2A and 3A) stand as four different examples of highly specific, close range signalling devices operated by polypeptide mediators at biological reaction sites involved in tissue injury. For communication with neural biological units, e.g. the hypothalamus, a chemostasis mechanism (temperature regulation) has been shown, for example, to be operated by a leucocyte-derived polypeptide effector, Figure 4B (1,6,8, 17-20, 33-35, 40, 44-47).

Concerning chemokinesis and chemotaxis, although of different efficiency for cell displacement, both mechanisms in principle may lead to the accumulation of leucocytes at the reaction site of inflammation. Obviously, the migration of cells is intimately associated with the mechanisms governing cellular adhesion and aggregation (Figure 5A). Their possible intimate relationship has been reflected also in Carter's hypothesis on haptotaxis and chemotaxis (67) (section 4.2.2). Furthermore, whether or not leucocyte mobilization from the bone marrow storage pools into the blood circulation should be a special case of chemokinesis or chemotaxis, and, thus, would follow the same mechanisms operating in the emigration of leucocytes from the blood circulation into tissues, are questions that find their answers in the evaluation of the specificity of chemical signals by which these and the other mentioned mechanisms are effected.

Thus, the recognition of reaction- and cell-specific chemorecruitment effectors which e.g. do not display chemokinetic and/or chemotactic activity on the cells to be mobilized from a storage pool, and vice versa, clearly distinguishes these from the other mechanisms. It answers those basic questions. In turn, the evaluation of the mechanistic specificity intrinsic to chemical effectors operating chemokinesis and chemotaxis of cells (section 4.2) allowed us to disclose in part the different nature of the two biologically intimately associated mechanisms shown schematically in Figure 5; and to bring about a notion as to how these two and the other described biological actions are discriminately functioning (6).

As mentioned, the definitions (Table 1) already show that e.g. chemorecruitment, chemokinesis, chemotaxis and chemotropism etc. are not special reactions of leucocytes or of other cells of the haematopoietic and immune systems in response to chemical stimuli. They are fundamental properties for displacement, motion and orientation of all living organisms and cells (3-6, 28-32, 52,58,65,67, 79-87). Historically, taxis and kinesis together with tropism were the first cellular reactions to environmental stimuli known and distinguished (52,65,82, 87-91). Engelmann (87) who detected the taxis reaction of cells in 1880, and Rothert (52) already found that various stimuli in the proximal cellular environment may cause cells to express different migratory behaviour: Apart from directed locomotion to chemical stimuli (chemotaxis), it is also possible to influence chemically the motility of cells migrating at random (chemokinesis) in terms of inhibition (apo-chemokinesis) or activation (pros-chemokinesis), (52). From investigations of the free migration of different organisms, Pfeffer (88) first concluded that cell taxis in general is subject to a special recognition process of the direction in which the cell finally moves. This same conclusion was drawn by Menkin (65) concerning the chemotaxis of leucocytes which was detected by Leber (90) in 1888. According to Delbrueck (83), the recognition and discrimination of specific signals comprises e.g. the information residing in the attracting molecules and their solutions, the mechanisms of transmembrane and specific transmission of this information into and within the cells, the translation of the environmental signal into distinct cellular responses (e.g. directional locomotion). In general, the term "specific chemical signal" has the meaning that a distinct cellular response is evoked by a chemical under negative exclusion of other effects. As to how far different, but often structurally similar polypeptides may elicit "specific" cellular responses, has been recently discussed by other investigators, too (94-96). Delbrueck stated that such signals and their processing remain, in general, a basic major concern of present research. They figure largely as "terra incognita of molecular biology" (83) and as the central problem to be solved. It concerns the behaviour of all organisms, cells and the specific mechanisms in the organization and function of molecular structures operated by them (5,6,8,11, 16,19,60,63-66, 71-73, 76-80, 83-86, 92-106).

Concerning the operation of chemical mechanisms for the organization of life-compatible patterns of molecular structures and cells in regenerative morphogenesis of tissues by inflammation and healing processes, on one hand, a large number of (about 1.0 x 10E04) specific signals are estimatedly necessary (40,156). They have to be transmitted into specific cellular reactions (with a maximum information of about 13-30 bits per specific response) (40,156). On the other hand, the limited space available at cell interfaces makes a general model in terms of a "one specific effector - one specific receptor molecule interaction" unlikely as the ONLY existing discrimination mode for evoking specific cellular reactions. Such unique, discrete sensory molecular structures which fit exclusively to one of the numerous effector molecules for specific interaction, may have evolved indeed in organisms in the special case of highly differentiated, specific sensory cells (or tissue units). An example for this case is discussed below and is illustrated in Figure 10. However, notably for leucocytes and other single, related cells involved in regenerative morphogenesis, the problem is, as to how an amoeboid-like, single cell by its unique membrane may handle at once reliable and efficient discrimination of numerous signals for display of a certain biological reaction.

Since the detection of specific cellular reactions to environmental stimuli, and, especially, since specific recognition processes intrinsic to chemotaxis of cells have been emphasized (88), a considerable number of models and mechanisms have been postulated for biological signalling devices in this and other biological phenomena (5,31,50, 64-67, 76-86, 88, 92-112). Most of the models and mechanisms so far evaluated consider and explain the responses of the cell, or the reactions of molecular structures, to one distinct biological signal under investigation. The mechanisms operating discrimination of different, concomitantly or consecutively emitted and received signals by cells and molecular structures, however, have been approached in only a few cases (detailed or summarized in 5,6,64, 65, 76-79, 8,93,96,100,112). The evolution theory of Eigen (77) stands as an example of such an approach. In order to understand the cellular and structural organization in inflammation and regenerative morphogenesis, models for recognition mechanisms of single (so far defined) chemical signals have also been developed as a first approach. Most of them were concerned with the chemotaxis of leucocytes (6,8,9,11,19,46, 70-73, 80-82, 108-111, 113-120), chemotropism and growth in three dimensions (1,3, 28-32, 92, 93, 101). Only recently, investigations were performed on the discrimination of chemical signals operating different chemical mechanisms for distinct cellular reactions. Thus, e.g., mechanisms involved in chemokinesis, chemotrapping and chemotaxis of leucocytes have been comparatively well investigated (6,8, 10-17, 60-63, 70-74, 80).

4.3.2 Discriminative recognition in cell taxis and kinesis: Model

This and the next section summarize our recent experimental studies and our (still fragmentary) model of the mechanisms of discriminative recognition and biological information transmission in cellular stimulation by "specific" chemical signals (in the form of the so far isolated endogenous polypeptide effector substances). In essence, it is a molecular model of cellular recognition in mediator-operated chemotaxis and of discrimination of cellular locomotion effects in chemokinesis. The information terms residing in solutions of biologically active endogenous polypeptide mediators shall be detailed. Their discrimination will be described in the processing of information by topochemically distinct multivalent binding patterns of effectors at (different sites of) cell interfaces, and by the separation of extracellular signal reception from intracellular transmission through cellular asymmetry centres. Since no comprehensive model of molecular mechanisms is available (so far) to detail the specificity of all the very different biological reactions communicated by the highly selective polypeptide effector molecules of inflammation and during the healing processes, further considerations still have to be restricted mainly to to chemokinesis, chemotaxis, chemorecruitment and chemotropism of the cells of the haematopoietic and immune systems (Figure 1).

Recognition is processing of information in a signalling device (Figure 6), consisting of a transmission channel and a receiver to which the emitted signal should be reliably and efficiently conveyed (122-124). For the chemotaxis of leucocytes as a basic mechanism in leucocyte infiltration and as a classical model for studying cellular recognition, the leucotaxin is the signal, the cell membrane the channel for transmission, and the receiver is the cell itself. It is instructed to direct its otherwise random locomotion to the emitting source (other cell or wound plasma) of the biological signal. Similarly, this applies to the chemotropism of endothelial cells which are instructed by another biological signal to grow hyperplastically in a certain direction. For chemokinesis of leucocytes, the distinct response of the cells to the chemical signals is a change in motility when migrating at random. In recruitment of the cells into the blood circulation, where they are in functional readiness, the distinct response of the cells to the chemical signal is the mobilization from quiescent residence storage pools (Figure 1).

Initially this investigation was aimed at the evaluation of structural equivalents of information terms residing in polypeptide effectors, and of the mechanisms of processing of those information terms in the same or different (ontogenically related) types of cells. For chemotaxis of neutrophil leucocytes, this investigation was directed toward the nature of the signal for direction finding (recognition of direction) conveyed to the cells by the isolated humoral leucotactic binary peptide system (anaphylatoxin and cocytotaxin) and the cytokine chemotaxins (6,8, 17-20, 37, 44-46, 51,125,126). Two basically different information terms were found to be distinguishable (schematically shown in Figure 5):

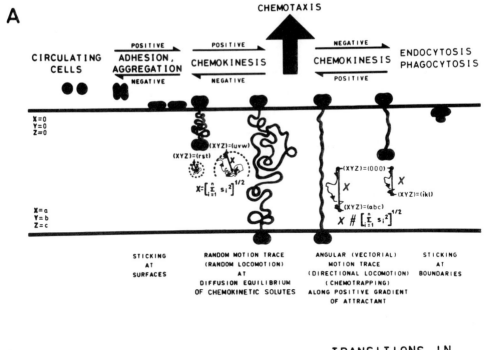

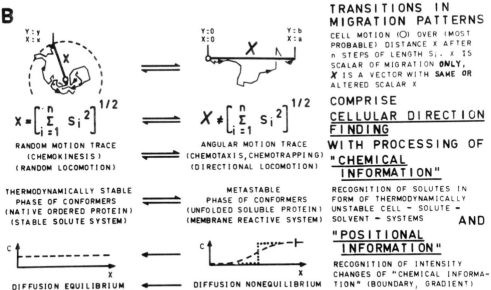

Fig. 5. Chemokinesis and chemotaxis of leucocytes by endogenous polypeptide effectors: Cellular reactions and recognition processes for transitions in the patterns of displacement and migration of leucocytes.

Schematic representations of:

A.
Cellular reactions of circulating leucocytes in response to and regulated by natural polypeptide effectors AFTER their chemorecruitment from their storage pools (Figure 1), for the emigration and accumulation at reaction sites in the tissue.

B.
Cellular recognition of information residing in dissipative (metastable) chemical and physical structures for finding of the direction by a locomoting (chemokinetically stimulated) cell. The terminology of Peterson and Noble (66) is adapted to describe the cell paths in taxis and kinesis by highly purified endogenous polypeptide mediators. The description shows that the efficiency of locomotion in direction is dependent on the influence of chemokinesins on the cells.

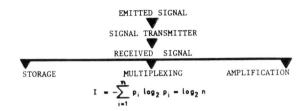

Fig. 6. Schematic presentation of structure and functions of a simple signalling device. The transmitted information I (expressed in binary digits or bits) is dependent on the number of different signals n emitted by the source and on the probability p(i) by which the ith signal occurs in the message. If the various probability states are all equally likely, maximum information is conveyed by the system. Then, I(max) is equal to the logarithm (base 2) of the number n of the various signals produced by the source (122-124). Discrimination may be achieved by separation of signal reception from signal processing. It may be exemplified by two different, formally limiting models, namely, transmission of messages through different, separated channels, or through a ratio detector in a receiver (filter effect).

4.3.2.1 The first information term

For directional locomotion without change of cellular motility (locomotion) scalars, the cell must be provided with a "positional information" (8,19,113,114). The positional information is conveyed by a concentration gradient, or a concentration boundary (concentration or diffusion non-equilibrium) of the "chemotactically active solute" (topic: second information term, see below). Without these dissipative physical structures, leucocytes cannot "migrate directionally"; or cannot be "trapped directionally", as they would be in case of a concentration boundary (Figure 5B, lowest panel). A concentration boundary is a concentration (stepwise) "gradient" at time zero $(T = 0)$, having an extension distance of zero $(x = a = 0)$. However, even without this positional information, the processing of the second information term ("chemical information", see below) which is necessary for recognition of direction, occurs independently. This, for instance, is the case at a concentration (diffusion) equilibrium of the chemotactic solute, when the physical structure intrinsic to the gradient or boundary is dissipated (6,9,15, 19,46,113,114). The used relationships between information and entropy terms intrinsic to dissipative or metastable physical and chemical structures are further detailed in the references (78,92, 122-124, 127-130), and, in part, schematically in Figures 5 to 7.

4.3.2.2 The second information term

For recognition of direction, the cell needs "chemical information". For a critical evaluation of the concept of "chemical information" used here for reasons of briefness, see reference (130). The question was about the nature of this term in solutions of polypeptide molecules of non-antibody structure which can exist in physico-chemically and biologically different forms (6,8, 108-110, 113-116, 136-138). Thus, e.g., investigations on the mutual structural influences of classical anaphylatoxin and cocytotaxin polypeptides combined in the function as leucotaxin

(6,8, 19,20, 44-46), have shown that in the presence of cocytotaxin, anaphylatoxin acquires a less compact polypeptide conformation than in its isolated, crystalline, native state. This and other terms used here are defined as follows:

"Native conformation" or "native state" is used to indicate a state (or phase) of many microscopic conformers, making up the macroscopically apparent native conformational state of a polypeptide, as generated within the normal physiological micro-environment and having a most compact three-dimensional spatial arrangement of amino acid residues. "Conformational state" or "conformer phase" is used to express the thermodynamic, macroscopic average properties determined by many microscopic states allowed for the system at a given temperature, pressure, etc. The term "unfolding" is used for reasons of briefness for a conformation less compact than the native state, as obtained by entropic parameters measured e.g. by viscosity, density, etc.

In this native state, anaphylatoxin is chemotactically inactive for neutrophil leucocytes at the same physiological concentrations as compared with the anaphylatoxin-cocytotaxin (leucotaxin) combination. In this binary polypeptide combination, anaphylatoxin in its less compact conformer phase plays the chemotactically active part (6,8,19,126). Similar findings on biological (chemotactic) activity to be acquired in anaphylatoxin when interacting within binary or oligodisperse polypeptide systems have been recently evaluated in several other laboratories (111, 131-135). The partial "unfolding" of anaphylatoxin, and thus, its transfer from a chemotactically inactive to a conformer phase chemotactically active for neutrophil leucocytes, can be measured by changes in viscosity, density and by fluorescence (6, 113-116). Changes in fluorescence are brought about by marker dyes of hydrocarbon regions on protein surfaces on exposition of the hydrophobic residues in the polypeptide chain of anaphylatoxin to the surrounding water molecules in which the polypeptide is dissolved. In addition, anaphylatoxin may acquire chemotactic activity for neutrophil leucocytes at comparable physiological concentrations in the absence of cocytotaxin, if transformed by non-physiological conditions in the solution into less compact conformer phases than in the native state. They are constrained by thermodynamic and kinetic criteria (6,9, 113-115, 136) and may be maintained for a longer period in restored, physiological media as ("metastable") thermodynamically unfavoured conformer phases. These metastable, dissipative conformer phases of anaphylatoxin under physiological conditions are the reactive phases of the cellular recognition process. Hence, as in the reactive, metastable conformer phases of this monodisperse anaphylatoxin solution, dissipative conformer phases of anaphylatoxin are the reactive, chemo-attractive principle for neutrophil leucocytes in the leucotactic binary polypeptide system under physiological conditions and concentrations of anaphylatoxin and cocytotaxin. Figure 7A schematically describes these relationships.

It shows that it may apply to other chemotactic substances of polypeptide or non-polypeptide structure of monodisperse or oligodisperse composition. This holds for any substance that forms in aqueous, physiological solution distinctly constrained, thermodynamically unfavoured, kinetically stable, dissipative states; e.g. by having exposed to surrounding water molecules a number of hydrophobic groups, yet not undergoing phase separation (6,8,19,44,45, 113-116). That conformational alterations in anaphylatoxin may be associated with the expression of its biological functions, has also recently been shown by others (119,120). This supports our original finding that it is a very fragile structural entity the biological functions of which are highly susceptable to changes of its conformational state, as is the case with other polypeptides (8,108-110,137,138).

From these results can be concluded that the structural equivalent of the "chemical information" (to be recognized and processed by the cell for direction finding) in the reactive, dissipative conformer phases of leuco-attractants is represented by negative entropic interactions of the polypeptide solute with solution (water) molecules. The information term intrinsic to this solute-solvent interaction is schematically shown in Figure 7B. This second information term (6, 113-115) is clearly distinct from Wilkinson's postulate (108-110, 137,138) that structureless (information-devoid random coil) conformations are recognized by the cell for direction finding. Nevertheless, both of our theorems agree in that conformational changes and exposition of hydrophobic groups in polypeptides in solution may cause them to acquire chemotactic activity for neutrophil phagocytes.

4.3.2.3 Information processing and psychophysics in chemotaxis

A phase separation process occurs on contact between the cell membrane and the dissipative conformer phase of a polypeptide. It is to be considered as the first reactive step and provides the driving force (about 33-50 kJ/mol) in the recognition process for processing of the intrinsic information. No postulate of a stereospecific receptor entity at the cell surface is a priori necessary for the operation of this recognition process for direction finding of neutrophil leucocytes (19, 113,114,136), as similarly suggested by Wilkinson (137,138). This lack of a requisite of a stereochemically specific receptor in this model does not ignore that such specific sensory receptor molecules may have also been evolved and exist: They are obvious e.g. in recognition and chemotaxis of sensitized leucocytes to appropriate antigens (Figure 10, section 4.3.3.).

The processing mechanisms of the two terms of information described above for direction finding are characterized by a non-linear relationship between the intensity of the stimulus (concentration of leucotaxin) on one hand, and the chemotactic response of the cell on the other hand (8,19,117,118,125,126, 136). The same results were obtained by Fernandez and Perez et al. (133,134). Keller et al. (10-12) found that this relationship conforms to known psychophysical laws (Weber-Fechner law) (105). It is characterized by a semi-logarithmic relationship, i.e. by a proportionality of the response (cellular directional locomotion) to the logarithm of the intensity of the stimulus (concentration of leucotaxin). This shows that information processing systems present in the membrane of the unicellular leucocytes (representing a primitive organism) have the characteristics of specific receptors in specialized sensory organs of higher organisms (105).

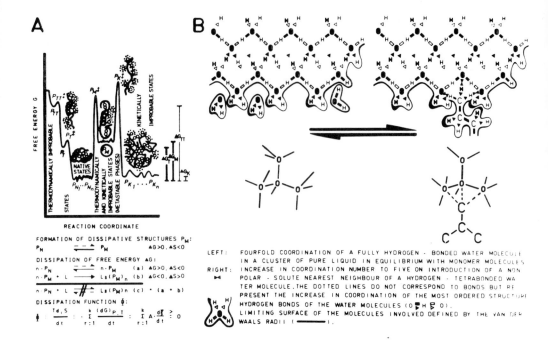

A

FREE ENERGY G

REACTION COORDINATE

FORMATION OF DISSIPATIVE STRUCTURES P_M:

$P_N \rightleftharpoons P_M$ $\Delta G > 0, \Delta S < 0$

DISSIPATION OF FREE ENERGY ΔG:

$n \cdot P_N \rightleftharpoons n \cdot P_M$ (a) $\Delta G > 0, \Delta S < 0$

$n \cdot P_M + L \longrightarrow L_a(P_M)_n$ (b) $\Delta G < 0, \Delta S > 0$

$n \cdot P_N + L \not\longrightarrow L_a(P_M)_n$ (c) $\cdot (a + b)$

DISSIPATION FUNCTION ϕ:

$$\phi : \frac{T_d, S}{dt} : -\sum_{r:1}^{k} \frac{(dG)_{P,T}}{dt} : \sum_{r:1}^{k} A \cdot \frac{d\xi}{dt} \geq 0$$

B

LEFT: FOURFOLD COORDINATION OF A FULLY HYDROGEN - BONDED WATER MOLECULE IN A CLUSTER OF PURE LIQUID IN EQUILIBRIUM WITH MONOMER MOLECULES

RIGHT: INCREASE IN COORDINATION NUMBER TO FIVE ON INTRODUCTION OF A NON POLAR - SOLUTE NEAREST NEIGHBOUR OF A HYDROGEN - TETRABONDED WATER MOLECULE. THE DOTTED LINES DO NOT CORRESPOND TO BONDS BUT RE PRESENT THE INCREASE IN COORDINATION OF THE MOST ORDERED STRUCTURE HYDROGEN BONDS OF THE WATER MOLECULES (O⫶H⫶O).

LIMITING SURFACE OF THE MOLECULES INVOLVED DEFINED BY THE VAN DER WAALS RADII (▬▬▬).

Fig. 7. Schematic representation of reactive chemical solute conformer phases and information terms for the cellular recognition of locomotion direction in the chemotaxis of neutrophil leucocytes (as shown in Figure 5).

A.

The free energy (G) profile of (polypeptide) solute transconformations and dissipative solute structures: Conformer phases P and their interaction with the leucocyte membrane (L) in the form of a simplified, general model for a polypeptide as a dynamic, flexible structure (statistic distributions). However, basically, none of the principles is constrained to polypeptides only, but may also apply to other structures. P(M) represents a thermodynamically unfavoured (metastable), reactive phase of conformers (section 4.2.2 to 4.2.4). For information processing in chemotaxis of neutrophil leucocytes, at physiological pH and conditions, it is constrained by minus delta G greater than or equal to 33-50 kJ/mol, by relative kinetic stability and by solubility of conformers within the water without fast progression of phase separation which would reflect a too negative second virial coefficient of the virial expansion of the solvent chemical potential (6,8,113-116,136). P(N) represents low energy transconformations, e.g. in allosteric transitions. For reasons of the constraints described, such reversible allosteric transitions as they are basic e.g. to enzyme regulatory mechanisms (154), may not be subject to cellular recognition in the chemotaxis of "normal" leucocytes (Figure 10) as defense cells (8,113,114). For alternative interaction of P(N) [instead of P(M) phases] with specific sensory receptor molecules on cell surfaces, see Figure 10. Other terms are subject to standard nomenclatures (76,78,112,127-130).

B.
The chemical nature of the (second) information term for cellular direction finding in leucotaxis: Negentropy (information) (123,127,130) of dissipative solute-solvent phase systems (right) in terms of the statistical-mechanical model of water structure (148,149). A cross-section of an equilibrium between flickering clusters of fourfold coordinated, fully hydrogen- (tetra-) bonded (most ordered) water molecules of very short life times (148,149) and free unbonded water molecules in pure water liquid, on one hand (left); and between partial flickering cages of such clusters of tetrabonded (most ordered) water molecules around introduced hydrocarbon (sites) of solutes in phases P(M) or P(N), (see Figure 10), on the other hand (right). According to this model of water structure (148,149), this interaction stabilizes the most ordered flickering water structures through an increase in coordination number of the hydrocarbon solute-nearest neighbour water molecules from four to five (right). This increase in coordination is considered as one of the basic (second) information terms residing in chemotactic solutions. Patterns of multivalent binding of such repeating structures in e.g. a polypeptide backbone at cell interfaces, are possible by phase separation of the solute conformers from those organized water molecules around them (148,149). For transparency, the effect of ionic groups on water and on binding patterns is omitted from this figure, but shown in Figure 10. The visualized single term represents at least 2 bits of information. Multiples of this information term are indicated in Figure 9.

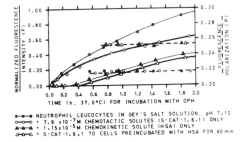

Fig. 8. Dynamics of membranes of viable leucocytes associated with recognition of direction in chemotaxis and promotion of locomotion in chemokinesis: Kinetics of uptake of hydrocarbon fluorophore probe (1,6-diphenyl hexa-1,3,5-triene, DPH) and mobility (microviscosity shown in terms of fluorescence polarization) (139) of hydrocarbon-lipid surface regions of membranes of chemokinetically (human serum albumin, HSA) and chemotactically (S-CAT-1.6.1) (44-46) stimulated cells. S-CAT-1.6.1 is a highly purified leucotaxin preparation with porcine anaphylatoxin and cocytotaxin in a molar ratio of 1 : 3.5 (44-46). The fluorescence intensities and the polarization were measured in a fluorescence spectrophotometer with correction modules for excitation and emission. Cuvettes with cells (1.25 x 10E07/ml) were stirred at 500 rpm during measurement. The kinetics of entry of the marker was measured by its addition at zero time to stirred cells at a final concentration of 1 umol/l from a dilute suspension of the marker of 2 umol/l in Gey's solution (46). The intensities were then measured by (1 s) pulse excitation of the probe. Polarization and other parameters were calculated according to Weber (139).

4.3.2.4 Discriminative recognition between taxis and kinesis

Discriminative information processing for chemotaxis and chemokinesis is mainly achieved by separation of extracellular signal reception and intracellular processing through cellular asymmetry centres on formation of topochemically distinct multivalent binding patterns of effectors at (different sites of) cell interfaces:

Investigations in our laboratory on the polarization of fluorescence intensities emitted by markers of specific membrane areas revealed (16,60,63,121) that no significant interactions occur between the membrane lipids and the polypeptide leucotaxin. The fluidity of the surface lipid layers of the membrane is not altered by the polypeptide(s) (Figure 8). In contrast, positively acting chemokinesins for leucocytes (leucoproskinesins like serum albumin, etc.) may interact with the surface lipid layers of the cell membrane. By this interaction, they shield superficial lipids of the membrane from exposure to surrounding water molecules: Leucoproskinesins like serum albumin reversibly adhere by their hydrophobic molecular sites to free membrane hydrocarbon regions. Thus, they lower the free energy required to expose cell surfaces or to maintain them uncovered (free) in aqueous solution: Adhesion on surfaces or aggregation of cells are phenomena which diminish the total free surface area of single cells from exposure to water. Thus, they are energetically favoured processes when free hydrophobic sites become covered, especially in the course of the spreading process (contact guidance). In contrast, this reaction would lower the tendency of the leucocyte to adhere onto surfaces, and increase its motility, when migrating at random. Studies on the exchange of hydrophobic markers between the cell membrane and the aqueous cellular environment showed (6,61) that the cell may also protect surfaces from exposure to water by intensified adhesion. Since e.g. serum albumin as pros-chemokinesin is always the natural proteinous constituent in the environment of the leucocyte, native cells normally may be reversibly coated entirely with serum albumin. It may function like a "shoe" or "coat" and as a transport vehicle permitting the extrusion of hydrophobic molecules from the cell into aqueous solution (e.g. in prostaglandin secretion). In contrast, negative chemokinesins (Figure 3A: Leuco-apo-kinesins) enforce the exposure of hydrophobic regions of the cell surface to water molecules. Hence, in this way, they bring about a higher tendency of the cell to adhere to surfaces or to aggregate with other cells. It is probably such a complex reversible interplay of positively and negatively acting chemokinesins at the cell surface, which, contrary to leucotaxins, regulate the locomotion of leucocytes migrating at random.

Within the reaction sequences triggered by cellular information processing, in contrast to chemokinesins, polypeptide leucotaxins interact with several independent, mobile membrane proteins and may form associates with them. These associates of independent, mobile membrane proteins may be considered as receptive units for direction finding. Their exact structure, however, has not been elaborated (16,63,121). This interaction is obviously independent of the reversible interaction of pros-chemokinesins (e.g. also serum albumin) with the membrane. Again in contrast to chemokinesins, within these reaction sequences of information processing for direction finding, polypeptide leucotaxins trigger a short transient (about one minute) rise in the intracellular concentration of cyclic AMP (14). A similar result was obtained for the interaction of the small exogenous peptide chemotaxins (formyl-methionine derivatives) by Jackowski and Sha'afi (140). Therefore, cyclic AMP may be considered as one of several possibly existing intracellular structural equivalents of the processing of extracellular information. However, as we found earlier (19,118), extracellular cyclic AMP is inactive in eliciting chemotactic responses in leucocytes. Therefore, the leucocyte membrane must be considered to have an asymmetry centre for cyclic AMP. For its turnover, vectorial catalytic processes (76, 141) are assumed: Thus, intracellular signal processing would be separated from extracellular signal reception. Such a separation, however, represents a basic principle of a discriminative system in any information processing of signalling devices (Figure 6) (6).

A further result of signal processing in chemotaxis is the measurable secretion or exudation of sets of effectors and enzymes of different activities from leucocytes. Some of them have been described also in this paper (156). This asymmetric reaction also points to an asymmetry centre in the leucocyte membrane apparent on leucotactic stimulation (6). Direction finding, but not locomotion, is subject to refractoriness (tachyphylaxis) on repeated exposure of cells to polypeptide leucotaxin activity (12). Hysteresis found on chemotactic stimulation of leucocytes (16,121) in terms of fluorescence signals emitted by membrane markers for protein sites can be considered as an expression of thermodynamically metastable membrane states and cooperative non-equilibrium transitions (142). They may indicate a physical basis of the memory and information storage of direction terms in chemotactically stimulated leucocytes (16,121) which, as biological effects, are apparent in terms of refractoriness and adaptation to different intensities of the stimulus (leucotaxin concentrations) (11,12). The directionality of hysteresis obtained on chemotactic stimulation of leucocytes, may produce periodicity on a molecular level by chemico-diffusional coupling, oscillations in chemical reactions of the multistage process of discriminative information transfer in relation to cellular position. It may also explain the evaluated asymmetry centres due to the observed transient changes in the level of intracellular cyclic AMP and extracellular secretion or exudation of biologically active effectors and enzymes on chemotactic stimulation (6,14,16,63). Hysteretic scanning loops might provide an answer to the question under debate (73) whether leucocytes process positional information (concentration gradient sensing) in leucotaxin solutions by a temporal or a spatial sensing mechanism: The mechanisms may not be different, but alike expressions of one physico-chemical phenomenon of macromolecules of cybernetic significance (6,16). Figure 9 schematically represents this description of recently elaborated molecular mechanisms of discriminative information processing in cellular recognition and the biological signal transmission for mediator-operated, reaction-specific chemotaxis and the chemokinesis of leucocytes.

4.3.3 Discrimination in chemotropism and chemorecruitment

Discriminative information processing mechanisms are operative for effector-elicited reaction-specific chemotropism and chemorecruitment of cells:

Similar principles as discussed in the preceding section may apply to the morphogenesis of blood vessel systems: Endothelial cells may be triggered to direction finding in chemotropism (directional hyperplastic growth) and to directional locomotion in terms of chemotaxis and chemokinesis as elaborated for leucocytes. However, these phenomena are far less well investigated, due to the difficulties in the preparation of highly purified, specific effector substances (1,6,7,156). It is noteworthy that there is no biological cross-reactivity (at physiological effector concentrations) between the chemotaxis of leucocytes and the chemotropism of blood vessel cells when operated by their respective highly purified mediators or effectors. On one hand, this might express differences in the (ontogenically related) cell types in terms of their discriminative receptive units at the cell membrane for different mechanisms of cellular displacement, motion and locomotion. On the other hand, this may be an expression of the information term(s) residing in the different effector molecules themselves: Whereas direction finding in chemotaxis probably (only) needs formation of certain asymmetric centres on the cell surface to direct a locomoting cell at the same locomotion scalar, direction finding in chemotropism requires a further cellular reaction to be induced by the extracellular signal polypeptide (e.g. monocyto-angiotropin, Figure 2B): Promotion of the endothelial cell to enter and pass through a mitotic cycle. Thus, it is conceivable that chemotropins, in principle, carry and constitute the two information terms as evaluated for chemotaxins of leucocytes. However, on the other hand, chemotropins have to carry further information term(s) making the polypeptide structure capable of forming a special pattern of multivalent binding on phase separation of the effector at the cell interface. The (additional) information terms would probably lead to other, topochemicaly distinct multivalent binding patterns which are different from chemotaxis: These terms might, in the case of chemotropins, be related to those residing in normal (chemopoietic) mitogens. We could not yet elaborate any clue as to the precise nature of these additional information terms. It is conceivable to assume additional interactions of the effector polypeptide with carbohydrate moieties at the cell surface, i.e. comparable to those known from other mitogens (94,143). On the other hand, reversible, also asymmetric, intracellular enzymatic reactions might be induced, e.g. glycosylation or phosphorylation-dephosphorylation reactions (144-146) which are basic to the viral transformation mechanisms in cells, too.

Whatever the differences in information residing in the effector molecules for sprout formation are, evidently, for the morphogenesis of closed circulation loops of blood vessels from endothelial sprouts, chemotropism, chemotaxis, chemokinesis and chemorecruitment of endothelial cells are necessary as separate mechanisms: Sprouting tips formed by chemotropism are not the only requisite for the formation of such closed loops of blood vessels (1,2). This mechanism is just the trigger to begin this morphogenetic reaction. In the beginning of sprouting, how does the tip of the sprout know not to combine with the tip of another adjacent sprout? What mechanism keeps them apart from each other and sprouting separately? Later on, how does the tip of the same (now elongated) sprout find the tip of some of its neighbours to unite for combined formation of a closed circulation loop of blood vessels with active biological (haemodynamic) functions (1,2,7,33,157)? Various hypotheses and models have been designed for the formation of patterns and network structures of biological units (3,31,32,89,91-93, 97-99, 101,147,158); in particular, too, as far as associated to tropism reactions (geotropism, phototropism, etc.) other than chemotropism. As to how they might be applied to the apparently very complex in-vivo situation, e.g. in terms of blood vessel system formation, no definite result is available: A suitable model can only be visualized when more is known about further effector entities operating cooperatively these most complex processes in morphogenetic reactions. Most likely, as demonstrated for leucocytes in this work, endothelial cells have their own effector network, by which they specifically operate such different categories of chemical mechanisms as chemotropism, chemotaxis, chemokinesis and the chemorecruitment of cells. This so far largely unknown effector network thus would be subject to activation by the network of specific leucocyte effectors. The isolated, leucocyte-derived chemotropins (Figure 2B) (1,7, 33-35,156) could be considered as one of its initial activation triggers.

A comparably complex situation for the elaboration of a detailed mechanism of information processing is represented in the chemorecruitment of cells of the haematopoietic and immune systems, being one of the classical reactions in Pathology and Physiology (21-27, 58). Peripheral leucocytes exposed to isolated leucorecruitins do not respond biologically in terms of chemotaxis or chemokinesis, nor in terms of chemopoietic reactions, etc. This lack of biological cross-reactivity may indicate that peripheral leucocytes are not at all responsive to information terms residing in leucorecruitins (6,7, 21-27, 40). On the other hand, although being responsive in terms of directional locomotion, stored bone marrow leucocytes are not mobilized and recruited into blood circulation by leucotaxins and leucokinesins, as judged by in-vitro and in-vivo assay systems (Figure 4A) (6,21,23,24,27,156). This confirms that chemorecruitment, chemotaxis and chemokinesis are dissimilar mechanisms and are operated by different effectors. However, the most limiting reaction parameters for a study of or an approach to a mechanism of this kind of cellular mobilization are currently unknown and remain as "terra incognita of molecular biology" (83): Although stored bone marrow leucocytes morphologically look like the corresponding circulating, peripheral white blood cells (56-58), they behave differently, giving rise to certain fundamental questions: What chemical or physical differences exist between a stored leucocyte type constrained to bone marrow "storage pools" (or "marginal storage pools") (Figure 1) on one hand, and the nascent, peripheral, circulating cell of the same phenotype on the other hand? Which physico-chemical reactions are induced at the "birth" of a new circulating leucocyte phenotype (in leucocyte storage pools); and what is the structural equivalent of the transition "barrier" between leucocyte storage pools in the bone marrow on one hand, and blood circulation on the other hand? Is it a glycosylation, a methylation, a hydrolase or a reversible phosphorylation- dephosphorylation reaction on the surface of leucocytes induced by leucorecruitins which makes nascent, circulating leucocyte types different from, or more matured than their stored phenotype precursors? Or is it a transient difference, just expressed and induced by leucorecruitins at the "birth" of a circulating leucocyte?

We do not yet know the answers to these fundamental questions, although they are of basic importance to haematology and immunology and their disorders, for instance leukemia. However, as judged from in-vivo and in-vitro assay systems, one of the obvious discrimination mechanisms operative in the chemorecruitment of leucocytes is endocrine (hormonal) information transmission (1,5,156). It is thus distinguished from the so far known effector-operated chemotaxis, chemokinesis, chemotropism and chemopoiesis of cells in which information is transmitted by paracrine or autocrine mechanisms (1,5,156). With reference to Figure 6, this discrimination of leucocyte chemorecruitment from other mechanisms operated by effectors at least in this respect represents a channel selection mode. The hope is that further work on the newly detected wound hormones will provide at least a partial answer in the near future. Nevertheless, for comparison, for about 60 years, we have known insulin as one of the classical hormones. We have known its primary structure for about 30 years. It was the first protein whose amino acid sequence was elucidated. Yet, the molecular mechanisms of the biological action of insulin and of the transmission of its specific information into cells are still a puzzle and the subject of intensive basic research (5,95). In view of the complexity of the leucocyte recruitment reaction, I assume that wound hormones will pose a similar puzzle in elaboration of their intimate mode of action.

4.4   MULTIVALENT BINDING AND DISCRIMINATIVE BIOLOGICAL SIGNALLING

The multivalent binding model serves as a basis for effector-operated discriminative biological signalling devices:

In summary, the data compiled from our work concern cellular recognition and discriminative mechanisms of information processing in cellular reactions as well as communication operated by the interactive endogenous effector networks derived from leucocytes, endothelial cells and wound plasma. Direction finding in chemotaxis and chemotropism, the regulation of locomotion in chemokinesis, the displacement and motion in chemorecruitment and chemopoiesis, and chemostatic mechanisms triggering cells of the haematopoietic and immune system, have been described.

Cellular recognition and the processing of information on direction finding in leucotaxis, and its discrimination from leucokinesis, leucorecruitment and the chemotropism of endothelial cells, suggest a multivalent binding process for the initial interaction of the reactive, chemotactically active conformer phases of the endogenous polypeptides with cell membrane proteins. The binding reaction and the information processing (Figure 9) can be explained on the basis of a multivalent model of a discriminative biological signalling device. The characteristics of such binding processes should most likely follow Jennissen's postulates (64) on the binding and the regulation of biologically active polypeptides on cellular interfaces. They were developed from laborious and detailed studies of polypeptide adsorption to hydrophobic binding sites in biolattices. Accordingly (64), the mechanism of binding for small molecules at interfaces is site-independent and follows a simple lock-and-key type model. In contrast, for a series of polypeptides, it was found site-dependent and follows a cooperative, multivalent binding pattern having between three and nine binding sites. Furthermore, this model of non-immunological recognition has considerable similarity to mechanisms of immune recognition, postulated independently by Lewin (112). Figure 10 schematically represents this similarity with reference to Lewin's work (112). This similarity is obvious in terms of the basic information evaluated

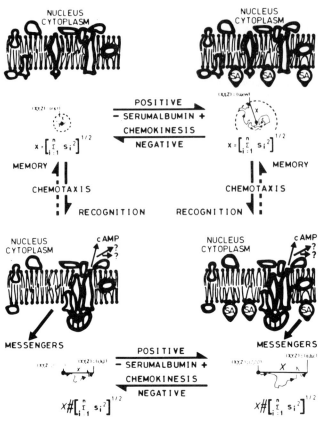

Fig. 9. Dynamics of membranes in viable leucocytes associated with recognition in the chemotaxis and promotion of locomotion in (pros-) chemokinesis. There are discriminative mechanisms of information processing for chemotaxis and chemokinesis by separation of extracellular signal reception and intracellular signal processing through cellular asymmetry centres: Cellular storage, amplification and multiplexing of signals (Figure 6). Increments of locomotion at random and in direction are used in the terminology of Peterson and Noble (66) and are further detailed in Figure 5. For reasons of transparency, carbohydrate moieties on cell surfaces are not shown, although they are probably essential in the complete consideration of the multivalent binding reactions of the polypeptides at the cell interface; especially in full description of the effective different modes of discrimination mechanisms of information terms

Hatched particles represent associates of classical anaphylatoxin solutes as chemo-attractant.

Serum albumin solutes as positive chemokinetic solute.

Thick arrow (thin arrow) indicates extracellular (intracellular) messengers produced as chemical equivalents in response to extracellular signal.

for achieving selective or specific cellular respones. Water molecules are ommitted for the same reasons, since their role in the mechanisms is detailed in Figure 7. Two topochemically distinct, limiting multivalent binding patterns have been elaborated for chemotaxis and chemokinesis and are shown: Firstly, the separation of a reactive phase (leucotaxin) at the cell protein interface from the leucotaxin solution, and, secondly, the multivalent interaction pattern of serum albumin (as proschemokinesin) with its hydrophobic groups (155) and with the lipid layer (as a major binding site). Apochemokinesins probably compete with this function of serum albumin and thus enforce the adhesion tendency of the cells (not shown in the figure). Each topochemically distinct and dependent contact point of solute with the cell interface represents a different pattern of multivalent binding. A further description is given in the text and Figure 10 (6,16,60,61,63). The two different multivalent binding patterns shown for chemotaxis and chemokinesis in principle represent one of the described (Figure 6), possible discrimination mechanisms, namely, transmission of information terms through different channels for elucidating specific cellular responses (chemotaxis OR chemokinesis). Modes of discriminative mechanisms by ratio detection in information terms are described in the text (section 4.4) and visualized in part in Figure 10.

Fig. 10. Models, information terms and reactive phases in non-immune and immune recognition for direction finding in leucotaxis.
Upper panel: Non-immune recognition and mechanism of information processing for chemotaxis of non-sensitized ("normal") leucocytes to endogenous leucotaxin effector molecules of non-antigen and non-antibody structure.
Lower panel: Model for immune recognition drawn similarly to Lewin (112) and adapted for direction finding in chemotaxis of sensitized leucocytes to appropriate antigens (113, 114,150-152). Dissipative physical structures (Figure 5) as positional (first) information terms (concentration gradients, boundaries, etc.) are omitted and not shown in this figure, although they are necessary as well for direction finding (see text). The similarities of the models shown are closer than being a formal relation only: Chemotaxis of non-sensitized ("normal") leucocytes to endogenous leucotaxins of non-antigen and non-antibody structure (Figure 9) as a formal case of non-immune recognition, is accomplished by the shown phenomenon of chemotaxis of sensitized cells to appropriate antigens ("antigen chemotaxis", "antigen recognition"), which is a formal case of immune recognition (113,114,150-152). In both cases, water molecule displacement provides the driving force of the recognition process (Figures 7 and 9). The latter is an example of interaction of thermodynamically stable conformer phases with evolved, discrete specific sensory receptor molecules as an alternative to the first given example (upper panel). It evaluates more [(greater than) 20-30] bits of information (102) and gains selection power for the cell. In principle, the different modes of recognition of same or similar information terms and their translation into specific cellular responses (e.g. chemotaxis) imply one limiting model form of ratio detection as discrimination mechanism in signal transmission. Thus, they distinguish themselves from discrimination of same or similar information terms (Figures 5-7) by their transmission in different channels (Figure 9) for obtaining specific cellular responses (e.g. chemotaxis OR chemokinesis). As well, discriminative ratio detection of information terms in membranes may lead to selective or specific cellular responses, as implied in the models described in section 4.3 for the other cellular responses discussed in this paper. Then, overlap of transmission or within one form of

discrimination mechanisms would result in cross-reactivity of
apparent cellular responses as produced by interaction with a
certain chemical stimulus: Thus, e.g., in complementing this
figure with the representation of Figure 9, chemicals which
multivalently interact at the cellular interface at a distinct
multivalent ratio of bonds and forces at topochemically restricted
hydrocarbon AND polypeptide regions may elicit concomitantly
cellular chemotactic AND chemokinetic responses.

NON-IMMUNOLOGICAL CELLULAR RECOGNITION:

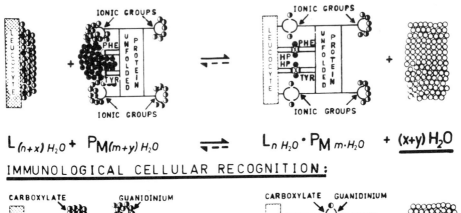

$$L_{(n+x)H_2O} + P_{M(m+y)H_2O} \rightleftharpoons L_{nH_2O} \cdot P_{M\,m\cdot H_2O} + \underline{(x+y)H_2O}$$

IMMUNOLOGICAL CELLULAR RECOGNITION:

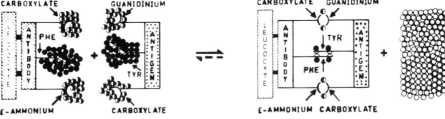

$$L\text{-}Ab_{(n+x)H_2O} + Ag_{(m+y)H_2O} \rightleftharpoons L\text{-}Ab_{nH_2O} \cdot Ag_{mH_2O} + \underline{(x+y)H_2O}$$

○ "NORMALLY" STRUCTURED WATER IN PURE LIQUID;
● "ORGANIZED" WATER MOLECULES AROUND HYDROPHOBIC
(NONPOLAR) PORTIONS ·(HP) OF SOLUTE MOLECULES;
◑ WATER AND IONIC SOLUTE ASSOCIATES AROUND IONIC
(POLAR) PORTIONS OF SOLUTE MOLECULES;
L : LEUCOCYTE; Ab : ANTIBODY; Ag : ANTIGEN;
P_M : METASTABLE, THERMODYNAMICALLY UNFAVOURED
PHASE OF PROTEIN CONFORMERS (CHEMOTACTIC SOLU-
TES); (n,m,x,y) : STOICHIOMETRIC INDICES;

Fig. 10

which are metastable, dissipative, physical and chemical structures. The latter information term can be visualized in negative entropic interactions (not bonds, but organization by higher coordination numbers) of the endogenous (polypeptide effector) solute with solution (water) molecules, when available theories of non-covalent interactions (148,149) are applied. On this basis, the close similarities between non-immunological recognition for direction finding in chemotaxis, and immune recognition become obvious: On one hand, there is chemotaxis of non-sensitized, "normal" leucocytes to endogenous leucotaxin effectors of non-antigen and non-antibody structure ("non-immunological recognition"). On the other hand, there is the phenomenon of chemotaxis of sensitized leucocytes to appropriate antigens ("antigen chemotaxis", "inadequate, antigen or immune recognition") (113, 114, 150-152). The latter phenomenon, first described by Jensen and Williams (152), represents a formal case of direction finding by immune recognition. It occurs through interactions of evolved, discrete and defined, specific sensory receptor molecules (units) (36,76,94,102,113,114, 150-152) with a thermodynamically and kinetically stable phase of a conformer (e.g. polypeptide antigens like ovalbumin). In both limiting cases i.e. non-immune and immune recognition, displacement of water molecules and phase separation provides a driving force for the recognition processes; the information terms may be based on features of the organization of water structure around solutes. In addition, both limiting cases complement each other: "Normal" leucocytes may be chemo-attracted for the infiltration at sites of still soluble, but damaged "self" components, e.g. "unfolded" protein conformer phases, on one hand. Sensitized cells may infiltrate by "immune chemotaxis" at sites of intrusion of foreign matter with appropriate antigenic character, on the other hand (113,114). Non-immunological chemotaxis may play a prominent role in the handling of newly intruded foreign matter as prospective antigens: Non-sensitized macrophages may be chemo-attracted in order to activate the immune network in lymphocytes and production of the appropriate antibodies (76, 96, 102).

The model visualized further suggests that within multivalent binding patterns, the number, the dynamics AND the topochemistry of the interactions of effector ligands at the cell surface (e.g. to lipid, polypeptide and/or carbohydrate moieties), determine the cellular function: The response to a certain effector molecule expresses the ability of the cell to discriminate. This is visualized in the model by the demonstrated, discriminative information processing mechanism by which selected multivalent binding sites lead to specific, independent cellular reactions (direction finding in chemotaxis and promotion of locomotion in chemokinesis). Possible cross-reactivity in cellular functions emerge from cross-reactivity of binding patterns of effector ligands in terms of valence and site overlap. Further discriminative mechanisms of information processing are evident on the basis of this model in which discrimination is achieved by separation of extracellular signal reception from intracellular signal processing through obvious cellular assymetry centres for chemical and physical reactions induced by the recognition process (discrimination in the form of filter effect selection modes) (Figure 6). As a general explanation, this model says, that not every exogenous or endogenous effector a priori needs and meets an already evolved, discrete and defined, specific, sensory receptive molecule (unit) at the membrane to elicit a specific biological response. More primitive, but still specific, discriminative processing mechanisms may also be operative by patterns of multivalent binding of effector sites to topochemically distinct surface areas or structures (discrimination in the form of channel selection modes) (Figure 6).

The signalling device (Figure 6) of leucocytes for the extracellular direction finding in the form of dissipative physical and chemical structures is a complete, efficient and reliable cellular information processing system: The extracellular information residing in the leucotaxin solution is received asymmetrically in the leucocyte membrane (channel) and, thereby, transformed into dissipative membrane-structural equivalents (metastable membrane protein associations). They are further processed in the membrane by transiently asymmetric, vectorial catalytical changes in the intracellular concentrations of substances; e.g. by transiently formed concentration gradients of cyclic AMP as one of the dissipative intracellular structural equivalents of the extracellularly provided information. Asymmetric reflexes (directional migration) of the cell without change of the total intrinsic locomotor capacity (motility as locomotion scalar) are induced following other directional increments formed on other asymmetric events (hysteresis). The signal is stored (refractoriness or tachyphylaxis and adaptation). Amplification and multiplexing of the signal are further expressions of the signal processing mechanisms and its translation into cellular responses (Figures 6 and 9). They are obvious by transiently asymmetric extracellular secretion of a variety of substances, including enzymes and a new set of effector molecules; e.g. a network of other (leucocyte-derived) leucotaxins (Figure 3B). Circumstantial evidence suggests (6,153,156) that the secretion of at least some effectors follows mechanisms which are comparable to neurotransmitter release reactions (107). They accomplish this type of biological information transmission system of leucocytes which is initially triggered by the original leucotaxin signal. In due course, the result is a physiologically organized formation of a secretory leucocytic tissue. It has capabilities for further cellular communication: It may trigger various networks of chemical effector systems of other proximate and remote biological target units (e.g. blood vessel cells, neural units, bone marrow) for the regulation of the body's systemic and local defense state. It may probably also interact with other, so far not considered information networks which serve to form new life-compatible morphogenetic patterns at the reaction site of tissue injury.

Acknowledgements:

I thank Mr. H. Renner for his skilful cooperation in this research subject. I am very grateful to Prof. Dr. H.P. Jennissen, University of Bochum, and Prof. Dr. J. Jensen, University of Miami, for numerous helpful discussions, recommendations and for their cooperation with which they contributed to this work.

90

SUMMARY

This contribution describes the properties of some highly
purified endogenous polypeptide effector substances as chemical
signals for triggering mechanisms of cellular reactions and
communication in regenerative tissue morphogenesis by inflammation
and healing processes. In special consideration are humoral and
cellular (plasma- and leucocyte-derived) effectors with activities
basic to functional expressions of the immune, haematopoietic and
cardiovascular system in situations which lead to changes in
tissue patterns. They operate passive and active displacement,
motions and organization of patterns of leucocyte phenotypes,
blood vessel (endothelial) cells and biological units in the form
of chemopoiesis, chemokinesis, chemotaxis, chemorecruitment,
chemotropism and chemostasis as main categories of chemical
mechanisms for cellular reactions and communication in
regenerative morphogenesis. Examples of autocrine, paracrine,
endocrine and neural information transmission mechanisms are given
for cellular communication among leucocytes, and leucocytes and
endothelial cells, as close range biological signalling devices,
on one hand; and between leucocytes and their bone marrow storage
pools, and leucocytes and thermoregulatory centres of the body
(hypothalamus), as signalling devices targeting remote cell units,
on the other hand. At proximate and remote sites, by such
leucocyte-emitted chemical signals, specific cellular reactions
are expressed in the form of regulation of random and directional
hyperplastic growth, mobilization and recruitment, random and
directional locomotion, and increase in temperature in cells and
biological units. Such reactions are instrumental in the
formation, organization and maintenance of cellular distribution
patterns in homeostasis of the number and phenotypical variety of
circulating leucocytes (i.e. leucocytosis and leftward shift
reactions), of structures of new blood vessels (angiogenesis) with
active biological (haemodynamic) functions, of motile secretory
leucocytic tissues, and of fever. They are examples of elementary
functional expressions of pathophysiological processes.
Investigations by physico-chemical and biological methods on the
molecular characteristics of effectors, and their interaction with
target cells, so far provided some relationships on the mechanisms
of action in cellular chemotaxis, chemokinesis and other reactions
for cellular displacement, motion and locomotion (with emphasis on
chemorecruitment and chemotropism). They are exemplified in the
biological specificity of action of endogenous polypeptide
effectors in operation of basic chemical mechanisms for cellular
reactions and communication in regenerative tissue morphogenesis,
the selectivity of mechanistic action of endogenous polypeptide
leucotaxins, the regulation of random locomotion (chemokinesis) of
leucocytes by endogenous polypeptide chemokinesins and the obvious
existence of discriminative receptive units or reactions on cells
as a basis for evoking biologically specific cellular responses.
Discriminative mechanisms in effector-operated cellular reactions
and communication are described and models of molecular mechanisms
of cellular recognition are presented. In special consideration is
a molecular model for cellular recognition in mediator-operated

chemotaxis of leucocytes which discriminates cellular locomotion effects in chemokinesis. The physical and chemical information terms residing in solutions of biologically active mediators are detailed. Their discrimination is described in the processing of information by topochemically distinct multivalent binding patterns of effectors at different sites of cell interfaces, and by the separation of extracellular signal reception from intracellular transmission through cellular asymmetry centres. They exemplify discrimination in terms of channel selection and filter effect modes. From these mechanisms, possible discriminative information processing mechanisms for effector-operated, reaction-specific cellular chemotropism and -recruitment are deduced. A multisite, multivalent model of binding patterns is shown as a basis for effector-operated discriminative biological signalling devices in which the number, dynamics and the topochemistry of the interaction of the effector ligands at the cell surface determines the cellular function. Cross-reactivity in cellular functions is expressed on cross-reactivity of binding patterns in valence and site terms. Non-immune (non-antigen) and immune (antigen) recognition mechanisms in chemotaxis of "normal" (non-sensitized) and immune (sensitized) cells to non-antigen (self) and antigen (foreign) matter are considered as related, limiting examples for primitive, but specific sensory receptive units and for evolved, specific sensory receptor molecules, respectively. One of their common (chemical) information terms which is processed in both mechanisms is visualized in negative entropic interactions of the (endogenous polypeptide effector or exogenous antigen) solute with solution (water) molecules. By the statistical-mechanical model of water structure, this information term may be visualized by an increase in the coordination number (not bond) to five on introduction of a non-polar solute-nearest neighbour of a hydrogen-tetrabonded water molecule. It is shown that the signalling device of leucocytes is a complete, efficient and reliable information processing system: The extracellular information residing in effector solutions may be discriminately received, processed, stored, amplified and multiplexed. It is capable of further cellular communication by triggering various networks of chemical effector systems of other proximate and remote biological target units (e.g. blood vessel cells, neural units, bone marrow, etc.) which are instrumental in formation, organization and maintenance of new life-compatible morphogenetic patterns at the reaction site of tissue injury.

REFERENCES

1. Wissler J.H.: Inflammatory mediators and wound hormones: Chemical signals for differentiation and morphogenesis in tissue regeneration and healing. In: Proc. 33th Mosbach Colloquium 1982: Biochemistry of Differentiation and Morphogenesis, edited by L. Jaenicke, pp.257-274. Springer Verlag, Heidelberg, 1982.

2. Gottwik M., H. Renner and J.H. Wissler: Biochemical neovascularization of muscles by leukocyte-derived polypeptide effectors: Morphogenesis and turnover of blood vessel patterns with active hemodynamics in vivo. Z. Physiol. Chem. 363:938-939, 1982.

3. Liebow A.A.: Situations which lead to changes in vascular patterns. In: Handbook of Physiology, Section 2: Circulation, Vol. 2, edited by W.F. Hamilton and P. Dow, pp.1251-1276. Amer. Physiol. Soc., Washington D.C., 1965.

4. Bloom W. and D.W. Fawcett (Eds.): Textbook of Histology, 10th ed. W.B. Saunders Company, Philadelphia, 1975.

5. Karlson P.: Was sind Hormone? Der Hormonbegriff in Geschichte und Gegenwart. Naturwissenschaften 69:3-14, 1982.

6. Wissler J.H.: Entzuendungsmediatoren: Chemische Anlockung, Motilitaetsbeeinflussung und molekulare Mechanismen biologischer Nachrichtenuebertragung bei der Ansammlung von Leukozyten. Habilitationsschrift, Ruhr-Universitaet Bochum, 1980; Forschungsberichte aus Technik und Naturwissenschaften 3:10, pp.1-36. Technische Informationsbibliothek Hannover 06A 2154, Physik Verlag, Weinheim, 1982.

7. Wissler J.H.: Biotechnik der Gewinnung leukozytaerer Entzuendungsmediatoren und Wundhormone. In: BMFT-Statusseminar: Tierische Zellkulturen, Juelich 1981, edited by Bundesministerium fuer Forschung und Technologie (BMFT), pp.293-303. Projekttraeger Biotechnologie Kernforschungsanlage, Juelich, 1982.

8. Wissler J.H.: Evaluation and action of biological mediators generated from normal serum by interaction with foreign macromolecules. In: Proc. Immunosymp. Wien 1973: Gram-negative Bacterial Infections and Mode of Endotoxin Actions; Pathophysiological, Immunological and Clinical Aspects, edited by B. Urbaschek, R. Urbaschek and E. Neter, pp.91-105. Springer Verlag, Wien, 1975.

9. Keller H.U. and M. Bessis: Migration and chemotaxis of anucleate cytoplasmic leukocyte fragments. Nature 258: 723-724, 1975.

10. Keller H.U., J.H. Wissler, M.W. Hess and H. Cottier: Chemokinesis and chemotaxis of phagocytes. In: Proc. 1st Eur. Conf. Biochemistry of Phagocytes Trieste 1976: Movement, Metabolism and Bactericidal Mechanisms of Phagocytes, edited by F. Rossi, P.L. Patriarca and D. Romeo, pp.15-20. Piccin Medical Books, Padova, 1977.

11. Keller H.U., J.H. Wissler, M.W. Hess and H. Cottier: Relation between stimulus intensity and chemotactic response. Experientia 33:534-536, 1977.

12. Keller H.U., J.H. Wissler, M.W. Hess and H. Cottier: Distinct chemokinetic and chemotactic responses in neutrophil granulocytes. Eur. J. Immunol. 8:1-7, 1978.

13. Keller H.U., J.H. Wissler and J. Ploem: Chemotaxis is not a special case of haptotaxis. Experientia 35:1669-1671, 1979.

14. Keller H.U., G. Gerisch and J.H. Wissler: A transient rise in cyclic AMP levels following chemotactic stimulation of neutrophil granulocytes. Cell Biol. Int. Rep. 3:759-765, 1979.

15. Keller H.U., J.H. Wissler, B. Damerau, M.W. Hess and H. Cottier: The filter technique for measuring leukocyte locomotion in vitro. Comparison of three modifications. J. Immunol. Meth. 36:41-53, 1980.

16. Wissler J.H. and E. Logemann: Biological memory and metastable membrane states associated with recognition and information processing in directional locomotion (chemotaxis) of leukocytes. Z. Physiol. Chem. 360:1204-1205, 1979.

17. Wissler J.H., M. Arnold, U. Gerlach and W. Schaper: Leukocyte-derived protein hormones for tissue repair (lympho-, mono- and leucokines): Large scale production, isolation and properties of cell-derived cytotaxins, cytokinesins, cytotoxins and mitogens. Z. Physiol. Chem. 361:351-352, 1980.

18. Wissler J.H.: Chemokinesins and chemotaxins of leukocytes and inflamed tissues: Natural mediator proteins for reversible promotion of random and directional locomotion (chemokinesis and chemotaxis) for accumulation of specific leukocyte types, process of their biotechnical preparation and pharmaceutical compositions. Eur. Pat. Publ. EP 0 061 141 A2 Bull. 82/39, DOS DE 31 10 610 Al, pp.1-82. Max-Planck-Gesellschaft zur Foerderung der Wissenschaften, Muenchen, 1982.

19. Wissler J.H., V.J. Stecher and E. Sorkin: Biochemistry and biology of a leucotactic binary serum peptide system related to anaphylatoxin. Int. Arch. Allergy 42:722-747, 1972.

20. Wissler J.H.: A process for producing and obtaining anaphylatoxin- and cocytotaxin-containing leukotaxin preparations and anaphylatoxin and cocytotaxin proteins in molecularly homogeneous, biologically active form. Eur. Pat. Publ. EP 0 042 560 A2 Bull. 81/52, DOS DE 30 22 914 Al, pp.1-53. Max-Planck-Gesellschaft zur Foerderung der Wissenschaften, Muenchen, 1981.

21. Rother K.: Leukocyte mobilizing factor: A new biological activity derived from the third component of complement. Eur. J. Immunol. 2:550-558, 1972.

22. Ghebrehiwet B. and H.J. Mueller-Eberhard: An acidic fragment of human C3 with leukocytosis-inducing activity. J. Immunol. 123:616-621, 1979.

23. Wissler J.H., B. Pfefferkorn, K. Rother, U. Rother, L. Schramm, H. Renner, H. Renker, A.M. Wissler and W. Schaper: Inflammation and the leukocytosis reaction: Purification, crystallization and properties of a serum-derived protein mediator with bone marrow leukocyte-mobilizing activity. Z. Physiol. Chem. 361:1358, 1980.

24. Wissler J.H.: Leukorekrutin: Ein Entzuendungsmediatorprotein aus Saeugerserum zur Induzierung einer Leukozytosereaktion, Herstellungsverfahren, Gewinnung in molekular einheitlicher, kristallisierbarer und biologisch spezifisch wirkender Form und Leukorekrutin enthaltendes Arzneimittel. German Patent DE 30 34 529 C2, Eur. Pat. Spec. EP 0 047 979 Bl Bull. 82/12, pp.1-44. Max-Planck-Gesellschaft zur Foerderung der Wissenschaften, Muenchen, 1982.

25. Wissler J.H., H. Renner, U. Gerlach and A.M. Wissler: Inflammation, cell mitosis and differentiation signals: Novel hormones in homeostatic regulatory mechanisms of hematopoiesis and left shift recruitment of leukocytes. Z. Physiol. Chem. 362:244-245, 1981.

26. Wissler J.H., H. Renner, U. Gerlach, M. Gottwik and A.M. Wissler: Cell division, differentiation signals and chemorecruitment of leukocytes: Isolation of novel monokine and leukocyte-derived hormones ("leuko- and metamyelorecruitins") regulating homeostasis of hematopoiesis and left shift of white blood cells in circulation and at tissue repair sites. Immunobiology 159:121-122, 1981.

27. Wissler J.H.: Chemorecruitins of leukocytes and inflamed tissues: A new class of natural leukopoietin proteins for chemorecruitment of specific leukocyte types from the bone marrow into blood circulation (leukocytosis and leftward shift reactions), process for their biotechnical preparation and pharmaceutical compositions. Eur. Pat. Publ. EP 0 061 140 A2 Bull. 82/39, DOS DE 31 10 561 Al, pp.1-72. Max-Planck-Gesellschaft zur Foerderung der Wissenschaften, Muenchen, 1982.

28. Algire G.H., H.W. Chalkley, F.Y. Legallais and H.D. Park: Vascular reactions of normal and malignant tissues in vivo. I. Vascular reactions of mice to wounds and to normal and neoplastic transplants. J. Natl. Cancer Inst. 6:73-85, 1945.

29. Warren B.A.: In vivo and electron microscopic study of vessels in a haemangiopericytoma of the hamster. Angiologica 5:230-249, 1968.

30. Cliff W.J.: Observations on healing tissue: A combined light and electron microscopic investigation. Phil. Trans. Royal Soc. London Series B 246:305-325, 1963.

31. Folkman J. and M. Hochberg: Self-regulation of growth in three dimensions. J. Exp. Med. 138:745-753, 1973.

32. Peterson H.-I. (Ed.): Tumor Blood Circulation: Angiogenesis, Vascular Morphology and Blood Flow of Experimental and Human Tumors. CRC Press, Boca Raton, 1979.

33. Wissler J.H. and H. Renner: Inflammation, chemotropism and morphogenesis: Novel leucocyte-derived mediators for directional growth of blood vessels and regulation of tissue neovascularization. Z. Physiol. Chem. 362:244, 1981.

34. Wissler J.H. and W. Schaper: Angiotropins of leukocytes and inflamed tissue: A new class of natural chemotropic protein mitogens for specific induction of directional growth of blood vessels, neovascularization of tissues and morphogenesis of blood vessel patterns, process for their biotechnical preparation and pharmaceutical compositions. Eur. Pat. Publ. EP 0 061 138 A2 Bull. 82/39, DOS DE 31 10 560 A1, pp.1-64. Max-Planck-Gesellschaft zur Foerderung der Wissenschaften, Muenchen, 1982.
35. Wissler J.H.: Richtungswachstum von Blutgefaessen und Neovaskularisierung von Geweben durch natuerliche chemotropische Mitogene (Angiotropine) aus Leukozyten. Commun. 19. Hauptversammlung Gesellschaft Dtsch. Chemiker, p.186. Verlag Chemie, Weinheim, 1981.
36. Glynn L.E., J.C.Houck and G. Weissmann (Eds): Handbook of Inflammation; Vol.1: Chemical Messengers of the Inflammatory Process, edited by J.C. Houck; Vol.2: The Cell Biology of Inflammation, edited by G. Weissmann; Vol.3: Tissue Repair and Regeneration, edited by L.E. Glynn. Elsevier - North Holland, Amsterdam, 1979, 1980, 1981.
37. Logemann E. and J.H. Wissler: Humoral polypeptide mediators of inflammation (leukorecruitin, anaphylatoxin, cocytotaxin): Homogeneity criteria and separation of identified nutrition pollutants as companion products present in blood. Z. Physiol. Chem. 363:939-940, 1982.
38. Wissler J.H.: Process for obtaining intact and viable leukocytes and thrombocytes from blood. United States Patent 4,343,793, pp.1-10. Max-Planck-Gesellschaft zur Foerderung der Wissenschaften, Washington, 1982.
39. Wissler J.H.: Fully synthetic cell culture medium. Eur. Pat. Publ. EP 0 060 565 A2 Bull. 82/38, DOS DE 31 10 559 A1, pp.1-27. Max-Planck-Gesellschaft zur Foerderung der Wissenschaften, Muenchen, 1982.
40. Wissler J.H. and H. Renner: Specific polypeptide mediators and wound hormones of monocytes: Leukopoiesis, leukocytosis, leftward shift reactions, leukokinesis, leukotaxis, angiogenesis, and fever. Immunobiology 162:438, 1982.
41. Wissler J.H.: Mitogens of leukocytes and inflamed tissues: Natural leukopoietin proteins for specific induction of proliferation and differentiation of leukocytes, process for their biotechnical preparation and pharmaceutical compositions. Eur. Pat. Publ. EP 0 061 139 A2 Bull. 82/39, DOS DE 31 10 611 A1, pp.1-64. Max-Planck-Gesellschaft zur Foerderung der Wissenschaften, Muenchen, 1982.
42. Maurer H.R., M. Kastner, R. Maschler, R. Neumeier, M. Arnold, U. Gerlach, K. Glendinning, B. Pfefferkorn and J.H. Wissler: Biotechnologische Isolierung und Charakterisierung von Poetinen und Chalonen der Granulopoese. Z. Physiol. Chem. 361:221, 1981.
43. Neumeier R., H.R. Maurer, M. Arnold, U. Gerlach, K. Glendinning, H. Renner and J.H. Wissler: Identification of two granulocyte/macrophage colony stimulating factors from porcine leukocyte cultures. Z. Physiol. Chem. 363:193-195, 1982.

96

44. Wissler J.H.: Chemistry and biology of the anaphylatoxin-related serum peptide system. I. Purification, crystallization, and properties of classical anaphylatoxin from rat serum. Eur. J. Immunol. 2:73-83, 1972.
45. Wissler J.H.: Chemistry and biology of the anaphylatoxin-related serum peptide system. II. Purification, crystallization, and properties of a new basic peptide, cocytotaxin, from rat serum. Eur. J. Immunol. 2:84-89, 1972.
46. Wissler J.H., V.J. Stecher and E. Sorkin: Chemistry and biology of the anaphylatoxin-related serum peptide system. III. Evaluation of leukotactic activity as a property of a new peptide system with classical anaphylatoxin and cocytotaxin as components. Eur. J. Immunol. 2:90-96, 1972.
47. Burdach St.E.G., K.G. Evers and J.H. Wissler: Infantile genetische Agranulocytose (IGA). Leukorekrutin im diagnostisch-therapeutischen Versuch (Diagnostic-therapeutic trial in infantile genetic agranulocytosis with leukorecruitin). Monatsschr. Kinderheilkd. 130:789-792, 1982.
48. Jilek F. and H. Hoermann: Fibronectin (cold insoluble globulin). V. Mediation of fibrin-monomer binding to macrophages. Z. Physiol. Chem. 359:1603, 1978.
49. Maurer H.R.: Leukozyten-Chalone: Neuere Ergebnisse. Dtsch. Apoth. Z. 120:839-844, 1980.
50. Houck J.C. (Ed.): Chalones. Elsevier-North Holland, Amsterdam, 1976.
51. Wissler J.H., H.R. Maurer, M. Kastner, R. Maschler, R. Neumeier, M. Arnold, U. Gerlach, B. Pfefferkorn, H. Tschesche and W. Schaper: Lymphokines, monokines, leukokines: Large scale production, isolation and properties of porcine leukocyte-derived cytotaxins, cytokinesins, cytotoxins, mitogens, stimulators (CSF) and inhibitors (chalones) of colony formation. Eur. J. Cell Biol. 22:387, 1980.
52. Rothert W.: Beobachtungen und Betrachtungen ueber tactische Reizerscheinungen. Flora 88:371-421, 1901.
53. Rich A.R. and M.R. Lewis: The nature of allergy in tuberculosis as revealed by tissue culture studies. Bull. Johns Hopkins Hosp. 50:115-131, 1932.
54. Letter to the Editor: Revised nomenclature for antigen-nonspecific T cell proliferation and helper factors. J. Immunol. 123:2928-2929, 1979.
55. Letter to the Editor: A proposal for the definition of terms related to locomotion of leukocytes and other cells. J. Immunol. 121:2122-2124, 1978.
56. College of American Pathologists (Eds.): Quality Evaluation Program 1970-1978. Skokie Illinois, 1978.
57. Hallmann L. (Ed.): Klinische Chemie und Mikroskopie, 11th Ed. Georg Thieme Verlag, Stuttgart, 1980.
58. Whipple H.E., M.I. Spitzer and H.R. Bierman (Eds.): Leukopoiesis in Health and Disease. Ann. N.Y. Acad. Sci. 113:511-1092, 1964.
59. Eur. Vortragsreihe (Europarat) No. 50: Pruefung auf Pyrogene. Eur. Arzneibuch (Eur. Pharmacopoeia), Vol.2, pp.56-59. Deutscher Apotheker-Verlag, Stuttgart, 1975.

Medicine Commission, Medicine Act 1968: I. Test for Pyrogens, Appendix XIV I, p.A115. Her Majesty's Stationery Office, London, 1973.
The United States Pharmacopeia, 19th revision: Pyrogen Test, p.613. United States Pharmacopeial Convention USP, Rockville Maryland, 1975.

60. Wissler J.H.: Fluidity (microviscosity) of surface lipid hydrocarbon layers of membranes of chemokinetically and chemotactically stimulated neutrophil polymorphonuclear leucocytes. Z. Physiol. Chem. 359:339-340, 1978.

61. Wissler J.H., H.P. Jennissen and H.U. Keller: Regulation of cellular transport of lipid-hydrocarbon molecules and of cellular contact phenomena of viable adherent leucocytes by serum albumin. Z. Physiol. Chem. 359:1462, 1978.

62. Keller H.U., J.H. Wissler and B. Damerau: Diverging effects of chemotactic serum peptides and synthetic f-Met-Leu-Phe on neutrophil locomotion and adhesion. Immunology 42:379-383, 1981.

63. Wissler J.H.: Mode of action of chemotactic and chemokinetic solutes and physical properties of membranes of neutrophil leukocytes in relation to cellular recognition in chemotaxis and locomotion in chemokinesis. Z. Physiol. Chem. 359:1167-1168, 1978.

64. Jennissen H.P.: The binding and regulation of biologically active proteins on cellular interfaces: Model studies of enzyme adsorption on hydrophobic binding site lattices and biomembranes. Adv. Enzyme Regulation 19:377-406, 1981.

65. Menkin V. (Ed.): Dynamics of Inflammation, 2nd Ed. Thomas, Springfield Illinois, 1956.

66. Peterson S.C. and P.B. Noble: A two-dimensional random-walk analysis of human granulocyte movement. Biophys. J. 12:1048-1055, 1972.

67. Carter S.B.: Haptotaxis and the mechanism of cell motility. Nature 213:256-260, 1967.

68. Ward P.A., H.G. Remold and J.R. David: The production by antigen-stimulated lymphocytes of a leukotactic factor distinct from migration inhibitory factor. Cell Immunol. 1:162-174, 1970.

69. Schiffmann E., B.A. Corcoran and S.M. Wahl: N-Formylmethionyl peptides as chemoattractants for leukocytes. Proc. Nat. Acad. Sci. USA 72:1059-1062, 1975.

70. Becker E.L.: Some interrelations of neutrophil chemotaxis, lysosomal enzyme secretion, and phagocytosis as revealed by synthetic peptides. Amer. J. Pathol. 85:385-394, 1976.

71. Schiffmann E. and J.I. Gallin: Biochemistry of phagocyte chemotaxis. Cur. Top. Cell. Regulation 15:203-261, 1979.

72. Showell H.J., R.J. Freer, S.H. Zigmond, E. Schiffmann, S. Aswanikumar, B. Corcoran and E.L. Becker: The structure-activity relations of synthetic peptides as chemotactic factors and inducers of lysosomal enzyme secretion for neutrophils. J. Exp. Med. 143:1154-1169, 1976.

73. Zigmond S.H.: Chemotaxis by polymorphonuclear leukocytes. J. Cell Biol. 77:269-287, 1978.

74. O'Flaherty J.T., D.L. Kreutzer and P.A. Ward: Chemotactic factor influences on the aggregation, swelling, and foreign surface adhesiveness of human leukocytes. Amer. J. Pathol. 90:537-550, 1978.
75. O'Flaherty J.T., H.J. Showell, D.L. Kreutzer, P.A. Ward and E.L. Becker: Inhibition of in vivo and in vitro neutrophil responses to chemotactic factors by a competitive antagonist. J. Immunol. 120:1326-1332, 1978.
76. Marois M. (Ed.): From Theoretical Physics to Biology. Proc. 3rd Int. Conf. Versailles 1971. Karger Verlag, Basel, 1973.
77. Eigen M.: Selforganization of matter and the evolution of biological macromolecules. Naturwissenschaften 58:465-523, 1971.
78. Prigogine I.: Zeit, Struktur und Fluktuationen (Nobel-Vortrag). Angew. Chem. 90:704-715, 1978.
79. Jaenicke L.: Sex hormones of brown algae. Naturwissenschaften 64:69-75, 1977.
80. Gallin J.I. and P.G. Quie (Eds.): Leukocyte Chemotaxis: Methods, Physiology, and Clinical Implications. Raven Press, New York, 1978.
81. Ebert R.H. and L. Grant: The experimental approach to the study of inflammation. In: The Inflammatory Process, Vol.1, 2nd Ed., edited by B.W. Zweifach, L. Grant and R.T. McCluskey, pp.3-49. Academic Press, New York, 1974.
82. McCutcheon M.: Chemotaxis in leukocytes. Physiol. Rev. 26:319-336, 1946.
83. Delbrueck M.: Signalwandler: terra incognita der Molekularbiologie. Angew. Chem. 84:1-7, 1972.
84. Gerisch G., D. Malchow and B. Hess: Cell communication and cyclic-AMP regulation during aggregation of the slime mold, Dictostelium discoideum. In: Biochemistry of Sensory Functions. Proc. 25th Coll. Ges. Biol. Chem. Mosbach 1974, edited by L. Jaenicke, pp.279-298. Springer Verlag, Berlin, 1974.
85. Koshland jr. D.E.: Bacterial Chemotaxis as a Model Behavioral System. Distinguished Lecture Series Soc. Gen. Physiol., Vol.2. Raven Press, New York, 1980.
86. Perez-Miravete A. (Ed.): Behaviour of Microorganisms. Plenum Press, London, 1973.
87. Engelmann Th.W.: Bacterium photometricum. Ein Beitrag zur vergleichenden Physiologie des Licht- und Farbensinnes. Pfluegers Arch. Ges. Physiol. 30:95-124, 1883.
88. Pfeffer W.: Locomotorische Richtungsbewegungen durch chemische Reize. Unters. Botan. Inst. Tuebingen 1:524-533, 1884.
89. Pfeffer W.O.: Uebersicht ueber das Vorkommen der verschiedenen Tropismen. In: Pflanzenphysiologie, 2.Ed., edited by W.O. Pfeffer, pp.561-598. Leipzig, 1904.
90. Leber Th.: Ueber die Entstehung der Entzuendung und die Wirkung der entzuendungserregenden Schaedlichkeiten. Fortschr. Med. 6: 460-464, 1888.
91. Rosen W.G.: Cellular chemotropism and chemotaxis. Quart. Rev. Biol. 37:242-259, 1962.
92. Crick F.: Diffusion in embryogenesis. Nature 225:420-422, 1970.
93. Wolpert L.: Positional information and the spatial pattern of cellular differentiation. J. Theoret. Biol. 25:1-47, 1969.

94. Edelman G.M. (Ed.): Cellular Selection and Regulation in the Immune Response. Soc. Gen. Physiol. Ser., Vol.29. Raven Press, New York, 1974.

95. Bradshaw R.A. and J.S. Rubin: Polypeptide growth factors: Some structural and mechanistic considerations. J. Supramol. Struct. 14:183-199, 1980.

96. Jerne N.K.: The somatic generation of immune recognition. Eur. J. Immunol. 1:1-9, 1971.

97. Wolpert L., J. Hicklin and A. Hornbruch: Positional information and pattern regulation in regeneration of hydra. Symp. Soc. Exp. Biol. 25:439-453, 1971.

98. Crick F.H.C.: The scale of pattern formation. Symp. Soc. Exp. Biol. 25:429-438, 1971.

99. Munro M. and F.H.C. Crick: The time needed to set up a gradient: Detailed calculations. Symp. Soc. Exp. Biol. 25:439-453, 1971.

100. Doetsch R.N.: A unified theory of bacterial motile behaviour. J. Theoret. Biol. 35:55-66, 1972.

101. Nicholls J.G. (Ed.): The Role of Intercellular Signals: Navigation, Encounter, Outcome. Rep. Dahlem Workshop Berlin 1979, Life Sciences Res. Rep. 14. Verlag Chemie, Weinheim, 1979.

102. Ebringer A.: Information theory and limitations in antibody diversity. J. Theoret. Biol. 51:293-302, 1975.

103. Abercombie M. (Ed.): Locomotion of Tissue Cells. Ciba Foundation Symposium 14 (New Series). Elsevier-North Holland, 1973.

104. Carterette E.C. and M.P. Friedman (Eds.): Handbook of Sensory Perception, Vol.3: Biology of Perceptual Systems. Academic Press, New York, 1973.

105. Loewenstein W.R. (Ed.): Handbook of Sensory Physiology, Vol.1: Principles of Receptor Physiology. Springer Verlag, Berlin, 1971.

106. Poynder T.M. (Ed.): Transduction Mechanisms in Chemoreception. Information Retrieval, London, 1974.

107. Katz B.: Quantal mechanism of neural transmitter release. Science 173:123-126, 1971.

108. Wilkinson P.C. and I.C. McKay: The chemotactic activity of native and denatured serum albumin. Int. Arch. Allergy 41:237-247, 1971.

109. Wilkinson P.C. and I.C. McKay: The molecular requirements for chemotactic attraction of leukocytes by proteins. Studies of proteins with synthetic side groups. Eur. J. Immunol. 2:570-577, 1972.

110. Wilkinson P.C. (Ed.): Chemotaxis and Inflammation. Churchill Livingstone, Edinburgh, 1974.

111. Becker E.L. and T.P. Stossel: Chemotaxis. Fed. Proc. 39: 2949-2952, 1980.

112. Lewin S. (Ed.): Displacement of Water and its Control of Biochemical Reactions. Academic Press, London, 1974.

113. Wissler J.H.: Modes of cellular recognition governing migratory responses of leucocytes. Abstr. Commun. 9th FEBS-Meeting, p.300. Budapest, 1974.

114. Wissler J.H.: Nature of information and its perception in motion patterns of leucocytes. Z. Physiol. Chem. 357:286-287, 1976.

115. Wissler J.H.: Conformational alterations in classical anaphy-latoxin and chemoattraction of neutrophil leucocytes. Z. Phy-siol. Chem. 361:350-351, 1980.

116. Wissler J.H., V.J. Stecher and E. Sorkin: Secondary structur-al properties of anaphylatoxin preparations and chemotactic activity for neutrophils. J. Immunol. 111:314-315, 1973.

117. Wissler J.H., V.J. Stecher and E. Sorkin: Regulation of serum-derived chemotactic activities by the leukotactic bina-ry peptide system. Antibiotics and Chemotherapy 19:442-463, 1974.

118. Wissler J.H., V.J. Stecher and E. Sorkin: Cyclic AMP and che-motaxis of leukocytes. In: Proc. Conf. Cyclic AMP, Cell Growth and the Immune Response, Marco Islands Florida 1973, edited by W. Braun, L.M. Lichtenstein and C.W. Parker, pp.270-283. Springer Verlag, New York, 1974.

119. Hugli T.E.: The structural basis for anaphylatoxin and chemo-tactic functions of C3a, C4a, and C5a. In: Critical Rev. Im-munol., Vol.1, edited by M.Z. Atassi, pp.321-366. CRC Press, Boca Raton Florida, 1981.

120. Hugli T.E.: The complement anaphylatoxins. Behring Inst. Mitt. 68:68-81, 1981.

121. Wissler J.H.: Metastable membrane states and memory formation associated with information processing in chemotaxis of leu-cocytes. Fed. Proc. 38:1428, 1979.

122. Shannon C.E. and V. Weaver (Eds.): The Mathematical Theory of Communication. University of Illinois Press, Chicago, 1949.

123. Brillouin L. (Ed.): Science and Information Theory. Academic Press, New York, 1962.

124. Khinchin A.I. (Ed.): Mathematical Foundations of Information Theory. Dover Publications, New York, 1957.

125. Wissler J.H., V.J. Stecher and E. Sorkin: Regulation of che-motaxis of leucocytes by the anaphylatoxin-related peptide system. In: Proc. 20th Coll. Protides of the Biological Fluids, Brugge 1972, edited by H. Peeters, pp.411-416. Perga-mon Press, Oxford, 1973.

126. Wissler J.H.: A new biologically active peptide system relat-ed to classical anaphylatoxin. Experientia 27:1447-1448, 1971.

127. Morowitz H.J. (Ed.): Entropy for Biologists. An Introduction to Thermodynamics. Academic Press, New York, 1971.

128. Katchalski A. and P.F. Curran (Eds.): Nonequilibrium Thermo-dynamics in Biophysics. Harvard University Press, Cambridge Massachusetts, 1974.

129. Van Holde K.E. (Ed.): Physical Biochemistry. Prentice-Hall, Eaglewood Cliffs New Jersey, 1971.

130. Decker P. (Ed.): Evolution in offenen Systemen. Bioide, eine Verallgemeinerung des Darwin'schen Prinzips. Tieraerztliche Hochschule, Hannover, 1974.

131. Conroy M.C., J. Ozols and I.H. Lepow: Structural features and biologic properties of fragments obtained by limited proteo-lysis of C3. J. Immunol. 116:1682-1687, 1976.

132. Fernandez H., P. Henson and T.E. Hugli: A single scheme for C3a and C5a isolation and characterization of chemotactic be-haviour. J. Immunol. 116:1732, 1976.

133. Fernandez H.N., P.M. Henson, A. Otani and T.E. Hugli: Chemotactic response to human C3a and C5a anaphylatoxins. I. Evaluation of C3a and C5a leukotaxis in vitro and under simulated in vivo conditions. J. Immunol. 120:109-115, 1978.
134. Perez H.D., I.M. Goldstein, R.O. Webster and P.M. Henson: Enhancement of the chemotactic activity of human C5a des arg by an anionic polypeptide ("cochemotaxin") in normal serum and plasma. J. Immunol. 126:800-804, 1981.
135. Kay A.B., H.S. Shin and K.F. Austen: Selective attraction of eosinophils and synergism between eosinophil chemotactic factor of anaphylaxis (ECF-A) and a fragment cleaved from the fifth component of complement (C5a). Immunology 24:969-976, 1973.
136. Wissler J.H. and E. Sorkin: Nature and mechanism of cellular recognition and regulation of leucocyte migration. Nouv. Rev. Franc. Hematol. 13:893-895, 1973.
137. Wilkinson P.C. and P.C. McKay: Recognition in leucocyte chemotaxis. Antibiotics and Chemotherapy 19:421-441, 1974.
138. Wilkinson P.C.: Recognition of protein structure in leukocyte chemotaxis. Nature 244:512-513, 1973.
139. Weber G.: Rotational brownian motion and polarization of the fluorescence of solutions. Adv. Protein Chem. 8:415-459, 1953.
140. Jackowski S. and R.I. Sha'afi: Response of adenosine cyclic 3',5'-monophosphate level in rabbit neutrophils to the chemotactic peptide formyl-methionyl-leucyl-phenylalanine. Mol. Pharmacol. 16:473-481, 1979.
141. McLaren A.D. and L. Packer: Some aspects of enzyme reactions in heterogenous systems. Adv. Enzymol. 33:245-308, 1970.
142. Neumann E.: Molecular hysteresis and its cybernetic significance. Angew. Chem. Int. Ed. 12:356-369, 1973.
143. Baserga R. (Ed.): Tissue Growth Factors. Handbook Exp. Pharmacol., Vol.57. Springer Verlag, Berlin, 1981.
144. Erikson R.L., M.S. Collett, E. Erikson and A.F. Purchio: Towards a molecular description of cell transformation by avian sarcoma virus. Proc. Roy. Soc. London B 210:387-396, 1980.
145. Krebs E.G.: Phosphorylation and dephosphorylation of glycogen phosphorylase: A prototype for reversible covalent enzyme modification. Cur. Top. Cell. Regulation 18:401-419, 1981.
146. Heilmeyer jr. L.M.G., U. Groeschel-Stewart, U. Jahnke, M.W. Kilimann, K.P. Kohse and M. Varsanyi: Novel aspects of skeletal muscle protein kinase and protein phosphatase regulation by Ca-II-ions. Adv. Enzyme Regulation 18:121-144, 1980.
147. Meinhardt H. (Ed.): Models of Biological Pattern Formation. Academic Press, London, 1982.
148. Poland D. and H.A. Scheraga: Theory of noncovalent structure in polyamino acids. In: Poly-alpha-Amino-Acids. Protein Models for Conformational Studies. Biological Macromolecules, A Series of Monographs, Vol.1, edited by G.D. Fasman, pp.391-497. Marcel Dekker, New York, 1967.
149. Nemethy G. and H.A. Scheraga: Structure of water and hydrophobic bonding in proteins. I. A model for the thermodynamic properties of liquid water. J. Chem. Phys. 36:3382-3400, 1962.

150. Jensen J.A. and V. Esquenazi: Chemotactic stimulation by cell surface immune reactions. Nature 256:213-215, 1975.
151. Williams D., V. Esquenazi, R. Cirocco and J.A. Jensen: The chemoattraction of neutrophils by heterologous and homologous cytotoxic sera. J. Immunol. 116:554-561, 1976.
152. Jensen J.A. and D. Williams: Chemotaxis of human neutrophils induced by lymphocytoxic sera. Nouv. Rev. Franc. Hematol. 13:889-891, 1973.
153. Wissler J.H.: Cellular communication between leucocytes: Production from large scale cultures, isolation and properties of leucocyte-derived cytotaxins, cytokinesins, cytotoxins and mitogens. Abstr. Commun. 2nd Eur. Conf. Biochemistry of Phagocytes, p.5. Trieste, 1980.
154. Monod J., J. Wyman and J.-P. Changeux: On the nature of allosteric transitions: A plausible model. J. Mol. Biol. 12: 88-118, 1965.
155. Rosenoor V.M., M. Oratz and M.A. Rothschild (Eds.): Albumin Structure, Function and Uses. Pergamon Press, Oxford, 1977.
156. Wissler J.H.: Large scale techniques for production and isolation of cellular effector substances of regenerative tissue morphogenesis by culturing cells in serum-free, synthetic fluids: Design, preparation and use of a novel medium. See appendix, this book, pp.393-471.
157. Hoeckel M., W. Wagner, H.Renner and J.H. Wissler: Action of highly purified monocyte-derived polypeptide mediators of chemotropic blood vessel growth ("monocyto-angiotropin") in the skin of rabbits. Immunbiology 165:280, 1983.
158. Fishman A.P.: Endothelium. Ann. N.Y. Acad. Sci. 401:1-272, 1982.

5 THE SEPHADEX MODEL OF ACUTE INFLAMMATION

G. EGGER

5.1 INTRODUCTION

Generally speaking, an acute inflammation consists of three major events that take place at the site of inflammation: The exudation of plasma components, the egress of white blood cells from the vessels and the reaction of the connective tissue. The relative proportion of these three elements is the basis for the variability of the inflammatory processes. An investigator dealing with acute inflammation has to select which one of these elements he wants to investigate and has to choose the appropriate model accordingly. There is no one method suitable for the evaluation of the entire inflammatory process, but each single method aims specifically at the measurement of a particular element of inflammation.

5.2 SELECTION OF A MODEL OF ACUTE INFLAMMATION

Frequently used methods for studying special aspects of the inflammatory process are:
(a) the paw oedema test and the blue tests for inflammatory hyperemia and oedema;
(b) subcutaneously implanted polyester sponges (1) and the air pouch test for the composition of the humoral component of inflammatory exudates;
(c) the injection of irritants into body cavities, the injection of cells with radioactive labelling (2) and the implantation of Dacron mesh tissue (3) for the reaction of the white blood cells;
(d) the cotton pellet test and the air pouch test for the reaction of the connective tissue.

The performance and evaluation of these methods are described in a paper by Rocha e Silva et al. (4).

For an investigator who deals with the functions and the fate of the radioactively labelled leucocytes during inflammatory processes, models would be useful that enable him to measure the labelled cells as well as the radioactive debris after their death at the site of inflammation. Such models would facilitate the answering of topical questions such as the appearance of labelled cells at the site of inflammation after intravenous injection or other methods of application, or the life-span of the leucocytes at the site of inflammation. In our laboratory, we have developed and used for several years a method (described below) that serves this purpose.

5.3 THE SEPHADEX MODEL

This model is particularly apt for measuring the quantity and composition of inflammatory exudates, that is to say, the cellular as well as the humoral components. Its principle is based on the subcutaneous injection of swollen and sterilized Sephadex G 200 (Pharmacia Fine Chemicals), an uncharged Dextran gel widely used in gel chromatography. By injecting a definite quantity of Sephadex and by injecting the Sephadex to form a spherical implant, the size of the subcutaneous wound cavity and consequently the intensity of the experimental inflammation can be exactly reproduced. White cells immigrating from the surrounding connective tissue gather on and between the Sephadex beads. Sephadex G 200 can absorb in its inner volume proteins of a molecular weight up to 800 000 and, therefore, is capable of soaking up a considerable share of the humoral substances occurring during an acute inflammation (see below). At given intervals, the Sephadex implants may be removed and the cells and the humoral exudate can be rinsed out onto filters that retain the Sephadex beads but allow the cells to pass through. Then, both components are separated by centrifugation and measured.

Contrary to the relatively clear situation of the white cells, the humoral component of the exudate contains everything soluble that occurs during inflammation, as well as degradation products: substances from the blood and the surrounding connective tissue, products of the immigrant cells, and, after their death and disintegration, their debris. More details of the method have been described by Klingenberg (5) and Egger (6).

5.3.1 The cellular response to Sephadex irritation

The cellular reactions towards 5 ml Sephadex injected into the subcutis of the dorsal right lower quadrant of Sprague-Dawley rats consists of the following elements: The major part of the cellular response occurs during the first five days. Different lots of animals often show marked differences in the course and the intensity of the inflammatory reaction. This variability has to be taken into account when experiments carried out with different lots are to be compared.

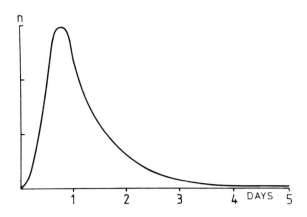

Fig. 1. Number of Neutrophils found in 5 ml of injected Sephadex. Ordinate: Number of cells. It would be useless to indicate concrete numbers, since the reactions of different groups of animals vary. Strong reactions may reach a peak of 50 million cells and more. Abscissa: Time. For further explanations see text.

Neutrophils (Figure 1): The immigration occurs as a rush soon after the injection of Sephadex which is typical for the neutrophil response. Their number reaches a maximum after about 18 hours and, thereafter, decreases exponentially.

Eosinophils (Figure 2): They usually develop two peaks around the first day and the third or fourth day. Some groups of the experimental animals lack the first peak.

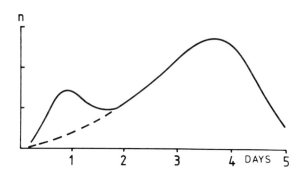

Fig. 2. Number of eosinophils. For symbols see Figure 1. The peaks usually do not exceed half a million cells.

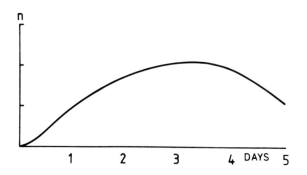

Fig. 3. Number of lymphocytes. For symbols see Figure 1. Their number at the climax varies between about 2 and 7 million.

Lymphocytes (Figure 3): The number increases moderately and, in most cases, shows a maximum around the fourth day. Before the lymphocytes disintegrate in the Sephadex implants, they develop marked stigmata of degeneration such as pyknotic or segmented nuclei, nuclei which merge with the cell membrane, and a vacuolized and expanded cytoplasm (7)

Monocytes appear only in modest numbers. The reaction of the connective tissue is discrete. The Sephadex inflammation subsides during the acute stage and does not develop a chronic phase. It is a model of an aseptic, traumatic inflammation. These data refer exclusively to the reaction to pure Sephadex G 200. Any substance, however, can be added and measured (8,9).

5.4 PECULIARITIES OF THE SEPHADEX MODEL

5.4.1 Test animals

An important factor is the quality of the animals since particular strains show their own typical inflammatory reaction. We usually use Sprague-Dawley rats from the Forschungsinstitut fuer Versuchstierzucht der Universitaet Wien, Himberg. S.-D. rats develop a swift and marked reaction towards Sephadex, thus shortening the duration of the experiments and facilitating their statistical evaluation. We found that Wistar rats show a slower and less distinct inflammatory response than S.-D. rats. Test animals ought to be bred under specific pathogen-free conditions that favour uniform inflammatory reactions. After delivery, the animals spend a 3 to 6 day interval of adaptation in our animal quarters. Subsequently, to keep the period of bacterial invasion as short as possible, they are subjected to the experiment. We use male rats since females tend to bite out the Sephadex implants. Other laboratory animals were not tested.

5.4.2 The site of inflammation

Another important issue is the selection of the site where an inflammation is to be induced. Specific questions require, of course, specific localizations. We usually inject 5 ml of Sephadex G 200 into the subcutis of the right lower quadrant of the back. With subcutaneous application, the reactions of different areas of the body must be taken into consideration. Even bilaterally-symmetrical sites show significant differences. We found that Sephadex implants in the left lower quadrant of the back contain more plasma proteins during the first 3 days of an inflammation than implants in the right side, and that, on the left, the lymphocyte reaction occurs earlier than on the right. The neutrophil and eosinophil reactions do not show differences. The same site therefore has to be treated throughout one experiment.

5.4.3 Yield of cells and proteins by filtration

We rinse the excised Sephadex implants with the four-fold quantity of a 0.9% NaCl solution through Schleicher and Schuell "black ribbon" filters. Rinsing 5 ml of Sephadex with 20 ml NaCl solution results in a yield of 77.28% of standard error of mean (SEM) +/- 1.38 cells and 89.19% SEM +/- 0.58 proteins. Total of cells respectively proteins recovered from multiple washings are taken as 100%. If the absolute contents of cells and proteins are sought, however, laboratory conditions should be standardized by repeatedly rinsing the removed Sephadex implants through the same filters to approximately zero-values, thus establishing the 100% values of the individual methodical processing. Once calibrated, the true values may be extrapolated in further experiments.

5.4.4 The number of cells at inflammatory sites

It is essential to know that neutrophil granulocytes do not leave a site of inflammation but die there and disintegrate. Therefore, the number of cells found at any time point in the Sephadex lesion is the result of immigrant minus dead cells, and the period of the cells' presence is determined by their life-span. As fast as the cells disintegrate, the Sephadex implants are enriched with their debris. The dynamics of this complex situation can be plausibly illustrated by a graphic model:

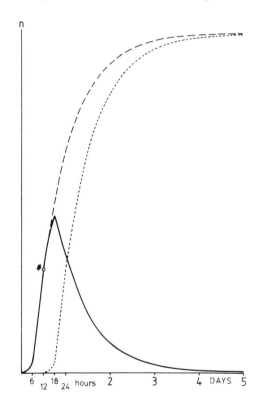

Fig. 4. Hypothetical model for an analysis of the number of neutrophils found in the Sephadex implants as shown in Figure 1. Ordinate: Number of cells. Abscissa: Time. The broken curve represents the total of cells that have immigrated into the Sephadex implants. During the first 12 hours before cell death starts, this curve is identical to the curve formed by the number of cells actually found in the Sephadex (full stroke, see below). The ingress develops its full intensity after 6 hours and then is linear until 12 hours. After 12 hours (arrow), the ingress decreases exponentially. This decrease is regulated at least in part by endogenous substances that curb the ingress of cells into the Sephadex implants (9). The dotted curve represents the total number of cells that have died and disintegrated. It has the same course as the curve of the immigrant cells, but is shifted according to the 12-hour life-span

of the cells. The number of immigrant cells minus the number of disintegrated cells results in the number of cells actually found in the Sephadex implants (full stroke). The number peaks after 18 hours. Since the three curves (immigrant, disintegrated and actually found cells) are mutually dependant, two of them are enough for a reconstruction of the entire process.

Figure 4 is an attempt to analyze the changes in the number of the neutrophils as shown in Figure 1. This model has to be considered to be a mere visual aid, since such important data as the constant 12-hours' life-span of the cells in the Sephadex, or the extent of the decrease in the cellular ingress into the Sephadex were only estimated. But whatever the real conditions were in a specifically investigated case, the number of cells found after some definite time interval is always the difference between the total number of immigrant cells and the total of the dead cells. Regarding labelling experiments, labelled cells (Figure 4, full stroke) as well as their radioactive debris after death (Figure 4, dotted) can be harvested from the Sephadex implants. With these data, the reconstruction of the total of immigrant cells (Figure 4, broken line) and, in consequence, the estimation of the life-span (= the distance between the immigrant and the perished cells on the abscissa) is feasible. A possible loss of cell debris by diffusion into the surrounding connective tissue or by phagocytosis by following cells has to be taken into consideration. The same principles apply to other cell types.

5.4.5 White cells in blood and inflammatory exudate

The white blood count is considered to be an essential indicator of an inflammatory process, and the number of white cells in the blood is taken to be a kind of mirror for the events at the site of inflammation. Actually, in the case of the Sephadex inflammation in rats, there is no correlation between the white blood count and the number of white cells at the site of inflammation as shown by the following experiment: Sephadex injected into rats was removed after 3,5,7,10,14,17 and 21 days and the cell contents were counted. Simultaneously, blood was sampled from carotid incisions and white blood counts were made. The results showed that the number of neutrophils and lymphocytes, though elevated above the normal level, did not correspond to the changes in the number of cells contained in the Sephadex (Figures 5 and 7). The blood level of the eosinophils was not altered at all (Figure 6). We also checked at daily intervals during the first five days of inflammation and found the same result, namely, no correlation.

Since white cells on their way from the site of origin to the site of inflammation are transported by the blood, this incongruity proves that their ingress into the vessels and/or their duration of stay in the blood have undergone considerable change during the course of inflammation.

112

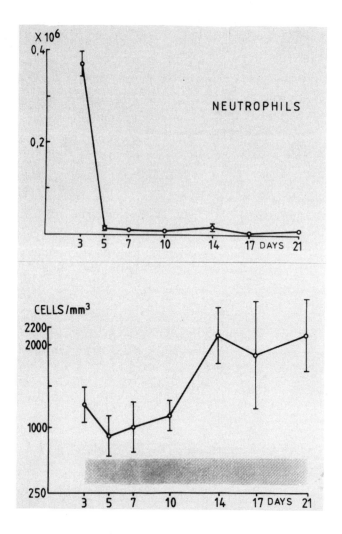

Fig. 5. Comparison between the cells found in the Sephadex implants (upper diagram) and in the blood (below). The normal blood values (animals without inflammation) are represented by the shaded line (= arithmetic mean +/- SEM). Ordinate: Number of cells +/- SEM. Abscissa: Time. The number of the neutrophils in the Sephadex drops on the fifth day to a value of about 15 000 cells. This level remains until the end of the experiment. The blood neutrophils are above normal, they increase during the experiment and show their highest level when the neutrophil invasion into the Sephadex implants has long since subsided.

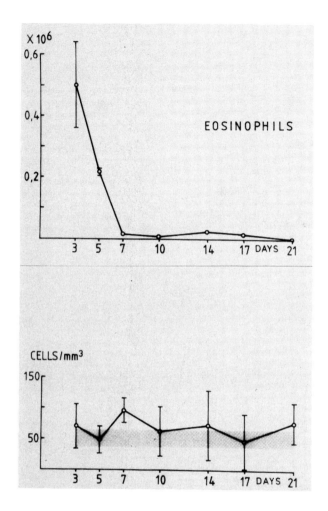

Fig. 6. For symbols see Figure 5. The eosinophils in the Sephadex decrease until the seventh day to a level of about 20 000. The blood values are normal during the entire experiment.

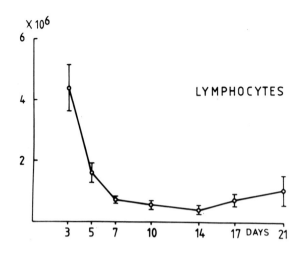

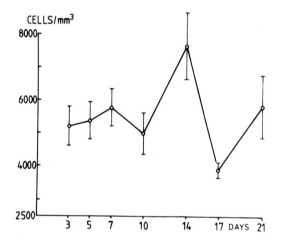

Fig. 7. For symbols see Figure 5. The number of the lymphocytes in the Sephadex decreases during the experiment to less than a million and does not correspond to the elevated blood counts.

SUMMARY

The choice of an animal model of acute inflammation depends on the topic to be investigated, e.g.
(a) the exudation of plasma components,
(b) the egress of white blood cells from the vessels, or
(c) the reaction of the connective tissue
    Frequently used methods to imitate experimental inflammation are:
for (a) the paw oedema, the blue tests and the subcutaneous implantation of polyester sponges,
for (b) the injection of irritants into the body cavities, the intravenous injection of labelled leucocytes and the implantation of DACRON mesh tissue,
for (c) the cotton pellet test and the granuloma pouch test.
    A new method for the accurate measurement of a) and b) involves subcutaneous injection of swollen Sephadex G 200.
    Considering the methodology and interpretation of experiments with Sephadex in rats emphasis of the following points is required: The quality of the test animals for experimental inflammation is crucial, since particular strains show their own typical variety of inflammatory reactions. Specific pathogen free breeding promotes uniform responses. Different sites of the body, even in a bilateral-symmetrical position, react differently. There is no correlation between the number of white cells in the blood and their appearance in the focus of inflammation; blood counts do not reflect the events at the site of inflammation.

116

REFERENCES

1. Robinson B.V. and J.M. Robson: Further studies on the anti-inflammatory factor found at a site of inflammation. Brit. J. Pharmacol. 26:372-384, 1966.
2. Perper R.J., M. Sanda, V.J. Stecher and A.L. Oronsky: Physiologic and pharmacologic alterations of rat leukocyte chemotaxis (Cx) in-vivo. Ann. N.Y. Acad. Sci. 256:190-209, 1975.
3. Senelar R. and J.P. Bureau: Inhibitory effect of pregnancy on the migration of the inflammatory cells: A quantitative histological study. B. J. exp. Path. 60:286-293, 1979.
4. Rocha e Silva M. and J. Garcia Leme: Chemical mediators of the acute imflammatory reaction, pp.49-99. Pergamon Press, Oxford, 1972.
5. Klingenberg H.G. and H. Dorner: Sephadexentzuendung bei der Ratte. Exp. Path 10:333-337, 1975.
6. Egger G. and S. Porta: The influence of a permanent Isoproterenol (ISO) application on the dynamics of the Sephadex inflammation. Exp. Path. 17:12-17, 1979.
7. Egger G., S. Porta and D. Gollmann: Antiinflammatory substances appearing during an acute inflammation and the alteration of their properties by Isoproterenol (ISO). An in-vivo investigation in rats. Exp. Path. 17:327-333, 1979.
8. Klingenberg H.G. and H. Dorner: Mikroskopische Unter-suchungen zur "gefaessabdichtenden" Wirkung der Kalziumionen. Experientia 32:1561-1562, 1976.
9. Egger G.: In-vivo demonstration of endogenous substances regulating the regression of the acute inflammation. Exp. Path. 20:175-181, 1981.

6 TECHNIQUES OF CELL HANDLING AND VIABILITY TESTING

N. COLAS-LINHART

6.1 INTRODUCTION

Several authors have used labelled leucocytes to detect inflammatory foci in cases of infection. 51-Cr was the first marker used for in-vivo detection but its high photon energy, the high rate of conversion and its long physical halflife are obvious disadvantages. Other gamma emitters such as 67-Ga have also been suggested for human leucocyte labelling and for direct intravenous administration in abscess detection (1). Since the development of 111-In-hydroxyquinoline (i.e. oxine resp. oxinate in the case of the salt), as described by Thakur et al. (2), several centres have used it for the clinical detection of abscesses and many variations of the technique have been tried (3).

The criteria for a good labelling technique are the following:

(a) high labelling efficiency;

(b) high stability, i.e. the activity should remain attached to the labelled cells;

(c) high cell specificity, i.e. only the desired cells, e.g. polymorphonuclear phagocytes, should be labelled and

(d) normal maintenance of cellular function, especially with regard to chemotaxis (4). In other words, labelled cells should be able to infiltrate infectious foci as effectively as unlabelled cells.

The most important factor to control is the cell viability because neutrophil polymorphonuclear cells have a short halflife and are liable to deterioration.

6.2 TECHNIQUES OF CELL SEPARATION

Twenty ml of human venous blood were collected and allowed to sediment in a dextran suspension (Pharmacia, Sweden). The WBC rich supernatant was separated and the remaining red blood cells were then removed by adding ammonium chloride solution 0.7 g/l (5). The final suspension consisted of about 80% polymorphs (PMN) and 20% mononuclear cells and eosinophils. The leucocytes were then washed and concentrated by centrifugation (300 g for 5 minutes) and resuspended in NaCl (9 g/l), and were finally suspended in Hank's balanced salt solution (HBSS, pH 7.4) before labelling. Three populations of PMN were studied.
1) PMN kept in Krebs' medium, referred to as "control" cells.
2) PMNs processed for labelling without exposure to any of the the tracers, referred to as unlabelled "reference" cells.
3) PMNs after labelling with 111-In, 99m-Tc, or 51-Cr, referred to as "labelled" cells.

Another technique was assayed using Plasmagel and Ficoll Paque. Red cell lysis was obtained by NaCl 0.2% and NaCl 1.2%.

6.3 LABELLING METHODS

We have developed a new leucocyte labelling technique derived from that used earlier for red cell labelling. The method was described in detail in a previous paper (4), but briefly it consists of "in-vitro pretinning", i.e. preincubation of the white cells in a "cold" tin pyrophosphate solution before labelling with 99m-Tc-pertechnetate. This method will be referred to as the Sn-pyrophosphate/99m-Tc-pertechnetate method (PYPE). To assess the cell viability during the labelling procedure we used several functional tests, migration studies and electron microscopic studies. Five leucocyte labelling techniques (111-In-oxinate, 111-In-oxinate without extraction, 99m-Tc-oxinate, Sn-pyrophosphate/99m-Tc-pertechnetate, 51-Cr) were also compared using the same separation methods, conservation medium, viability assays, migration and electron microscopic studies.

6.3.1 111-In-oxinate (2)

This technique has already been described in detail (2), but the oxinate concentration was reduced to 1 mg/ml in ethanol according to recent papers (6). The enriched white blood cell (WBC) suspension was incubated with the 111-In-oxinate solution for 15 minutes at room temperature. We used two oxinate concentrations:
a) 2.5 ug oxinate for 1.0 x 10E07 cells
b) 0.5 ug oxinate for 1.0 x 10E07 cells.

This concentration of cells seemed to be the standard in current use.

6.3.2 111-In-oxinate without extraction

This modification of Thakur's technique needed no extraction of the radioactive chelating agent nor a pure alcohol solution (7).

6.3.3 99m-Tc-oxinate (8)

This technique used a solution prepared by adding to the oxinate solution of 5 ug oxinate 0.1 ml of a tin pyrophosphate solution and 20 mCi pertechnetate.

6.3.4   Sn-pyrophosphate preincubation/99m-Tc-pertechnetate PYPE (5)

The cell suspension was incubated for 15 minutes at 37 deg.C with a stannous pyrophosphate solution (59.4 mg pyrophosphate and 1.3 mg stannous chloride in a 3 ml solution) using 150 ul/2.0 x 10E07 leucocytes. ("in-vitro pretinning"). Free pyrophosphate was removed by centrifugation and washing of the cells. The resulting sediment was labelled by incubation in 1 ml of a high specific activity pertechnetate solution (20 to 30 mCi/ml) for 10 minutes at 20 deg.C.

6.3.5   51-Cr-chromate (9)

This technique required 7.5 to 30 uCi of 51-Cr to be added to 1.0 x 10E08 WBCs. The cells were incubated for one half hour at 37 deg.C.

6.4   IN-VITRO TESTS OF THE LABELLED CELLS

6.4.1   Radioactive label: efficiency, stability

The labelling efficiencies were calculated by measuring the radioactivity of the suspension before centrifugation and that of the pellet and the supernatant after centrifugation at 300 g for 5 minutes. The efficiency was calculated in classical fashion as the ratio (percentage) of the activity of the pellet to that of the total.

The stability of the radioactive label was tested by repeated measurement of the free 99m-Tc in the supernatant after centrifugation. The supernatant activity (free label) was counted three times: at 5 minutes, 3 and 24 hrs after labelling. At the same times electrophoresis was performed on the supernatant using veronal buffer, pH = 6.8, Whatman paper no. 1 in methanol 35% water solution.

6.4.2 Labelled cells: selectivity and homogeneity

Firstly, it was important to know the composition of the cell preparation and the affinity of the different cells for the tracer. Secondly, was it nessecary to verify the labelling homogeneity by histo-autoradiography. To determine the cellular uptake of 99m-Tc by white blood cells, we used a new "track" autoradiographic method which visualized the materialized tracks of 99m-Tc internal conversion and Auger electrons (10).

6.4.3 Labelled cells: chemotaxis, phagocytosis

Chemotaxis was assayed by the Cutler and Nelson technique under agarose. Leucocyte migration was observed using a light microscope, after 2.5 hrs incubation at 37 deg.C. This test was also performed after each labelling step simultaneously with the stability test described above.

Phagocytosis and metabolic tests: There are many metabolic tests for the study of the biochemical phenomena associated with phagocytosis and the death of pathogenic agents (e.g. bacteria) caused by polymorphonuclear cells. Of these, the following were applied:
- spontaneous or stimulated oxygen production (by Zymosan)
- oxyperoxide anion production measured by nitroblue tetrazolium reduction.
- hydrogen peroxide production
- iodination by 125-I.

6.4.4 Labelled cells: electron microscopic studies

The cell morphology was examined by electron microscopy after the cells had been fixed with 2.5% glutaraldehyde and embedded in epoxy resin (EPON). To assess each labelling procedure, a series of photographs of the labelled cells was taken and compared with unlabelled cells from the same blood sample (control cells). Triplicate blood samples were used for each experimant. To control PYPE labelling, microscopic studies were performed at each step of the preparation (5). The role of oxinate in the technique using 111-In-oxinate was assessed by comparing results obtained from cells incubated with the 111-In-oxinate complex in the same concentration.

6.5 IN-VIVO TESTS OF THE LABELLED CELLS

Polymorphonuclear cellular viability cannot be assessed completely by only using in-vitro tests. In order to obtain blood kinetic data in-vivo, the PYPE method was applied to canine white cells. These leucocytes were labelled and reinfused in normal or abscess-bearing dogs (11).

6.6 RESULTS

Since each step in the leucocyte labelling technique involves some degree of functional damage, it cannot be discussed without reference to cell viability and specificity.

6.6.1 Effects of sedimentation and lysis of erythrocytes

There was no completely perfect method of obtaining a pure PMN cell population without damaging them, and in practice it appeared also impossible to lyse the red cells without concomitant damage to the leucocytes.

Several methods of removing red cells without damaging white cells have been described in the literature. We tested some of them with a chemotaxis method and the results are shown here (Table 1).

Table 1.   Effect of Red Cell Lysis upon Lycocytes

Method for RBC lysis	Mean WBC number/l	Chemotaxis (0 to +++)
1 Immunological (anti-A serum)	5.6 x 10E06	+
2 Hypotonic dilution (water) (in dextran suspension)	15.0 x 10E06	+
3 Hypotonic dilution (water) (after centrifugation)	30.0 x 10E06	0
4 Ammonium chloride 0.87% solution	27.5 x 10E06	+++
5 No RBC removal	30.0 x 10E06	+++

Immunological and various hypotonic methods of RBC lysis were used and chemotaxis was assayed simultaneously (4 experiments)

The best result, i. e., RBC disappearance, preservation of all WBC and normal chemotaxis was obtained in experiment 4

124

Lysis of the erythrocytes by addition of ammonium cloride was considered best since it did not reduce the number of leucocytes and did not impair their chemotaxis. Some of the other methods greatly reduced the number of white cells, others impaired chemotaxis. The most satisfactory was the ammonium chloride method as described by Gray et al. (12).

Electron microscopic studies were performed at each step of the procedure and confirmed other test results.

After dextran sedimentation numerous membranous filaments were observed on the cell membrane (Figure 1).

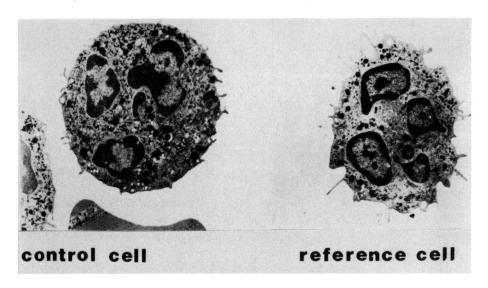

control cell   **reference cell**

Fig. 1. The reference cell (x 2 750), obtained after the cellular separation, shows long membrane projections when compared with a control cell (x 3 700).

This irregular morphology of the membrane was confirmed by scanning electron microscopy (Figure 2).

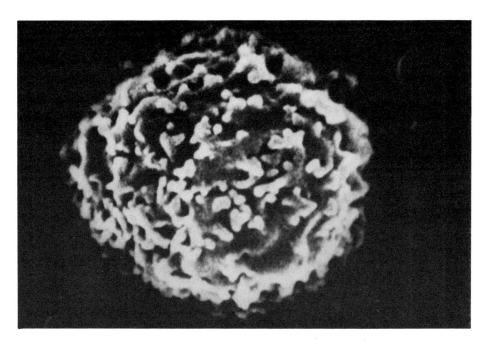

Fig. 2. A reference cell is shown by scanning electron microscopy.

After ammonium chloride some cytoplasmic vacuoles could be seen in some cells. Other methods of lysis were even more damaging.

From photomicrographs we could appreciate the cellular composition. But it was necessary to study the affinity of different cells to the tracer. The results are shown on Table 2 with the PYPE method. The number of platelets was relatively high but their uptake of 99m-Tc was minimal. So there was no need for extra effort to remove them from our preparation. The problem was different with the 111-In-oxinate since the labelling efficiency of the platelets is high with this tracer. With Plasmagel and Ficoll Paque separation we obtained a very pure PMN preparation (95%) without cell alterations.

126

Table 2.   Relative Importance and Labelling
                          Efficiency of   Labelled   Cells

                   Percent   Labelling   Activity per
                   after   efficiency   10 mCi 99m-Tc
                   separation

Red cells   1/10 G.B.   90%   300   uCi

Platelets   1/3 G.B.   10%   1   mCi

Lymphocytes   1-2/10 G.B.   10%   25   uCi
Monocytes

PMN   80-85%   40%   8.7   mCi

6.6.2 Effects of the labelling procedures (12)

6.6.2.1 Chemotaxis -
     Spontaneous random migration and chemotaxis of "reference"
and "control" cells were not significantly different (Student's
test). The chemotactic indices of PMNs labelled either with PYPE
or 51-Cr (2.37 +/- 0.43 and 2.45 +/- 0.63 respectively) were
analogous to those of unlabelled cells. Other chemotactic indices
were very close to 1.0, demonstrating that such labelled cells
moved in all directions without preferential orientation.

6.6.2.2 Phagocytosis and metabolic tests –

PMN cells labelled with 111-In-oxinate showed a diminished stimulated oxygen consumption and decreased ingestion rates and iodination. The results obtained with the other 111-In-oxinate procedure (without extraction) were slightly different: late ingestion and iodination were also decreased, but spontaneous and stimulated oxygen consumption were normal. The 99m-Tc-oxinate labelling method resulted in a very poor oxygen consumption of stimulated PMN, but iodination and ingestion rates were increased. Using pyrophosphate and 99m-Tc (PYPE), both spontaneous and stimulated oxygen consumption remained within normal limits, as did iodination; only ingestion tests showed slightly diminished values. These PYPE results were similar to those obtained using 51-Cr-labelling, which was shown to be a valuable reference, since all the functional tests remained normal.

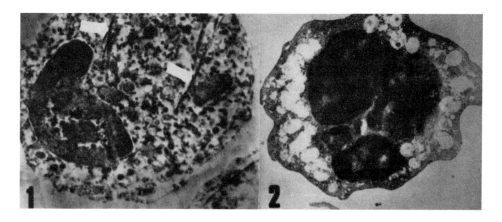

Fig. 3. Cells are damaged by oxinate in procedures 1 and 2.   On photograph 1 actine filaments are clearly visible.

6.6.2.3 Electron microscope studies of labelled PMN cells –

Electron microscope studies provided two kinds of information. The first was qualitative, showing directly the degree of cell damage. The second was quantitative as the proportion of damaged cells could easily be established. It

128

clearly demonstrates the toxicity of 111-In-oxinate to labelled cells in procedures (1) or (2). (Figure 3)

6.6.2.4 Autoradiographic studies –
    Labelled polymorphonuclear cells were very easily seen on the slides (Figure 4). The length of the materialized tracks varied considerably. Most of them originated obviously from the cells. Quantitative data were also derived from the examination of 1000 labelled cells. 75% to 80% of the cells appeared to be labelled.

Fig. 4.   Results from auto-
           radiographic studies
           with 99m-Tc-labelled
           cells.

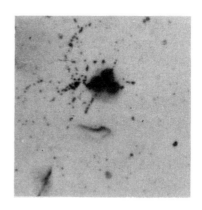

6.6.2.5 Biological tests in dogs –
    We could easily and consistantly detect inflammatory foci using scintigraphic techniques (Figure 5). The focal activity accumulation in infectious tissues seemed to be lower than that previously reported by In-oxinate methods (6,13).

129

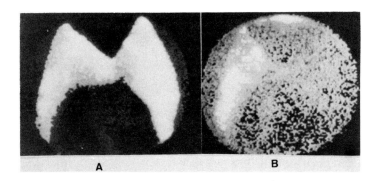

Fig. 5. 99m-Tc visualization (a) of leg abscess compared with hypoactivity using 113m-transferrin injection after 6 hours.

6.7 DISCUSSION

6.7.1 Discrepancies with other published results

Our results are quite different from those published by Thakur et al. (13) concerning the function of WBC labelled by the 111-In-oxinate method and question the in-vivo usefulness of these labelled leucocytes. Each labelling technique could alter PMN function due to one or more of the following:
a) physical damage resulting from excessive handling of the cells during the isolation, washing or labelling procedures;
b) direct chemical damage by oxinate or ethanol used in the technique (1) or tin pyrophosphate in the PYPE method;
c) damage due to intracellular radiation from 111-In or 99m-Tc (see Hofer, Chapter 12, biological cell damage from Auger electrons).

In contrast to 32-P-DFP which irreversibly binds to neutrophils, the tracers we studied were bound less tightly and were furthermore not specific for granulocytes. There is no rapid and efficient method for separating granulocytes from small

volumes of blood while preserving their viability completely.
However, electron microscopic studies did not show cell
alterations after our separation technique and lysis of red blood
cells (5). Control techniques of assessing phagocytic and
enzymatic activity of leucocytes are numerous and the tests that
we used differ from those of other authors.

Limitation of the in-vitro studies: The in-vitro methods of
assessment of neutrophil function unfortunately cannot adequately
predict the in-vivo behaviour of these cells after labelling and
reinjection into the bloodstream. So, with intact in-vitro
function, labelled neutrophils are rapidly removed from the
circulation by uptake into the liver, spleen or lungs. We
confirmed this in studies carried out with PYPE in dogs (5).
Similar results were obtained by others using 111-In-oxinate.

6.8 CONCLUSIONS

The following conclusions may be drawn from our experiments:
1) Some labelling methods result in a low labelling
efficiency of the granulocytes and an important loss of the
cell-bound radioactivity in-vitro. Therefore, they are of only
limited usefulness in order to predict the in-vivo behaviour of
labelled WBCs.

2) A good correlation was found between viability, chemotaxis
tests, and electron microscopic studies in the three other methods
of WBC labelling by 111-In-oxinate, 51-Cr-chromate, or
Sn-pyrophosphate/99m-Tc-pertechnetate. None of these however,
showed completely normal results. Among them, the best results
in-vitro were obtained using the 51-Cr method, the
Sn-pyrophosphate/99m-Tc-pertechnetate (PYPE) technique being a
close runner-up.

3) The "gold standard" for the evaluation of labelled PMN
cells remained the assessment of the in-vivo distribution and
accumulation of labelled cells in foci of septic pathology by
scintigraphy.

SUMMARY

Radioactively labelled leucocytes have been suggested for the detection of inflamatory foci for several years. Before routine use in man, it is necessary to check the viability of labelled cells. Five leucocyte labelling techniques, i.e. 111-In-oxinate, 111-In-oxinate without extraction, 99m-Tc-oxinate, Sn-pyrophosphate/99m-Tc-pertechnetate, 51-Cr, were compared using the same separation methods, conservation medium, viability assays and migration studies. Electron microscopic studies allowed the assessmant of cellular damage induced by the labelling techniques as well as the calculation of the percentage of cells disrupted during preparation. With 99m-Tc-pyrophosphate, the labelling homogeneity was tested using a new autoradiographic method, and the viability of the labelled cells in-vivo was confirmed by animal studies in dogs and rats. A good correlation was found between viability, chemotaxis tests and electron microscope studies among each of the various labelling methods used, but none showed completely normal results. So, while in-vitro studies offer much information concerning labelled cells, they are unable to predict the in-vivo behaviour of these cells.

132

REFERENCES

1. Dhawan V.M., J.J. Sziklas and R.P. Spencer: Localization of Ga 67 in inflammations in the absence of circulating polymorphonuclear leucocytes. J. Nucl. Med. 19:292-294, 1978.
2. Thakur M.L., R.E. Coleman and M.J. Welch: Indium 111 labeled leucocytes for the localization of abscesses: Preparation, analysis, tissue distribution, and comparison with gallium-67 in dogs. J. Lab. Clin. Med. 89:217-22ᴿ 1977.
3. McAfee J.G.: Importance of cell labeling techniques. In: Indium 111 labeled neutrophils, platelets and lymphocytes, edited by M.L. Thakur and A. Gottschalk, Trivirum Publishing Company, New York, p. 1, 1980.
4. Tubiana M.: La cinetique des populations de cellules. Annales de Biologie Clinique 7-9:793-822, 1968.
5. Linhart N., ᴿ. Bok., M. Gougerot, M.T. Gaillard and M. Meignan: Tc 99m labelled human leucocytes: an in vitro functional study. Acta Haemat. 63:71-80, 1980.
6. Segal A.W., R.N. Arnot, M.L. Thakur, et al: Indium 111 labelled leucocytes for localization of abscesses. Lancet 2:1056-1058.
7. Ducassou D. and J.P. Nouel: Le marquage des elements figures du sang par l'indium radioactif - methodologie - resultats - indications. XVIIIe Colloque de Medecine Nucleaire, II. pp.18-22, 1977 (Abstract).
8. Bernard P., D. Coornaert, C. Laporte and F. Roux: Utilisation des leucocytes autologues techneties dans la detection des absces. J. Franc. Biophysique Med. Nucl. 2:1105-109, 1978.
9. Dresch C. and Y. Najean: Etude de la cinetique des polynucleaires apres marquage "in vitro" par le radiochrome. I. Etude critique de la methode et resultats obtenus chez les sujets normaᵘˣ. Nouv. Reᵛ. Franc. Hemat. 7:27-48, 1967.
10. Barbu M., N. Colas-Linhart and A. Petiet: 99m-Tc radioautography of labeled white cellˢ. Acta Haemat., (accepted for publication July 1983).
11. Linhart-Colas N., M. Meignan, B. Bok, N. Rotman and M. Gougerot: "In vivo" kinetics of 99 Technetium labelled leucocytes in dogs and the effects of an abscess. Biomedicine 32:133-139. 1980.
12. Gray H.W., M.F. Tsan and H.N. Wagner jr.: A quantitative study of leucocyte cohesion Effects of divalent cations and pH. J. Nucl. Med. 18:147:150, 1977.
13. Linhart-Colas N., M. Barbu, M.A. Gougerot and B. Bok: Five leucocytes labelling techniques: a comparative in vitro study. Br. J. Haemat. 53:31-41, 1983.
14. Thakur M.L., R.E. Coleman and M.J. Welch: Indium 111 labeled leucocytes for the localization of abscesses: Preparation, analysis, tissue distribution, and comparison with gallium-67 citrate in dogs. J. Lab. Clin. Med. 89:217-228, 1977.

6.9 EDITOR'S NOTE: ASSAYS OF MIGRATORY ACTIVITY

The mobility of migratory blood cells under experimental conditions has been studied by the Boyden chamber system (1) or the more recently introduced Zigmond chamber (2).

The modified Boyden chamber system consists of two opposing chambers on top of each other separated by a filter; it measures enhanced migration due to either an increase in random locomotion or in directed migration or both. The Zigmond chamber is formed between a cover glass on top and a beam between two troughs below; the troughs run parallel to each other in a lucite slide separated by a beam which is slightly lower than the outside shoulders so that a gap is formed between the cover glass and the beam separating the throughs. Cells may migrate on the underside of the cover glass from one trough toward the other across the separating beam. The Zigmond chamber tests the directional mobility of migratory cells, if they adhere to the cover glass. Zigmond and Hirsch (3) have pointed out that an observed increased migration could result from a response directed by the chemical gradient, that is from chemotaxis, or from increased random locomotion, chemokinesis, or both. The synthetic peptides stimulate both forms of movement, radioactive labelling of the cells may impair both forms of movement. Therefore the observed altered cellular activity is best described as "enhanced respectively diminished migration" or "stimulated respectively depressed movement", whereas "chemotaxis" or "chemokinesis" should be reserved to experimental circumstances where the precise nature of the cellular movement is demonstrably clear.

In the modified Boyden chamber system 1 ml of washed neutrophil leucocytes containing about 2.5 x 10E06 cells is added to the upper compartment of the chamber separated from 1 ml of peptide solution by a 25 mm diameter filter of 0.6 um average pore size (e.g. Schleicher + Schuell). The loaded chambers are incubated at 38 deg.C for 30 minutes. The time interval is chosen to give, for a particular batch of filters used, the greatest difference between the number of cells moving into the filter with no test substance in the lower compartment (background) and the maximum number of cells moving into the filter when stimulated by a test substance (e.g. a stimulating peptide). At the end of the incubation period the filters are removed and stained and the number of cells in 5 high-power (400 magnification) fields are counted and averaged. Increased penetration of cells into or through the filter of a Boyden chamber system under the stimulus of a chemical agent is generally taken as indicating the chemotactic activity of the agent. Zigmond and Hirsch (3) have described a technique for determining if the movement of the cell into the filter of a Boyden chamber system under the influence of different gradients is greater than could be expected on the basis of increased rates of locomotion alone and is therefore due to a true chemotactic response.

The test of whether or not a peptide (or other substance) stimulates chemotaxis, i.e. directionally oriented migration, the distance is measured from the top of the filter to the farthest plane of focus still containing two cells using the micrometer adjustment of the microscope. This distance is to be determined across five fields and averaged, and filters from duplicate chambers are to be examined.

The cells are suspended in Hank's balanced solution containing 0.01 M tris(hydroxymethyl) aminomethane, pH 7.2, 1 mg/ml of glucose, and serum albumin. A number of 0.5-1.0 x 10E07 cells are placed in the upper compartment of a modified Boyden chamber. The cells are separated from the bottom compartment by a 3.0 micrometer pore size filter (Millipore Corp.). Duplicate chambers are incubated for 60 to 90 minutes at 37 deg.C. The medium used to fill the compartments (with cells above, without cells below the filter) may contain the same or varying concentrations of the substance (radioactive label, peptide) thought to stimulate or impair chemotaxis in the upper and lower chambers.

For reversibility studies the cells are incubated for 30 minutes at 37 deg.C in varying concentrations of a given peptide or other substance before washing with buffer or saline and testing in fresh medium.

If substances stimulate random movement of the neutrophil, this is shown by the penetration of the filter obtained when no gradient is present. When the concentration of a substance expected to stimulate or depress migratory activity is greater below than above the filter the gradient is termed positive; when the concentrations of the test substance are reversed (higher concentration in the cell suspension) the gradient is termed negative.

The Zigmond chamber represents a new system to study cell migration under direct observation by phase contrast microscopy. The cells can be viewed as they are exposed to controlled concentrations and concentration gradients of chemotactic factors. Using this system it was shown that cell orientation depends on the mean concentration as well as the concentration gradient of factors, thus deviating from the classical Weber-Fechner law of sensory physiology (2).

A lucite (plexiglass) slide (1 in. x 3in. x 0.125 in.) was cut across its width to have two troughs 4 mm wide and 1 mm deep, separated by a beam 1 mm wide. A chamber is formed by placing a glass cover slip (22x40 mm) over the slide covering troughs and beam. Thus a fluid layer may develop between the under-surface of the cover slip and the surface of the beam when the troughs are filled with fluid. The thickness of the fluid layer is to be measured by the micrometer on the fine focus knob of the microscope; it should not exceed a range of 3 to 10 micrometer on either side. This range of thickness can be accomplished if the cover slip and the shoulders bearing it are clean and dry as the cover glass is placed on the slide. The resistance to flow across the beam is sufficiently great so that no trypan blue will be detectable in the other trough containing water when solution of that dye is first introduced into the first trough. Some flow occurs as time goes on, yet the original trypan blue solution remains distinctly darker than that of the other trough even after 72 hrs at room temperature.

It has been calculated that in the absence of flow a linear gradient of a molecule of about 450 molecular weight should be established to 99% completion across the beam in 76 minutes. Since in practice some perturbation occurs when the troughs are filled, the formation of the desired gradient of a chemical between the two sides of the chamber develops faster than theory predicts, namely between 15 and 30 minutes. The gradient will remain steep (at room temperature) until about 90 min after the initial filling; thereafter the gradient begins to decay and becomes less and less steep as time goes on.

The migratory blood cells to be studied are brought into the chamber by bringing a drop of whole blood or white blood cell suspension onto the cover glass in the centre. The cell suspension is allowed to dry for 10 to 15 minutes before the cover slip is inverted with the cell bearing side toward the lucite slide. The granulocytes and monocytes adhere to the cover slip and may be rinsed with a suitable solution prior to inversion. If a drop of whole blood is dried onto the cover slip in its centre this is done in a moist chamber with 5% carbondioxyde at 37 deg.C for 1 hour. Gentle washing of the cell bearing side with saline after the clot has retracted will remove fibrin, red cells and mononuclear cells leaving granulocytes and monocytes attached to the cover slip. The glass cover slip is held tightly in place by brass clips.

The scoring of the cell orientation is done viewing the cells in the centre microscope field of the beam with a x 40 phase objective field diameter 0.4 mm. The direction of locomotion is judged morphologically; the front of a moving cell can be identified by its pseudopod and the rear by its knob-like tail. Cells are scored as either moving into the 180 deg. sector toward the high concentration of a chemotactic factor or into the 180 deg. sector toward the low concentration. Only cells with pseudopods and tails and whose direction of movement can be evaluated are to be scored. Immobile cells and cells moving perpendicularly (about 10 deg.) to the gradient are not counted. The unscored population was usually less than 20% of the total in Zigmond's original work (2). The beam is scanned across the slide until at least 100 cells are scored. The results are expressed as a percentage, i.e. the number of cells moving toward the high concentration (times 100) divided by the total number of scorable cells, i.e. all cells moving toward or away from the high concentration of the chemotactic factor.

REFERENCES

1. Boyden S.: Chemotactic effect of mixtures of antibody and antigen on polymorphonuclear leucocytes. J. Expl. Med. 115:453:466, 1962.
2. Zigmond S.H.: Ability of polymorphonuclear leukocytes to orient in gradients of chemotactic factors. J. Cell Biol. 75:606-616, 1977.
3. Zigmond S.H. and J.G. Hirsch: Leukocyte locomotion and chemotaxis. New method for evaluation and demonstration of cell-derived chemotactic factors. J. Expl. Med. 137:387, 1973.

7 RADIOLABELLING NEUTROPHILS
CURRENT ACCOMPLISHMENTS AND FUTURE POSSIBILITIES

M.L. THAKUR

7.1 INTRODUCTION

The past few decades have been exciting for those who have been interested in the study of neutrophil granulocytes and their function. Originating from bone marrow, neutrophils have the ability to migrate toward bacterial invasion or tissue necrosis in the body. Such migration is initiated by the generation of a large number of substances that have characteristics to attract neutrophils. The development of ingeneous techniques for isolating neutrophils free of contaminating platelets and erythrocytes, light microscopy, histochemical staining and electron microscopy have facilitated such studies of neutrophils, their ultrastructure and function. In addition to these techniques, studies with radio-labelled neutrophils have made a substantial contribution to our understanding of the neutrophil function and its life span in mammals.

In the initial attempts, suitable radioactive tracers were given in-vivo and allowed to be incorporated into neutrophils. Most of the radioactive tracers used emitted beta rays and necessitated isolation of neutrophils from whole blood for the determination of radioactivity associated with the cells. Such assessment of radioactivity allowed scientists to determine the cell maturation cycle and their life span in-vivo.

The next generation of radioactive compounds were aimed at labelling isolated neutrophils in-vitro. This allowed investigators to label neutrophils under controlled conditions with a radionuclide of choice. Due to the relative inconvenience of counting the disintegration rate of beta rays, radionuclides decaying with the emission of gamma rays were chosen. The subsequent refinement in labelling techniques, and the availability of external detection devices, such as scintillation cameras, have enabled scientists to study in-vivo cell kinetics and the cellular accumulation at unknown and deep sites of infection or inflammation. The technique is facilitated by the use of a radionuclide that can be employed to label neutrophils effectively and be monitored externally after labelled cells have been administered in-vivo. This volume is designed to discuss prospects of this technique and to highlight the underlying problems. In this article, I have attempted to give a very brief account of the previous and the current approaches, and the future possibilities that might further simplify the radiolabelling of neutrophils.

7.2   TRACERS FOR IN-VIVO LABELLING

Initially the radiolabelling was accomplished by the in-vivo administration of certain radioactive tracers (Table 1). Broadly, these have been classified as: a) DNA or cohort labels, and b) non-DNA or random labels (1). The DNA labelling was achieved by the administration of either 32-phosphorous as sodium phosphate, 14-carbon labelled nucleic acid precursors such as adenine, guanine and orotic acid or tritiated thymidine. The tracers thus became available to bone marrow stem cells and were incorporated into DNA during maturation of the cell cycle. The process thereby provided investigators with a true cohort cell label (2,3).

Among non-DNA labels, 75-Se-selenomethiomine and 32-phosphorous diisopropyl fluorophosphate were the most prominent compounds (4-11). With the use of these compounds, many studies have been performed. These have resulted into the contribution of the most basic information in neutrophil kinetics (11-13). These compounds, however, were non-specific and labelled neutrophils, lymphocytes as well as platelets. The studies were further complicated by the difficulties in beta counting, the toxicity of some compounds, and the reutilization of the tracer after cell destruction (7,14).

Table 1.   Physical Characteristics of Radio-
             Nuclides Employed for Cell Labelling

Radionuclide	Physical halflife	Measured emission	Energy	(MeV)
3-H	12.3 y	beta	0.0186	(max)
14-C	5730.0 y	beta	0.1561	(max)
32-P	14.3 d	gamma	1.7100	(max)
51-Cr	27.7 d	gamma	0.3200	(10%)
75-Se	120.0 d	gamma	0.2646	(57%)
99m-Tc	6.0 h	gamma	0.1405	(88%)
111-In	67.0 h	gamma	0.1720	(90%)
		gamma	0.2470	(94%)

Data from Dillmann and Von der Lage (32).

7.3   TRACERS FOR IN-VITRO LABELLING

The radioactive agents explored thereafter were aimed at
labelling neutrophils in-vitro. These were all gamma emitting
radionuclides (Table 1) and labelled cells non-specifically. The
agents primarily included 51-Cr sodium chromate, 99m-Tc-
pertechnetate, other 99m-Tc-labelled compounds, 67-Ga-citrate and
111-In labelled compounds. Labelling neutrophils with these
radionuclides required cells to be isolated in-vitro from whole
blood and suspended in a suitable medium.

7.4   99m-TECHNETIUM

Labelling neutrophils with 99m-Tc involves "pretinning", i.e.
incubating cells with stannous chloride before
99m-Tc-pertechnetate is added to the cell suspension (15). The

exact mechanism by which neutrophils are labelled with 99m-Tc is not clear. However, labelling efficiencies of 70-80% have been reported. 99m-Tc has a suitable halflife for studies involving neutrophils (Table 1). The radionuclide emits gamma photons that can be efficiently detected externally and is available world wide at a modest cost. These qualities make the tracer highly desirable. However, a high percentage of spontaneous release of radioactivity from labelled cells has prevented the use of this tracer. Assuming the spontaneous release may have been due to the adherence of the tracer on the cell surface, scientists have investigated labelling neutrophils by phagocytosis. In this technique either 99m-Tc sulphur colloid or 99m-Tc phytate, which forms colloid in the presence of plasma calcium, is incubated with the neutrophil suspension (16). The technique resulted in approximately 40% of the radioactivity in cell association but met with several practical difficulties. Unengulfed radioactive particles could not be isolated without affecting cell viability. Many particles, apparently considered phagocytosed, remained on the cell surface and released radioactivity on addition of fresh non-radioactive colloid. Furthermore, subsequent to this stimulation, the full preservation of physiological functions of the labelled neutrophils remained doubtful.

In this volume Oberhausen and colleagues have described a technique to label monocytes by allowing them to phagocytose 99m-Tc-Sn-colloid in whole blood. The radioactive colloid was incubated for 30-40 min in whole blood and the unengulfed particles (10-20%) were dissolved by addition of Na-citrate. It has been claimed that cells labelled in this manner and administered back to patients, accurately diagnosed abscesses on 85% of the occasions. However, there was a rapid loss of 50-70% of the administered radioactivity in the liver and spleen. This loss is much greater than that observed when cells are labelled with a non-phagocytotic technique.

142

7.5 51-CHROMIUM, 67-GALLIUM

51-Cr sodium chromate is a frequently employed blood cell
tracer in non-imaging applications. These include the
determination of erythrocyte mass and survival, neutrophil
survival and chemotactic functions. The long shelf life of the
tracer makes the use of this agent attractive. However, draw
backs associated with the low labelling efficiency, the
spontaneous release of radioactivity and the weak gamma ray
emission, weigh heavily against the use of this tracer,
particularly in imaging procedures.

67-Ga citrate has been investigated as a possible tracer for
neutrophils (17). The poor labelling yields, however, have
prevented any further use of 67-Ga, as a neutrophil tracer.

7.6 111-In-OXINATE

The availability of lipid-soluble agents of 111-In has
generated impetus in the field of neutrophil studies. 111-In has
a desirable halflife and emits gamma rays suitable for external
detection (Table 1). 111-In in an ionic form, such as chloride,
does not label cells. However, when chelated with certain
compounds to form a neutral complex, 111-In becomes an excellent
tracer for neutrophils. First such a complex was prepared with
8-hydroxyquinoline (oxinate) in 1975 (18). When 111-In oxinate
(Figure 1) is incubated with cells suspended in a suitable medium,
a high proportion (90%) of the compound diffuses passively through
the cell membranes, and transfers the radioactivity to cytoplasmic
components (19).

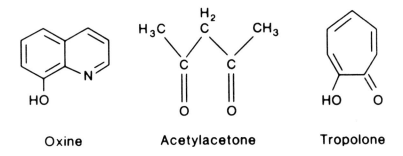

Fig. 1. Structural formulae of compounds that produce lipid
soluble complex with 111-In for cell labelling

The association of the radioactive tracer with cytoplasmic
components prevents the spontaneous elution of radioactivity from
the labelled cells. This together with the high labelling yields
and the desirable physical characteristics have, thus far, made
111-In a useful tracer for neutrophils. During the past few
years, much has been achieved by non-invasive means using
111-In-labelled neutrophils in the determination of neutrophil
kinetics and in the localization of inflammatory lesions (20-22).
Nevertheless, some disadvantages of the compound and the labelling
procedures have become evident.

111-In oxinate is a non-specific agent. It labels all types
of blood cells and thereby necessitates the isolation of the
desired cell type from whole blood. 111-In oxinate is also a weak
complex and dissociates in the precence of plasma transferrin.
111-In then binds to the protein. This process lowers the
labelling efficiency. The use of balanced salt solutions for cell
suspension produces a high labelling efficiency but may alter the
cell viability. An excess of oxinate can also affect cell
viability. These drawbacks indicate that there is a compelling
need for a radioactive agent that will: 1) allow efficient cell
labelling in plasma and 2) preferably, label neutrophils
specifically in whole blood, which will eliminate the need for
cell separation. Aspiration for such refinements in the cell
labelling technique has fostered the investigation of several new
agents (23-26).

144

7.7   111-In-ACETYLACETONE

Acetylacetone (Figure 1) chelates 111-In in aqueous medium, produces a lipid-soluble complex and labels neutrophils efficiently (24). Acetylacetone was considered to be less toxic than oxinate (23). Comparative studies, however, have revealed that to obtain labelling yields close to those of 111-In -oxinate, the acetylacetone concentration must be 120 times greater than that of oxinate. Since acetylacetone is only 21 times less toxic than oxinate, the actual toxicity to cells from the new agent is no less than that from oxinate. Like 111-In oxinate, 111-In acetylacetone is also a weak complex and does not permit efficient cell labelling in plasma.

7.8   111-In-TROPOLONE

111-In-tropolone (Figure 1), yet another lipid-soluble complex of indium, has been introduced recently (25,26). Tropolone is less toxic than both oxinate and acetylacetone. Tropolone also forms a saturated complex with 111-In in an aqueous system. Although the stability constants of 111-In tropolone have not been determined, it has been shown that the agent labels cells in plasma and yields an incorporation of radioactivity into cells higher than that with 111-In oxinate and acetylacetone in the same medium. Recently, however, it has been observed that exposure of neutrophils to tropolone, at concentrations required for efficient labelling, resulted in a marked impairment of chemotaxis (27).

7.9 111-In-MERC

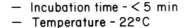

— Incubation time - < 5 min
— Temperature - 22°C

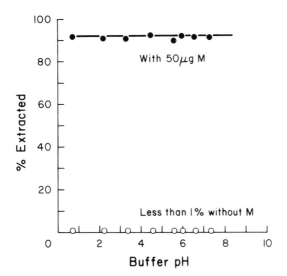

Fig. 2. Preparation of 111-In-Merc (M); Influence of pH
        (The complex was extracted into chloroform)

Recently, we have prepared a new lipid-soluble agent namely 111-indium-2-mercapto pyridine-n-oxide (Merc). Merc can also exist as pyrithione [1-hydroxy-2 (1 H) - pyridinethione]. The compound is known as omadine to Biochemists. The two functional groups, SH and OH, make the compound an excellent metal chelating agent. Merc, when dissolved in a suitable solvent, forms a complex with ionic 111-In over a wide range (2-12) of pH at room temperature (Figure 2).

Indium with six co-ordination numbers is expected to bind to three molecules of Merc and produces a neutrally charged lipid soluble complex of the type shown in Figure 3. The complex is extractable in chloroform and similar solvents. Different chemical conditions are reqired for chelation with 99m-Tc and radioactive ruthenium. These are discussed elsewhere (28).

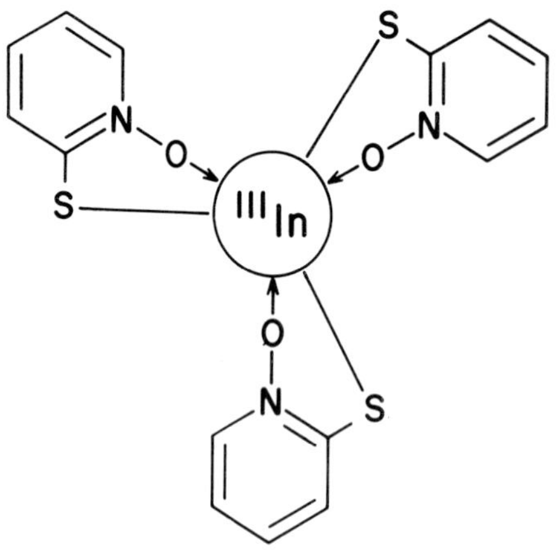

146

^{III}In Merc

Fig. 3. Schematic diagram of a saturated (1:3) 111-In-Merc complex

    A microgram quantity of Merc chelates no-carrier-added-111-In almost quantitatively and obviates the need for solvent extraction. The ability of Merc to form the complex in an aqueous medium at a physiological pH allows us to use the agent conveniently. Furthermore, the complex labels cells efficiently in plasma. A comparative study, using 111-In complexes of oxinate, acetylacetone, tropolone, Merc and 99m-Tc and Ru-105 Merc, revealed that 111-In Merc incorporated the highest quantity of the radioactivity into an equal number of platelets suspended in plasma (Table 2).

Table 2. Percentage Radioactivity in Platelets
----
15 Min Incubation. Platelets - 5.0 x 10E08/ml

Agent	111-In Merc	99m-Tc Merc	103-Ru Merc	111-In Oxin	111-In Trop	111-In AA *)
Temp.	22 deg.	22 deg.	22 deg.	22 deg.	22 deg.	22 deg. C
In Saline		54.5				
In Plasma	57.6	28.3	8.3	5.4	2.2	2.6
----

*) Oxin = Oxinate, Trop = Tropolone, AA = Acetylacetone

White blood cells labelled with 111-In Merc have been shown to accumulate into experimental abscesses (28). The ability of the agent to effectively label cells in plasma is regarded as a considerable improvement in the cell labelling technique. However, the fact remains that the agent labels all types of cells and the need for cell isolation still persists.

7.10 SELECTIVE NEUTROPHIL LABELLING

An agent that would allow cell labelling selectively in whole blood would be most desirable. Our preliminary investigations in this direction have generated promising results (29).

Certain synthetic peptides have been shown to be chemo-attractant to human neutrophils (30). The process of chemo-attraction has been attributed to the existence of specific receptors, possess the ability to absorb chemo-attractive substances and to regenerate new receptors. Among synthetic peptides formyl-methionyl-leucyl-phenylalanine (FMLP) has been shown to have a very high potency (30). In order to be able to label FMLP with 111-In, we have covalently attached the peptide to

148

human transferrin (TF), which acts as an effective chelating agent
for 111-In. Peptides attached to proteins have been shown to
retain their chemo-attractive ability. Under certain experimental
conditions, 60% of the added 111-In TF-FMLP can be taken up by
human neutrophils. Previous data have demonstrated the ability of
neutrophils to absorb such molecules, yet to still respond
normally to other chemotactic stimuli (31). This ability may
allow 111-In TF-FMLP labelled neutrophils to retain their normal
physiological functions. The higher 111-In TF-FMLP specific
activity than that achievable currently, is expected to yield a
higher than 60% labelling efficiency.

In future, therefore, selective labelling of neutrophils with
111-In in whole blood may be feasible. Such a procedure will make
the neutrophil labelling technique simple and convenient.
Furthermore, the technique may provide investigators with a
reliable tool to perform studies of in-vivo neutrophil kinetics
and that of locating inflammatory lesions with radiolabelled
neutrophils which may have suffered only a minimal alteration of
physiological functions.

Acknowledgement
I thank Ms. Iris Molina and Ms. Cathie Cooper who took great
care in typing this article.

SUMMARY

Initially the radiolabelling of white blood cells was accomplished by the in-vivo administration of certain radioactive tracers. Broadly, these have been classified as: a) DNA or cohort labels or b) non-DNA or random labels. The DNA labelling was achieved by the administration of either 32-phosphorous as sodium phosphate, 14-carbon labelled nucleic acid precursors such as adenine, guanine and orotic acid or tritiated thymidine. The tracers were injected to become available to stem cells in bone marrow and were incorporated into DNA during maturation of the cell cycle. The process thereby provided investigators with a true cohort cell label.

Among non-DNA labels, 75-Se selenomethiomine and 32-phosphoruous diisopropyl fluorophosphate were the most prominent compounds. The use of these compounds yielded most of the basic information on neutrophil kinetics. These compounds, however, were non-specific and labelled neutrophils, lymphocytes as well as platelets.

Radioactive agents which emit gamma rays and label cells non-specifically primarily include: 51-Cr-sodium chromate, 99m-Tc-pertechnetate, other 99m-Tc-labelled compounds, 67-Ga-citrate and 111-In-labelled compounds. Labelling neutrophils with these radionuclides requires cells to be isolated in-vitro from whole blood and suspended in a suitable medium.

Lipid-soluble chelates of 111-In, which has a desirable half life, may form a neutral complex and thereby become excellent tracers for neutrophils. First such a complex was prepared with 8-hydroxyquinoline (oxinate) in 1975. A significant advance was represented by 111-In-tropolone which has been shown to label cells in plasma and at efficiencies higher than that of 111-In-oxinate and acetylacetone in the same medium.

Recently, we have prepared a new lipid-soluble agent namely 111-indium-2-mercapto pyridine-n-oxide (Merc). Merc can also exist as pyrithione [1-hydroxy-2 (1 H) - pyridinethione]. This compound is known as omadine to Biochemists. The two functional groups, SH and OH, make the compound an excellent metal chelating agent. Merc, when dissolved in an aqueous medium, forms a complex with ionic 111-In at a physiological pH at room temperature and labels all types of blood cells in plasma very effectively, at a favourably low molar ratio Merc/111-In. The need for cell isolation persists, however.

REFERENCES

1. Thakur M.L. and A. Gottschalk: Role of radiopharmaceuticals in nuclear hematology. Radiopharmaceuticals II, 349-359 Society of Nuclear Medicine, New York, 1979.
2. Perry S., H.A. Goodwin and Zimmerman: Physiology of granulocytes - Part I. JAMA 203:937-944, 1968.
3. Rubini J.R., E. Westcott and S. Keller: In vitro DNA labelling of bone marrow and leukemia blood leukocytes with tritiated thymidine-II. H-᠑ thymidne biochemistry in vitro. J. Lab. Clin. Med. 68:566-576, 1966.
4. Cooley H. and F.H. Gardner: The use of selenomethionine (Se-75) as a label for canine and human platelets. Am. Soc. Clin. Inv. 44:1036-1037, 1965 (Abstract).
5. Penner J.A. and M.C. Meyers: Methionine-Se-75 uptake in circulating blood cells and plasma proteins. J. Lab. Clin. Med. 68:1005 1966 (Abstract).
6. McIntyre P.A., B. Evatt, B.A. Hodkinson, et al: Selenium-75, selenomethionine as a label for erythrocytes, leukocytes and platelets in man. J. Lab. Clin. Med. 74: 472-480, 1970.
7. Grobb D., J.L. Lilienthal Jr., A.M. Harvey, et al: The administration of diisopropyl fluorophosphate (DFP) to man. Bull. John Hopkins Hospital, 81:217-243, 1947.
8. Cohen J.A. and M.G.P.J. Warringa: The effect of P-32 labeled diisopropyl fluorophosphate in the human body and its use as labelling agent in the study of the turnover of blood plasma and red cells. J. Clin. Inv. 33:459-467, 1954.
9. Leeksma C.H.W. and J.A. Cohn: Determination of the life span of human platelets using labeled DFP. J. Clin. Inv. 35:964-969, 1956.
10. Athens J.W., A.M. Mauer, H. Ashenbrucker, et al: Leukokinetic studies I. A method for labelling leukocytes with DF-32P Blood 14:303-333, 1959.
11. Mauer A.M. Athens J.W., Ashenbrucker H., et al: Leukocyte kinetics II. A method for labelling granulocytes in vitro with radioactive DFP-32. J. Clin. Inv. 39:1681-1686, 1960.
12. Athens J.W., O.P. Haab, S.O. Raab, et al: Leukokinetic studies IV. The total blood, circulating and marginal granulocytes, turnover rate in normal subjects. J. Clin. Inv 40:989-995, 1961.
13. Raab S.O., J.W. Athens, O.P. Haab, et al: Granulokinetics in normal dogs. Am. J. Pathology 206:83-88, 1964.
14. Mizuno N.S., V. Perman, F.W. Bates, et al: Lifespan of thrombocytes and erythrocytes in normal and thrombopenic calves. Blood 14:708-719, 1959.
15. Linhart N. B. Bok, M. Mergman, et al: Technetium-99m labeled human leukocytes: in vitro and animal studies. In: Indium-111 Labelled Neutrophils, Platelets and Lymphocytes, pp.69-78, edited by Thakur M L. and A. Gottschalk, Trivirum Publishing Company, New York, 1980.

16. McAfee J.F. and M.L. Thakur: Survey of radioactive agents for in vitro labelling of phagocytic leukocytes II - particles. J. Nucl. Med. 17: 488-492, 1976.
17. Burleson R.L., B.L. Holman and D.E. Tow: Scintigraphic demonstration of abscesses with radioactive labeled leukocytes. Surg. Gyn. Obstet. 14: 379-382, 1975.
18. Thakur M.L., R.E. Coleman and M.J. Welch: Indium-111 labeled human leukocytes for abscess localization: preparation, analysis, tissue distribution and comparison with Ga-67 citrate in dogs. J. Lab. Clin. Med. 89: 217-228, 1977.
19. Thakur M.L., A.W. Segal, L. Louis, et al: Indium-111 labelled cellular blood components - mechanism of labelling and intracellular location in human neutrophils. J. Nucl. Med. 18:1020-1024, 1977.
20. Thakur M.L. and A. Gottschalk (Eds): Indium-111 labeled neutrophils, platelets and lymphocytes. Trivirum Publishing Company, New York, 1980.
21. Proceedings of the British Institute of Radiology: Cell labelling with gamma emitting radionuclide for in vivo study. Br. J. Radiol. 53: 9??-993, 1980.
22. Hardeman M.R., W.B. van der Pompe and E.A. von Royen (Eds:) Proceedings of Symposium on Cell Labelling. Nuclear Geneeskundig Bulletin, Academic Medical Center, University of Amsterdam, Jaargang 4, Supplement, 1982.
23. Goedemans W.T.H.: Simplified cell labelling with In-111 acetyl acetone and indium-111 oxinate. Br. J. Radiol. 54: 636-637, 1981.
24. Sinn H. and D.J. Silvester: Simplified cells labelling with In-111 acetyl acetone. Br. J. Radiol. 52:758-759, 1979.
25. Dewanjee M.K., S.H. Rao and P. Didisheim: Indium-111 tropolone, a new high-affinity label: preparation and evaluation of labelling parameters. J. Nucl. Med. 22: 981-987, 1981.
26. Danpure H.J., S. Osman and F. Brady: The labelling of blood cells in plasma with In-111 tropolonate. Br. J. Radiol. 543:247-249, 1982.
27. English D., Private communications.
28. Thakur M.L.: In preparation
29. Zoghbi S.S., M.L. Thakur, A. Gottschalk, et al: Selective cell labelling; a potential radioactive agent for labelling of human neutrophils. J. Nuc. Med. 22:32, 1981 (Abstract).
30. Schiffman E., B.A. Corioran and S.M. Wahl: Formylmethionyl peptides as chemo-attractants for leukocytes. Proc. Natl. Acad. Sci., USA 72:1059-1062, 1975.
31. Goldstein I.M.: Chemotactic factor receptors on leukocytes; scratching the surface (Editorial). J. Lab. Clin. Med. 97: 599-601, 1981.
32. Dillman L.T. and F.C. Von der Lage: Radionuclide decay schemes and nuclear parameters for use in radiation - dose estimation. MIRD pamphlet 10. Society of Nuclear Medicine, New York, 1975.

7.1 EDITOR'S NOTE: CHEMOTACTIC AGENTS AS CELL SPECIFIC LABELS

A large number of substances have been reported to induce chemotaxis in neutrophils (1). Wissler's article (Chapter 4) yields insight into the mechanism of chemical attraction. It is therefore not surprising that substances of widely variable composition and molecular size will induce chemotaxis or chemokinesis. Schiffmann et al.(2) reported that simple, synthetic N-formyl methionyl peptides cause chemotaxis in neutrophils and monocytes. Systematic studies of this group of investigators have shed light on the structure-activity relations of such synthetic peptides as inducers of chemotaxis and lysosomal enzyme secretion (3,4,5,6).

Table 1. Comparison of Chemotactic Activities of Peptides Measured by Maximally Effective Concentration and Efficacy at that Concentration

Peptides	No. of dose-response experiments	Maximally eff. molar concentr. (median value)	Efficacy expr. as chemotactic ratio (peptide/control) mean +/- SEM *
a) Tripeptides and larger peptides			
f-Met-Leu-Phe	8	10E-08	1.85+/-0.12
F-Met-Met-Phe	5	10E-09	1.63+/-0.14
f-tri-Phe	9	10E-09	1.46+/-0.05
f-tetra-Phe	3	10E-09	1.69+/-0.21
f-penta-Phe	3	10E-09	1.70+/-0.13
f-tri-Leu	3	10E-08	1.40+/-0.11
f-tri-Ala	3	10E-09	1.23+/-0.06
Ac-tri-Ala	4	10E-09	1.48+/-0.11
f-tri-Tyr	13	10E-09	1.45+/-0.07
f-tri-Tyr Me ester	3	10E-08	1.32+/-0.09
f-tri-Ser	3	10E-06	1.39+/-0.01
Glu-Gly-Phe	3	10E-04	1.43+/-0.13
f-Glu-Gly-Phe	2	10E-07	1.27, 1.33*
b) Dipeptides			
f-Met-Met	11	10E-05	1.82+/-0.16
f-Met-Phe	19	10E-05	1.52+/-0.07
f-Met-Leu	9	10E-05	1.44+/-0.07
butyryl-Met-Met	3	10E-07	1.46+/-0.16
f-Tyr-Phe	4	10E-07	1.60+/-0.15
f-Phe-Tyr	3	10E-05	1.50+/-0.3
f-L-leu-L-leu	3	10E-06	1.38+/-0.02
f-D-leu-D-leu	2	10E-06	1.50, 1.21*
f-Leu-Tyr	3	10E-07	1.58+/-0.04
f-Trp-Phe	2	10E-06	1.12, 1.23*
f-Trp-Trp	2	10E-06	1.12, 1.20*
f-Tyr-Tyr	3	10E-06	1.59+/-0.16
f-Ser-Met	3	10E-06	1.43+/-0.07
c) Protein controls			
Casein (800 ug/ml)	25	-	2.36+/-0.09
Alkali denatured HSA (1 mg/ml=1.4 x 10E-05M)	7	-	2.13+/-0.20

* Where only two dose-response experiments were done, the figure for each is given instead of a mean +/- SEM. (5)

154

Table 2.   Chemotactic Activity of Synthetic Peptides

		ED(50) +/- SE	Relative * Activity +/- SE
1.	f-Met	2.1+/-0.62x10E-03	0.0003 +/- 0.00017
2.	f-Met-Leu	4.0+/-0.45x10E-07	1.0
3.	f-Met-Leu-Phe	7.0+/-1.7 x10E-11	5,050.0 +/-820.0
4.	f-Met-Leu-Glu	1.3+/-0.38x10E-06	0.37 +/- 0.17
5.	f-Met-Leu-Ala	3.6+/-1.0 x10E-07	0.98 +/- 0.11
6.	f-Met-Leu-Leu	4.8+/-1.3 x10E-08	9.2 +/- 2.7
7.	f-Met-Phe	4.1+/-0.95x10E-07	1.3 +/- 0.33
8.	f-Met-Phe-Leu	5.4+/-1.9 x10E-08	10.0 +/- 2.4
9.	f-Met-Phe-Met	1.5+/-0.33x10E-09	169.0 +/- 50.0
10.	f-Met-Met	8.8+/-2.3 x10E-07	0.57 +/- 0.21
11.	f-Met-Met-Met	5.1+/-0.62x10E-09	70.0 +/- 32.0
12.	f-Met-Met-Met-Met	3.0+/-0.13x10E-10	760.0 +/- 82.0
13.	f-Met-Met-Ala	5.4+/-1.8 x10E-07	1.0 +/- 0.3
14.	f-Met-Met-Phe	2.1+/-0.49x10E-10	1,900.0 +/-260.0
15.	f-Leu-t-Met	2.5+/-1.5 x10E-08	17.0 +/- 5.6
16.	f-Leu-t-Met-Arg	1.1+/-0.4 x10E-06	0.25 +/- 0.06
17.	Met-Leu-Phe	6.7+/-1.9 x10E-07	0.48 +/- 0.08
18.	Met-Leu-Glu	2.7+/-1.0 x10E-03	0.00017+/- 0.00005
19.	Met-Leu-Leu	2.1+/-0.24x10E-04	0.0015 +/- 0.0003
20.	Met-Phe-Leu	2.4+/-1.1 x10E-04	0.003 +/- 0.0015
21.	Met-Met-Met	1.0+/-0.39x10E-04	0.003 +/- 0.0008
22.	Met-Met-Met-Met	1.3+/-0.29x10E-06	0.19 +/- 0.06
23.	Met-Met-Ala	1.9+/-0.39x10E-04	0.003 +/- 0.00008
24.	Met-Met-Phe	9.0+/-3.9 x10E-07	0.7 +/- 0.29

----
* Relative to f-Met-Leu = 1.0 (3)   ED = effective dose

The most active of the synthetic N-formyl-methionine peptides, formyl-methionyl-leucyl-phenylalamine, attracts cells maximally at concentrations of the order of 1.0 x 10E-09 molar (3). The migratory activities of the different peptides are reported as the ED(50), the concentration of chemotactic factor giving 50% of the maximum activity. The ED(50) value depends on the activity of the peptide and also on the cells used in testing. In order to ensure that the activities determined with different cells are always comparable, the peptide F-Met-Leu is used (based initially on an arbitrary choice) as the standard chemo-attracting peptide and is to be included in each assay. The migratory activity of each peptide is given as the ED(50) and as the relative activity or potency ratio, that is the ratio of the ED(50) of F-Met-Leu, run in the same experiment, to the ED(50) of the given peptide. Zoghbi et al. (7) developed a bifunctional chelate by conjugating covalently N-formyl-methyonyl-leucyl-phenylalamine to human transferrin, which will bind 111-In (2.4 x 10E02 Ci/m mole transferrin at pH 7 and 37 deg.C during a 30 minute incubation period) the coupling agent used was l-ethyl-3-(dimethylamino propyl) carbodiimide Hcl.

The synthetic N-formylpeptides do bind specifically to polymorphonuclear leucocytes and monocytes, but they activate them to perform multiple functions, chemotaxis, granule enzyme secretion (in the presence of cytochalasin B), aggregation, triggering of the respiratory burst etc. The naturally occurring bacterial chemotactic factors reacting with the neutrophil formyl-peptide receptor are believed to be N-formylated signal peptides (involved in the initiation of prokaryotic protein synthesis). Normally 111-In labelled F-Met-Leu-Phl conjugates of transferrin will activate neutrophils when binding to their receptor sites, thus setting off a series of events which on completion terminates the life and biological functioning of the polymorphonuclear migratory blood cell. Experimental validation of this shortening of neutrophil life span was carried out by McAfee et al.(8). Furthermore, the injection of activated neutrophils (chemotactic factors) causes severe neutropenia in rats as well as in dogs (8,9).

156

Autologous plasma, when exposed to complement-activating agents that generate leucotactic activity, induces transient neutropenia after infusion into rabbits. Tryptinized human C5 as well as the chemotactic fragment isolated from zymosan-activated human serum also induces transient neutropenia in rabbits, as do chemotactically active synthetic tripeptides. In each instance the neutropenia inducing agents parallel the chemotactic activity. Thus, neutropenia inducing activity and chemotactic activity seem to be related to the physiological responses of neutrophils. In-vivo margination and/or agglutination of leucocytes may underlie this phenomenon of neutropenia (9).

Substance P, a potent vasodilatory and smooth muscle contracting agent, binds specifically to the formyl peptide receptor of the rabbit neutrophil. It stimulates chemotaxis and induces lysosomal enzyme secretion in concentrations which similarly inhibit F-Met-Leu-(tritiated) Fc receptor binding. Competetive antagonists of the formyl peptide receptor also inhibit the activity of substance P (10).

It appears justified to generalize that binding of labelled synthetic chemo-attractants of neutrophils (and monocytes) will sufficiently alter biological function and effectiveness of the PMN cells, thus labelled, as to invalidate the purpose of the radionuclide procedure.

Van Epps et al.(11) demonstrated that neutrophils that either had been exposed to a chemotactic stimulus or had migrated in response to this stimulus were functionally more active in systems measuring stimulated chemiluminiscence, superoxide anion generation, and bactericidal activity than those that had not been exposed to chemotactic factors.

Recently specific antagonists of the synthetic chemo-attractants have been reported (6). These were, in general, structurally related to the antagonist series and were classic competitive antagonists at the receptor level. The first such antagonist reported was an amino-protected dipeptide, carbobenzoxy-phenylalamine-methiomine (Cbo-Phe-Met-OH). This was followed by several other amino-protected peptides. In contrast to the almost absolute requirement for the small formyl group in peptide linkage in the agonist series of chemo-attractant peptides, the antagonists tolerated large bulky groups present in a urethan linkage. Affinity to the receptor of antagonists is not a direct function of the amino protection by carbobenzoxy nor by terminal butoxy groups. The mere presence of a urethan linkage will not produce an antagonist, too. The primary sequence of amino acids, while crucial in chemo-attractant peptides, appears to be of little or no significance in the antagonist series. Correct steric configuration is a necessary prerequisite for agonists, but plays no role in antagonists. Carboxyterminal esterification may change biological activity; the latter was tenfold higher in the benzyl ester when compared to the parent compound CHO-Met-Leu-Phe-OH, whereas in t-butoxy-NCl-Leu-Phe-OH its inhibitory effect was reversed when it was benzylated to t-butoxy NCl-Leu-Phe-OBzl. (12)

It is clear that in the case of the positive chemo-attractant agents there are definite and precise structural requirements, whereas little certain knowledge exists of the structural requirements of antagonists, i.e. substances exhibiting classic competitive interactions in both radioreceptor and biological assays. It is obvious to explore granulocyte labelling by means of the antagonists of the synthetic chemo-attractants. The stability of their binding to the granulocytes, and their biological effects are not well known; results of preliminary exploratory studies do not appear promising (8).

Receptors:

Until recently there was no direct evidence for the existence of specific chemotactic receptors. Given the very great heterogeneity of chemotactic agents it appeared unlikely that there should be a single species of chemotactic receptors in neutrophil granulocytes. Wilkinson (1), Wissler, Stecher and Sorkin (13) have in the past argued against there being any specific chemotactic receptors. However, the recent work showing the very great specificity of endogenous leucocyte derived peptides (Wissler, Chapter 4), and of chemotactically active synthetic small peptides (3) and the low concentrations (1.0 x 10E-10 to 1.0 x 10E-12 M) at which some of them are effective, suggest that there is interaction with specific cell receptors (14), or that there is specific interaction with receptor-like sites in the cell membrane (Wissler, Chapter 4).

Tetramethylrhodamine (TMR) labelled N-formyl-NCl-Leu-Phe-NCl-Tyr-Lys is a potent chemo-attractant for human neutrophils. Binding of this peptide to living neutrophils was observed by means of video intensification microscopy. At 37 deg.C diffuse membrane fluorescence was seen initially, followed by rapid aggregation and internalization of the fluorescent peptide. These processes were dependent on specific binding to the formyl peptide chemotactic receptor (15).

Binding of two biochemically distinct chemotactic factors, FMLP and C5a, to their respective receptors on human granulocytes produces a transient severalfold increase in cAMP. To determine if arachnidonic acid metabolites were responsible for the increased cAMP concentrations, two inhibitors of arachnidonic acid metabolism, indomethacin and ETYA (5,8,11,14-Eicosa-tetraynoic acid), were incubated with granulocytes prior to exposure to FMLP or C5a. ETYA, but not indomethacin, inhibited both the cAMP and superoxide responses to a similar degree. However, the mechanism of this effect was found to be through inhibition of the binding of FMLP to its receptor rather than through inhibition of arachnidonate metabolism.

REFERENCES

1. Wilkinson P.C.: Chemotaxis and Inflammation. Churchill Livingstone, Edinburgh, London, 1974.
2. Schiffmann E., B.A. Corcoran and S.M. Wahl: Formyl-methionylpeptides as chemoattractants for leukocytes. Proc. Natl. Acad. Sci. USA 72:1059, 1975.
3. Showell H.J., R.J. Freer, S.H. Zigmond, E. Schiffmann, S. Aswanikumar, B. Corcoran and E.L. Becker: The Structure-Activity Relations of Synthetic Peptides as Chemotactic Factors and Inducers of Lysosomal Enzyme Secretion for Neutrophils. The Journal of Experimental Medicine, 143:1154:1169, 1976.
4. Day A.R., J.A. Radding, R.J. Freer, H.J. Showell, E.L. Becker, E. Schiffmann, B. Corcoran, S. Aswanikumar and C. Pert: Synthesis and Binding Characteristics of an Intrinsically Radiolabeled Chemotactic Acyl Tripeptide: N-alpha-formyl-norleucyl-leucy- phenylalanine. FEBS Letters 77:241:294, 1977.
5. Wilkinson P.C.: Synthetic peptide chemotactic factors for neutrophils: the range of active peptides their efficacy and inhibitory activity, and susceptibility of the cellular response to enzymes and bacterial toxins. Immunology 36:579:588, 1979.
6. Freer R.J.. A.R.Day, J.A.Radding. E. Schiffmann, S. Aswanikumar, H.J. Showell and E.L. Becker: Further Studies on the Structural Requirements for Synthetic Peptide Chemoattractants. Biochemistry 19:2404-2410, 1980.
7. Zoghbi S.S., M.L. Thakur and A. Gottschalk: A Potential Radioactive Agent for the Selective Labelling of Human Neutrophils. J. Nucl. Med. 22:32, 1981 (Abstract).
8. McAfee J.G., personal communication, 1983.
9. O'Flaherty J.T., H.J. Showell and P. Ward: Neutropenia induced by systemic infusion of chemotactic factors. J. Immunol. 118:1586-1589, 1977.
10. Marasco U.A., H.J. Showell and E.L. Becker: Substance P Binds to the Formylpeptide Chemotaxis Receptor on the Rabbit Neutrophil. Bioch. + Biophys. Research Communications 99:1065-1072, 1981.
11. Van Epps D.E. and M.L. Garcia: Enhancement of Neutrophil Function as a Result of Prior Exposure to Chemotactic Factor. J. Clin. Invest. 66:167-175, 1980.
12. Freer R.J., A.R. Day, N. Muthukumaraswamy, H.J. Showell and E.L. Becker: Antagonists of the Formylated Peptide Chemoattractants: Structure-Activity-Comparisons With Formyl-Methionyl-Leucyl-Phenylalanine-OH. In: Biochemistry of the Acute Allergic Reactions, pp.161-168, Publisher A.R. Liss, Inc., New York, 1981.
13. Wissler J.H., V. Stecher and E. Sorkin: Chemistry and biology of the anaphylatoxin related peptide systems. III. Evaluation of leucocyte activity as the property of a new peptide system with classical anaphylatoxin and cocytotaxin components. Europ. J. Immunol. 2:90, 1972.
14. Ward P.A. and E.L. Becker: Biology of Leucotaxis. Rev. Physiol. Biochem. Pharmakol.77:125-148, 1977.

15. Niedel J.E.,   I. Kahane   and   P. Cuatrecasas: Receptor-Mediated   Internalization   of Fluorescent Chemotactic Peptide by Human Neutrophils. Science 205:1412-1414, 1979.
16. Zigmond S.H.   and   J.G. Hirsch: Leukocyte   locomotion   and chemotaxis.   New   method for evaluation and demonstration of cellderived chemotactic factor.   J.   Exp.   Med.   137:387, 1973.
17. O'Flaherty J.T., H.J. Showell, D.L. Kreutzer, O.A. Ward and E.L. Becker: Inhibition of in vivo and in vitro Neutrophil Responses to Chemotactic Factors by a Competetive Antagonist. J.   Immunol. 120:1326-1332, 1978.

8 LABELLING BLOOD CELLS WITH 111-In-TROPOLONATE

H.J. DANPURE AND S. OSMAN

8.1 INTRODUCTION

111-In-tropolonate is the latest in a series of lipid-soluble metal chelating agents used to label blood cells for clinical and biological use. The series began in 1976 with 111-In-oxinate (1) and has now been extended to include 111-In-acetylacetonate (2,3) and 111-In-oxine-sulphate (4). 111-In-chelates are now widely used as tracers for platelets and granulocytes; labelled granulocytes have proved especially valuable in the non-invasive diagnosis of abscesses and other inflammatory lesions (5,6,7) and labelled platelets for locating vascular thrombi (8) and monitoring of human kidney transplants (9).

All the metal complexes reported so far, including 111-In-tropolonate, non-specifically label all cells they come into contact with as well as plasma proteins. However, a notable and most important difference between 111-In-tropolonate and its predecessors is that the competition between cells and plasma for 111-In can be manipulated so that the majority of 111-In labels the cells with the cell numbers available from 50-100 ml human blood, whereas with 111-In-oxinate and 111-In-acetylacetonate the reverse is true. Therefore, to achieve a labelling efficiency of 50% or more, blood cells are generally labelled with 111-In-oxinate and 111-In-acetylacetonate in a plasma-free medium. Removing cells from plasma is known to be detrimental to platelets (8,10) as well as granulocytes (11) so the ability of 111-In-tropolonate to label cells in plasma should reduce the cell damage as well as simplify and speed-up the isolation and labelling procedures; an important consideration to anyone who is routinely labelling cells for clinical use.

162

8.2 PROPERTIES OF TROPOLONE AND In-111-TROPOLONATE

Tropolone is the commonly used name for 2-hydroxy-2,4,6 cyclohepatrien-1-one, a 7-membered cyclic hydroxy ketone whose structure is shown in Figure 1.

Tropolone

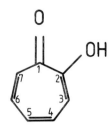

Fig. 1. Structural formula of Tropolone
(2-hydroxy-2,4,6-cycloheptatrien-1-one)

Tropolone is a water-soluble bidentate ligand with aromatic properties which was first synthesized by Cook et al. in 1951 (12). Its LD(50) in mice is 150mg/kg (13). Tropolone forms complexes with a number of metals including In, Ga, Cu, Fe, Cr (14) and has been found to promote excretion of iron in rats with iron overload (13).

The 111-In-tropolonate complex contains a central indium atom surrounded by three tropolone molecules; it is lipid-soluble, stable in acidic solutions but decomposes in basic solutions (14). The partition coefficient for 111-In-tropolonate between olive oil and buffer is greater than that for 111-In-oxinate and 111-In-acetylacetonate (15) whereas the stability constant is similar to that for 111-In-oxinate (16).

8.3 PREPARATION OF In-111-TROPOLONATE FOR CELL LABELLING

A stock solution of tropolone at 4.4 x 10E-03 M in Hepes-saline buffer pH 7.6, containing 20 mM Hepes and 0.8% w/v NaCl (17) is prepared, then filter sterilised, and stored at -20 deg.C in the dark. 111-In-chloride in 0.04 M HCl, kindly supplied by Amersham International at 10 mCi/ml (37 MBq/ml) is diluted in 0.04 M HCl as required, then 10-100 ul are added to 1 ml 4.4 x 10E-03 tropolone in Hepes-saline buffer, pH 7.6. One hundred microlitres of the 111-In-complex are then added to 1 ml of cells in plasma. For clinical use, where a total of 100-250 uCi (0.4-1.0 MBq) on the cells is required, the complex can be prepared by adding 10-50 ul 111-In-chloride in acid directly to cells in 1 ml plasma containing 4.0 x 10E-04 tropolone, provided the ratio of acid to plasma does not exceed 1 : 20. Further details will be given in the section on cell labelling.

8.4 CELL SEPARATION

Unfortunately all metal complexes investigated as cell labelling agents so far non-specifically label all cells they come into contact with, though with varying efficiency. Consequently, to study the fate of one particular type of blood cell in-vivo the cell type must be isolated from an aliquot of fresh blood before labelling.

It is essential that the viability of the cells is maintained during the in-vitro cell separation and labelling procedure if the indium-labelled blood cells are to behave in-vivo as normal blood cells. Loss of viability may arise from mechanical damage produced by centrifuging the cells for too long at too high a g-force or depletion of essential nutrients during any steps where the cells are removed from plasma. The latter problem should not arise when using 111-In-tropolonate to label blood cells as the required separation of all blood cells can be performed in plasma

(17). However, mechanical damage could still be a problem and so we have tried to use low g-forces for short spinning periods in order to achieve the required cell separation.

8.4.1 Erythrocytes

To separate erythrocytes from normal healthy volunteers, whole blood, anticoagulated with ACD (NIH formula A), is mixed with a sedimenting agent e.g. hydroxyethyl starch to give a final concentration of approximately 0.6% w/v. This accelerates the rate of sedimentation of the erythrocytes at 1 g so that after 30-60 minutes of incubation at room temperature or 37 deg.C a pellet of packed red cells and a supernatant of leucocyte-rich platelet-rich plasma (LRPRP) is obtained. The LRPRP is removed and the erythrocytes are diluted with cell-free plasma obtained by spinning LRPRP at 640 g for 10 minutes. The cells can then be labelled in plasma with 111-In-tropolonate. If the blood donor has a high erythrocyte sedimentation rate (ESR) the addition of a sedimenting agent is unnecessary.

8.4.2 Platelets

Platelets must be handled carefully otherwise they will spontaneously aggregate. The procedure we use involves centrifuging whole blood containing ACD (as above) at 640 g for 1-2 minutes to pellet the leucocytes and erythrocytes. The supernatant of platelet-rich-plasma (PRP) is removed, acidified with more ACD (1 part ACD to 10 parts PRP) which reduces the pH to 6.5, then centrifuged at 640 g for 5-10 minutes to pellet the platelets. The pellet of WBCs is resuspended in 0.5-1.0 ml ACD-plasma pH 6.5 for labelling with 111-In-tropolonate.

8.4.3 Mixed leucocytes and granulocytes

Leucocyte-rich platelet-rich plasma, obtained from whole blood after the removal of the erythrocytes, when centrifuged at 100 g for 5 minutes gives a pellet of 'mixed' leucocytes. The composition of the 'mixed' cells from normal volunteers was approximately 3.5 erythrocytes for each granulocyte as well as mononuclear cells and a few platelets. Although the 'mixed' leucocytes may be satisfactory for the detection of inflammatory lesions, they are not suitable for measurements of granulocyte kinetics. We therefore developed discontinuous density-gradients of Percoll (Pharmacia), which is composed of polyvinylpyrrolidone (PVP)-coated silica particles. The gradients are iso-osmotic and have a low viscosity which permits a rapid isopycnic separation of cells (18). Percoll does not impair the chemotactic response, bactericidal activity or generation of superoxide anion by granulocytes (19). Initially the appropriate densities of Percoll were made from iso-osmotic Percoll (IOP) (produced by adding 1 ml 1.5M NaCl to 9 ml Percoll, specific gravity approximately 1.13 g/ml), diluted with isotonic saline (Figure 2).

When we began to use 111-In-tropolonate in plasma as a cell labelling agent we modified the procedure so that the cells were maintained in plasma throughout their isolation by diluting iso-osmotic Percoll (IOP) with autologous plasma. We found that a three-step discontinous gradient of 50%, 60% and 65% v/v Percoll in plasma centrifuged at 150 g for only 5 minutes gave the required separation of granulocytes (17) as shown in Figure 2. Using 2 ml of each solution in a 10 ml conically based Sterilin test tube, granulocytes from approximately 25 ml blood could be separated without overloading the gradient. After centrifugation the granulocyte band, generally found at the interface between the 50 and 60% Percoll/plasma bands, was carefully removed with a wide-bore sterile Pasteur pipette, diluted five times with cell-free plasma and centrifuged at 100 g for 5 minutes to remove the Percoll. The pellet of granulocytes, which contained 80-95% granulocytes, no mononuclear cells or platelets and 5-20% erythrocytes, was resuspended in 0.5-1.0 ml cell-free plasma for

labelling with 111-In-tropolonate. When labelled in 90% plasma,
97% of the cell-bound 111-In was on the granulocytes making these
cells satisfactory for cell kinetic studies. Approximately 60-80%
of the granulocytes are recovered from the 'mixed' leucocytes
using the Percoll gradients. We also use a two-step discontinuous
density gradient of Metrizamide (Nyegaard) to separate the 'pure'
granulocytes. A sterile solution of Metrizamide at 350 g/l in
distilled water (100%) is diluted with autologous cell-free plasma
to give 40% v/v and 50% v/v Metrizamide in plasma. Two ml
aliquots of the 40 and 50% solution are used in a 10 ml Sterilin
test tube overlaid with about 2 ml of 'mixed' leucocytes in
plasma. The gradient is centrifuged at 150 g for 5 minutes and
the separation that is achieved is shown in Figure 2.

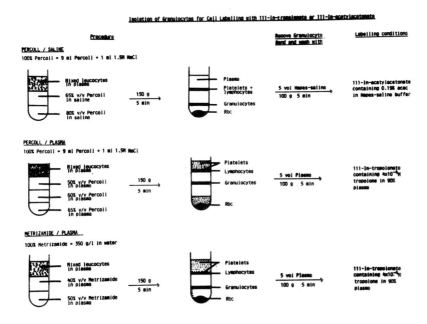

Fig. 2.

8.5   CELL LABELLING

8.5.1   Clinical studies

   To label 'mixed' leucocytes or 'pure' granulocytes, isolated
from 50-100 ml whole blood as described above, the cells are
resuspended in either 0.5 or 1.0 ml ACD-plasma pH 7.2 depending on
the number of cells obtained. Fifty to one hundred microlitres of
tropolone at 4.4 x 10E-03 M in Hepes-saline buffer is added,
followed immediately by 10-50 ul 111-In-chloride in 0.04 M HCl
containing 100-500 uCi (0.4-2.0 MBq) of 111-In, i.e. the
111-In-chloride is at 10 mCi/ml (370 MBq/ml). If the specific
activity of the 111-In-chloride is such that more than 50 ul is
required, then the volume of cells in plasma must be
proportionately increased, but this will reduce the labelling
efficiency. The cells are incubated at room temperature for
5 minutes, then 5 ml plasma is added and the cells are centrifuged
at 100 g for 5 minutes. The cells and supernatant are separated
and the activity in each fraction is measured in order to
determine the percentage of the 111-In bound to the cells. The
cells are resuspended in 5 ml fresh plasma and reinjected into the
patient as soon as possible after labelling. The procedure for
labelling platelets is the same except that the cells are
resuspended in 0.5 or 1.0 ml ACD-plasma pH 6.5 in order to
maintain their viability during labelling.

8.5.2   In-vitro studies

   For in-vitro studies the amount of 111-In required to be
present on the cells will be much lower than that needed for
clinical studies. In this situation the 111-In-tropolonate
complex can be formed before addition to the cells rather than in

situ as described above. 10-100 ul of 111-In chloride in acid are added to 1 ml 4.4 x 10E-03 M tropolone in Hepes-saline just before use, then 100 ul of the complex is added to 1 ml of cells in plasma at pH 7.2 for erythrocytes and leucocytes and at pH 6.5 for platelets. This results in the cells being labelled in 90% plasma with 111-In-tropolonate containing 4.0 x 10E-04 M, which is the optimum tropolone concentration for labelling blood cells in 90% plasma.

8.6   LABELLING EFFICIENCY OF 111-In-TROPOLONATE

8.6.1   Tropolone concentration

All solutions of 111-In complexes used to label cells need to contain a vast excess of the chelating agent relative to the amount of indium if the 111-In is to label the cells. The reason for this is unknown at present. To determine the effect of the tropolone concentration on the labelling efficiency of 111-In-tropolonate, 100 ul 111-In-tropolonate containing between 1.0 x 10E-05 to 4.0 x 10E-03 M tropolone was added to 1 ml of erythrocytes, platelets or 'pure' granulocytes in plasma or Hepes-saline and the cells were incubated at 37 deg.C for 15 minutes. The cells were separated from the plasma by centrifugation and the percentage of cell-associated radioactivity was measured. The results are shown in Figure 3. 4.0 x 10E-04 M was found to be the optimum concentration for labelling the 3 types of blood cells in 90% plasma, but for cells labelled in Hepes-saline buffer the optimum tropolone concentration was ten times lower (results not shown). Our value of 4.0 x 10E-05 as the optimum tropolone concentration for cell labelling in a plasma-free medium agrees with that of Burke et al. (20) for 'mixed' human leucocytes and Dewanjee et al. (15) for canine platelets, but disagrees with Rao and Dewanjee (16) for rabbit erythrocytes, where they find no peak value, only a reduction in labelling efficiency at concentrations above 6.5 x 10E-04 M. They did however use 500 times more cells than we did.

The optimum tropolone concentration for labelling human blood cells with 111-In-tropolonate in 90% plasma was 4.0 x 10E-04 M (17) which is higher than the value found by Dewanjee et al. (15) for canine platelets, but the final concentration of plasma used in the latter experiments is not given and may be less than 90%, in which case one would expect the optimum tropolone concentration to be lower. Alternatively, if the final plasma concentration was 90%, the difference in optimum tropolone concentration may reflect a species-specific difference in the ability of 111-In-tropolonate to label blood cells in plasma.

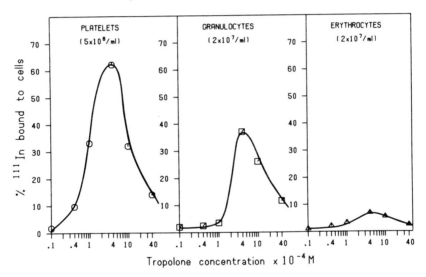

Fig. 3. Effect of tropolone concentration on the binding of 111-In-tropolonate to blood cells in 90% plasma

8.6.2 Plasma concentration

Table 1 shows the labelling efficiency of 'pure' granulocytes, platelets and erythrocytes labelled in 90% plasma or Hepes-saline buffer. The concentration of tropolone and acetylacetone associated with the 111-In-tropolonate and 111-In-acetylacetonate complexes was 4.0 x 10E-04 M and 1.9 x 10E-02 M respectively.

Table 1.

Total Volume of Labelling Medium (ml)	Labelling Efficiency	
	85% plasma	Hepes-Saline Buffer
1	47	86
2	28	85
5	11	85
10	5	85

Effect of labelling 1 million granulocytes in different volumes of 85% plasma or Hepes-saline buffer with 111-In-tropolonate containing 4.0 x 10E-04 M or 4.0 x 10E-05 M tropolone respectively.

With both cell labelling agents the labelling efficiency in Hepes-saline buffer was greater than in plasma but the values for cells labelled with 111-In-tropolonate in 90% plasma were much better than those for 111-In-acetylacetonate. We therefore conclude that with both compounds plasma proteins compete with the cells for 111-In and reduce the labelling efficiency. The competition between cells and plasma for 111-In-tropolonate is more favourable towards the cells, whereas with 111-In-acethylacetonate it is more favourable towards the plasma.

The low cell concentrations used in this experiment are approximately 5-10 times lower than those used clinically. Raising the cell concentration increases the labelling efficiency as described in the next section.

8.6.3 Cell concentration

The labelling efficiency of 111-In-tropolonate for blood cells labelled in 90% plasma increases dramatically as the cell concentration is increased (as shown in Figure 4).

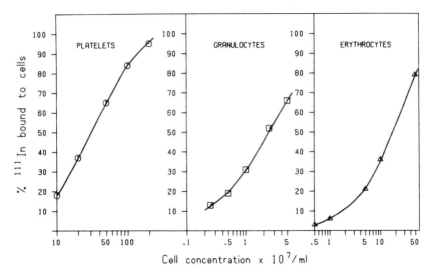

Fig. 4. Effect of cell concentration on the labelling efficiency of 111-In-tropolonate in 90% plasma

The effect is much smaller if the cells are labelled in buffer (results not shown) because the buffer does not compete with the cells for indium. But with cell labelling in plasma both the cells and the plasma bind the indium, so the ratio of cell volume to plasma volume is important. As the ratio increases, e.g. when the cell concentration is raised, so the amount of 111-In on the cells increases, but if the ratio decreases, e.g.

when a fixed number of cells is labelled in increasing volumes of plasma, the amount of 111-In on the cell decreases as shown in Table 2.

Table 2.   Labelling of Blood Cells with 111-In-Tropolonate and
           In-111-Acetylacetonate in Plasma or Hepes-Saline Buffer
----
   Cells   Labelling Efficiency

Type	Number	111-In-Tropolonate		111-In-Acetylacetonate	
		Plasma (90%)	Hepes-Saline	Plasma (90%)	Hepes-Saline
Gran.	2.0 x 10E07	36%	93%	7%	88%
Plat.	5.0 x 10E08	34%	83%	9%	64%
Ery.	1.0 x 10E08	32%	91%	6%	96%

This emphasizes the importance of having a high   cell concentration rather than large numbers of cells at a low concentration when labelling cells with 111-In-tropolonate in plasma, e.g. 1 million granulocytes in 0.1 ml plasma, i.e. 10 million cells/ml will give a better labelling efficiency than 10 million granulocytes in 10 ml plasma i.e. 1 million cells/ml. This demonstrates that quite small numbers of blood cells can be efficiently labelled with 111-In-tropolonate in plasma, provided the cell concentration is high.

In the paper by Dewanjee et al. (15) where platelet labelling in ACD-saline and plasma is compared, the same total number of cells is used in each case but the cell concentration in plasma is eight times greater than in saline, giving the impression that labelling in plasma is almost as good as that in saline.

8.6.4 Time and temperature

111-In-tropolonate rapidly labels cells in plasma with the maximum uptake occurring after 5 minutes incubation at room temperatures or 37 deg.C (17). The maximum uptake for canine platelets (15) and rabbit erythrocytes (16) labelled at 37 deg.C in ACD-saline with 111-In-tropolonate occurred after approximately 20 minutes and 5 minutes incubation respectively. In the latter studies the maximum uptake occurred at longer times when the cells were incubated at 25 deg.C or 4 deg.C.

8.6.5 pH

The highest labelling efficiency using 111-In-tropolonate in ACD-saline was obtained at pH 9 for canine platelets (15) and pH 6.5 for rabbit erythrocytes (16). We find that the labelling efficiency obtained with human platelets labelled with 111-In-tropolonate in plasma is lower at pH 6.5 than 7.2. However we recommend that platelets are labelled at pH 6.5 rather than 7.2 because the viability of the platelets is better at the lower pH.

8.6.6 Citrate ion concentration

Scheffel et al (21) demonstrated that citrate ion reduced the labelling efficiency of human platelets incubated with 111-In-oxinate in plasma or buffer. A similar reduction in labelling efficiency with increasing citrate concentration has also been reported for canine platelets (15) and rabbit erythrocytes labelled with 111-In-tropolonate in saline.

8.7   IN-VITRO VIABILITY OF LABELLED CELLS

Burke et al. (20) have measured the chemotactic response and phagocytic capacity of granulocytes in 'mixed' leucocyte preparations isolated and incubated in a plasma-free medium with $5.0 \times 10E-05$ M tropolone or 111-In-tropolonate containing $4.0 \times 10E-05$ tropolone. They found a small reduction in chemotaxis and phagocytosis of cells labelled with both agents but concluded that 111-In-tropolonate and tropolone impaired the in-vitro functions of granulocytes to a lesser extent than 111-In-oxine or 111-In-acetylacetone. In contrast, no reduction in random migration, chemotaxis and percent phagocytosis was observed with our 'mixed' leucocytes or 'pure' granulocytes isolated in Percoll/plasma before or after labelling with 111-In-tropolonate in plasma (A.J. Pinching, personal communication) nor with cells isolated in Percoll/saline and labelled with 111-In acetylacetonate.

The inability of these particular in-vitro tests to detect any difference between cells isolated and labelled in plasma with 111-In-tropolonate and those isolated and labelled in saline with 111-In-acetylacetonate cast doubt on the value of such tests in predicting the in-vivo function of labelled cells. The same cells which show no difference in in-vitro function show marked differences in-vivo as discussed in the next section.

8.8   CLINICAL RESULTS

Metrizamide/plasma or Percoll/plasma-separated granulocytes isolated as described earlier have been labelled with 111-In-tropolonate in 90% plasma and used for dynamic imaging of the lungs, spleen and liver and compared with granulocytes separated by Percoll/saline gradients and labelled with 111-In-acetyl-acetonate in Hepes-saline buffer. Granulocytes isolated and labelled in saline are sequestered in the lungs for at least 15 minutes before being slowly released, whereas cells isolated and labelled in plasma show a rapid transit through the lungs (11). The rapid transit through the lungs leads to a much faster accumulation in the spleen and liver than found with saline-labelled cells. In patients with inflammatory lesions the 'mixed' leucocytes or 'pure' granulocytes isolated and labelled in plasma with 111-In-tropolonate localize more rapidly than cells labelled with 111-In-oxinate or 111-In-acetylacetonate (22). Approximately 200 studies have now been carried out by Drs. Peters and Saverymuttu on patients with suspected abscesses or inflammatory bowel disease (mainly Crohn's disease and ulcerative colitis).

The average labelling efficiency was 50-80% depending on the number of cells used and the indium remained firmly associated with the cells after several washes in plasma or following reinjection into the patient. They found that 75% of the positive patients that were scanned for the first time at 40 minutes (27 studies) were positive and by 3 hours they were all positive. The clinical results show a specificity of 100% and a sensitivity of 96%. Two examples of the localization observed with granulocytes labelled with 111-In-tropolonate in plasma are shown in Figures 5 and 6.

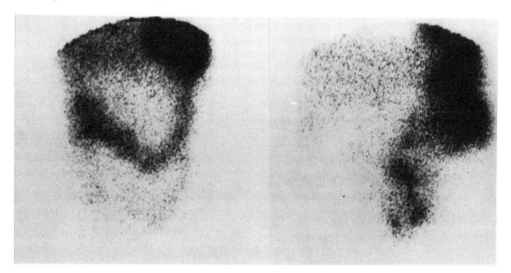

Fig. 5. Colon in patient with ulcerative colitis

Fig. 6. Paracolic abscess

8.9 FUTURE PROSPECTS

Our future aims for cell labelling should be to simplify the cell labelling procedure whilst maintaining the integrity and viability of the cells.

Although 111-In-tropolonate labels blood cells in plasma it does so less efficiently than in buffer, therefore it would be an advantage to be able to label cells with the same efficiency in plasma as in buffer i.e. to have cell-labelling agents which do not react with plasma proteins. This may not be possible as the mechanism of cell labelling may involve interaction with cellular proteins.

Another improvement would be to find agents which would deposit the radionuclide solely on or in the plasma membrane, rather than within the cell such as 111-In-BLEDTA (23). This would reduce the radiation damage to the cells. The radiation damage to cells labelled with indium-tropolonate can already be reduced by using the shorter half-life indium radionuclide In-113m rather than 111-In because of the rapid rate of localization observed with indium-tropolonate labelled leucocytes.

Simplification of the cell labelling procedure by using agents which selectively label particular blood cells in whole blood would also be an advantage provided that the agent did not damage the cells and that the cells could take up sufficient activity for clinical studies. A procedure for specific labelling of monocytes in whole blood using Tc-99m-tin-colloid has been developed by Schroth et al. (24) and preliminary in-vitro results on a selective agent for human neutrophils have been published by Zoghbi et al (25) (see Editor's Note on chemotactic agents as cell specific labels at the end of Chapter 7).

SUMMARY

lll-In-tropolonate is the latest in a series of metal chelating agents used to label blood cells for clinical diagnostic studies and measurement of cell kinetics. It has the advantage over other cell labelling agents e.g. lll-In-oxinate and lll-In-acetylacetonate that it efficiently labels blood cells in plasma, even at low cell concentrations, e.g. with 2.0 x 10E07 granulocytes the labelling efficiency in plasma is 52%. The labelling efficiency can, however, be increased to approximately 80% for the same number of cells if the plasma is replaced with Hepes-saline buffer pH 7.6 or if the cell concentration in plasma is raised. Labelling the cells in plasma, rather than buffer, has the advantage that it eliminates the need to wash the cells free of plasma and enhances their viability.

lll-In-tropolonate is rapidly formed by mixing the water-soluble ligand tropolone (2-hydroxy- 2,4,6-cyclohepta-trienone) with lll-In-chloride in acid; the resulting lipid-soluble complex is readily and non-specifically incorporated into all blood cells. It is therefore necessary to isolate the required cell type before labelling. Mixed leucocytes obtained from healthy donors by differential centrifugation following sedimentation of the erythrocytes with hydroxyethyl starch, contain approximately 3.5 red cells to each granulocyte as well as mononuclear leucocytes and a few platelets. To isolate "pure" granulocytes two density gradient systems using either a two-step discontinous gradient of Percoll diluted with autologous plasma or Metrizamide diluted with plasma have been developed. The resulting cells contain 80-95% granulocytes, no mononuclear cells or platelets and 5-20% erythrocytes. When these "pure" granulocytes are labelled with lll-In-tropolonate in plasma approximately 97% of the cell-bound indium is on the granulocytes. The optimum concentration of tropolone mixed with lll-In-chloride that is required to label granulocytes in 90% plasma is 4.0 x 10E-04 M but is reduced to 4.0 x 10E-05 M if the cells are labelled in Hepes-saline buffer.

At Hammersmith Hospital approximately 200 studies have been carried out by Drs. Peters and Saverymuttu using granulocytes labelled with lll-In-tropolonate in 90% plasma for measurement of cell kinetics or diagnosis of inflammatory lesions. The labelling efficiency was 50-80% depending on the number of cells obtained and the injected dose of lll-In was 150-250 uCi. Maintenance of the cells in plasma throughout the isolation and labelling phases results in labelled granulocytes which rapidly pass through the lung, show a low accumulation in the liver and rapidly localize in inflammatory sites. Approximately 75% of positive images were obtained by 40 minutes after reinjection of the labelled cells and the remainder by 3 hrs.

lll-In-tropolonate also labels platelets and erythrocytes in plasma but we have no information on their in-vivo distribution.

REFERENCES

1. McAfee J.G. and M.L. Thakur: Survey of radioactive agents for in vitro labelling of phagocytic leucocytes. 1. Soluble Agents. J. Nucl. Med. 17:480-487, 1976.
2. Sinn H., and D.J. Silvester: Simplified cell labelling with 111-Indium acetylacetone. Brit. J. Radiol. 52:758-759, 1979.
3. Danpure H.J. and S. Osman: Cell labelling and cell damage with 111-Indium acetylacetone - an alternative to 111-Indium oxine. Brit. J. Radiol., 54:597-601, 1981.
4. McAfee J.G., G.M Gagne, G. Subramanian, Z.D. Grossmann, F.D. Thomas, M.L. Roskopf, P. Fernandes and B.J. Lyons: Distribution of leucocytes labelled with 111-In-oxine in dogs with acute inflammatory lesions. J. Nucl. Med. 21:1059-1068, 1980.
5. Thakur M.L., J.P. Lavender, R.N. Arnot, D.J. Silvester and A.W. Segal: 111-Indium labelled autologous leukocytes in man. J. Nucl. Med. 18:1014-1021, 1979.
6. Ascher N.L., L. Forstrom and R.L. Simmons: Radiolabelled autologous leucocyte scanning in abscess detection. World J. Surgery 4:395-402, 1980.
7. Saverymuttu S.H., A.M. Peters, H.J. Hodgson, V.S. Chadwick and J.P. Lavender: 111-Indium autologous leucocyte scanning: comparison with radiology for imaging the colon in inflammatory bowel disease. British Medical Journal, 285:255-257, 1982.
8. Goodwin D.A., J.T. Bushberg, P.W. Doherty, M.J. Lipton, F.K. Conley, C.I. Diamanti and C.F. Meares: 111-Indium labelled autologous platelets for location of vascular thrombi in humans. J. Nucl. Med. 19:626-634, 1978.
9. Fenech A., A. Nicholls and F.W. Smith: 111-In-labelled platelets in the diagnosis of renal transplant rejection: preliminary findings. Brit. J. Radiol. 54:325-327, 1981.
10. Thakur M.L., L. Walsh, H.L. Malech and A. Gottschalk: 111-Indium-labelled human platelets: improved method, efficacy and evaluation. J. Nucl. Med. 22:381-385, 1981.
11. Peters A.M., S.H. Saverymuttu, H.J. Danpure, S. Osman, J.P. Lavender, V.S. Chadwick and H.J. Hodgson: Granulocyte (PMN) kinetics: isolation and labelling in plasma abolishes lung sequestration. Clin. Sci. 62:P.69 (Abstract), 1982.
12. Cook J.W., A.R. Gibb, R.A. Raphael and A.R.Somerville: Tropolone Part I. The preparation and general characteristics of tropolone. J. Chem. Soc., 503-511, 1951.
13. Grady R.W., J.H. Graziano, G.P. White, A. Jacobs and A. Cerami: The development of new ion-chelating drugs II. J. Pharmacol. and Exptl. Therapeutics 205:757-765, 1978.
14. Muetterties E.L. and C.M. Wright: Chelate Chemistry. I. Tropolone and aminotroponimine derivatives of the main-group elements. J. American Chem. Soc. 86:5132-5137, 1964.

15. Dewanjee M.K., S.A. Rao and P. Disisheim: 111-Indium-tropolone, a new high-affinity platelet label: Preparation and evaluation of labelling parameters. J. Nucl. Med. 22:981-987, 1981.
16. Rao S.A. and M.K. Dewanjee: Comparative evaluation of red cell-labelling parameters of three lipid-soluble-111-In-chelates: Effect of lipid solubility on membrane incorporation and stability constant on transchelation. Eur. J. Nucl. Med. 7:282-285, 1982.
17. Danpure H.J., S. Osman and F. Brady: The labelling of blood cells in plasma with 111-In-tropolonate. Brit. J. Radiol. 55:247-249, 1982.
18. Pertoft H. and T.C. Laurent: Isopycnic separation of cells and cell organelles by centrifugation in modified colloidal silica gradients. In: Methods of Cell Separation, Vol. 1, edited by N. Catsimpoolas, Plenum Press, pp.25-65, 1977.
19. Harbeck R.J., A.A. Hoffman, S. Redecker, T. Biundo and J. Kurnick: The isolation and functional activity of polymorphonuclear leucocytes and lymphocytes separated from whole blood on a single Percoll density gradient. Clinical Immun. + Immunopathology 23:682-690, 1982.
20. Burke J.E.T., S. Roath, D. Ackery and P. Wyeth: The comparison of 8-hydroxyquinoline, tropolone and acetylacetone as mediators in the labelling of polymorphonuclear leucocytes with 111-Indium. A Functional study. Eur. J. Nucl. Med. 7:73-76, 1982.
21. Scheffel U., M-F. Tsan and P.A. McIntyre: Labelling of human platelets with (111-In) 8-hydroxyquinoline. J. Nucl. Med. 20:524-531, 1979.
22. Saverymuttu S.H., A.M. Peters, H.J. Reavy, H.J. Danpure, S. Osman and J.P. Lavender: The clinical use of 111-Indium-tropolone leucocytes for the detection of sepsis. Nucl. Med. Comm. 3:100 (Abstract), 1982.
23. Goodwin D.A., L.F. Fajardo, K.L. Frank, C.F. Meares and V. Hughot: Receptor binding, transport and metabolism of 111-Indium-radiopharmaceuticals by electron microscope autoradiography. Nucl. Med. Comm. 3:99 (Abstract), 1982.
24. Schroth J.J., E. Oberhausen and R. Berberich: Cell labelling with colloidal substances in whole blood. Eur. J. Nucl. Med. 6:469-472, 1981.
25. Zoghbi S.S., M.L. Thakur and A. Gottschalk: Selective cell labelling: A potential radioactive agent for labelling of human neutrophils. J. Nucl. Med. 22:P.32 (Abstract), 1981.

9 A NEW GRANULOCYTE SEPARATION AND LABELLING TECHNIQUE

A. MOISAN AND J. LE CLOIREC

9.1   INTRODUCTION

Labelling blood granulocytes presents, in   our   opinion,   two fields of interest:

- granulocyte kinetics
-localization of deep-seated sites of infection

We have developed a new method of granulocyte separation   and labelling.   Its   validity   was   tested   in-vitro   by   a   scanning electron microscope and by bactericidal and chemotactic assays.

9.2   MATERIAL AND METHODS

9.2.1   Blood sampling

Fifty millilitres of whole blood were drawn   onto   500   iu   of heparin   or   8 ml   of   ACDA   using   a   hypodermic syringe, minimum diameter 0.9 mm.   The sample was divided into two batches:
- 10 ml to obtain a sufficient quantity   of   platelet-poor   plasma (PPP) or final suspension (by centrifugation 400 g, 10 mn),
- 40 ml, which were transferred into 2 conical tubes.

9.2.2 Sedimentation

Ten percent of Dextran (Dextran-clin 6%)) was added to the whole blood. If the sample is drawn onto ACD, then 10% of Plasmagel desode (Plasmagel desode R. Bellon) is added.

The preparations were mixed and then transferred into 2 sterile tubes to eliminate deposits which had formed on the sides of the first tubes.

Sedimentation was carried out at 37 deg.C in a hot water bath until a transparent plasma was obtained. The duration varied according to the sedimentation rate. The tubes were set at an angle of 15% to the vertical plane. The platelet-rich plasma (PRP) was removed by a pipette, collected in 2 tubes and diluted with an RMPI medium. Further preparations were carried out at room temperature.

9.2.3 Flotation

A pipette was used to add the preparation to 2 conical tubes containing 5 ml of Ficoll-metrizoate (Lymphoprep or MSP) gradient. The preparation was then centrifuged (200 g, 10 nm, 30 deg.C).

The lymphocyte ring, then the supernatant, were removed with a pipette. The gradient was only partially extracted to complete elimination of the lymphocytes. Ten millimetres of the medium were then added and the contents of the 2 tubes were collected in a single tube which was left for 5 minutes before centrifugation at 150 g, 2 mn, 30 deg.C. The button was resuspended in 3 to 5 ml of medium prior to labelling.

9.2.4 Labelling

For the kinetic study, 50 to 100 uCi of 111-In-oxinate complex were added, and 300 to 500 uCi were added for the detection of abscesses.

Labelling lasted a maximum of 5 minutes. The preparation was washed with 10 ml of culture medium before centrifugation at 150 g, 2 mn, 30 deg.C.

9.2.5 Resuspension

The supernatant was removed. The washed granulocyte button was resuspended in PPP before reinjection into the patient. The radioactivity of the resuspended supernatant and granulocyte button was measured with a radio-isotope calibrator to assess labelling efficiency which proved to be 89% for 62 preparations with a standard deviation of 5%.

9.2.6 Routine quality control

We controlled the purity of the preparation with a trypan blue dye and by staining live cells on a microscope slide. Absence of lymphocyte and platelet contamination and a low red blood cell (RBC) count confirmed the suspension was relatively pure. On average, 4 to 5 granulocytes per RBC were found.

A "pure" preparation fulfils two requirements: Firstly, as the oxinate-indium complex is non-specific as a tracer, a "pure" preparation is necessary, especially for cell kinetic investigation. Secondly, several authors have already shown that radiation from 111-In damages lymphocytes. We carried out in-vitro experiments ourselves and, in our opinion, only lymphocyte-free cell preparations should be used.

9.3   RESULTS

9.3.1

Fifty six post-operative cases were examined to detect
deep-seated sites of infection.

Post-injection scanning was performed with a gamma-camera at
90 minutes, 4 hours and, in the event of an early negative scan,
at 24 hours.

The overall results were as follows:
- true-positives: 19
- false-positives: 0
- true-negatives: 35
- false-negatives: 2

The true-positives were those patients who presented an
infected   fluid   collection,   confirmed   by surgery, and the
true-negatives were those patients who progressed favourably
without treatment.

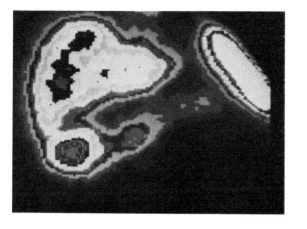

Fig. 1.
Scan performed 4 hours
after   injection   of
labelled granulocytes
to   locate   a   sub-
hepatic   abscess
following hemicolec-
tomy.

9.3.2 Kinetics

To date, we have studied 6 cases, 5 of which were controls. The kinetics were investigated by means of blood samples taken over a period of 72 hours and by dynamic scintigraphic imaging using a gamma-camera connected to a data processing system.

Given the small number of cases studied, we feel it is difficult to reach a meaningful conclusion with regard to the blood survival curve of the labelled granulocytes.

The other parameters obtained are given below:
- recovery of circulating cells 30 minutes after testing, expressed as a percentage,
- spleen and liver pools expressed as percentages 30 minutes following injection,
- half-clearance time in the lungs.

Table 1. Blood Survival Curve of Labelled Granulocytes

Case	Recovery % at 30 min	Spleen % at 30 min	Liver % at 30 min	T50 Lungs in min
1	35	12	9	18
2	40	13	12	15
3	37	13	10	16
4	42	14	9	12
5	24	15	10	17
6	30	33	10	13

Case 6 was a patient suffering from leucopenia and thrombopenia of immune origin who was cured after splenectomy.

The following documents give data concerning a healthy subject.

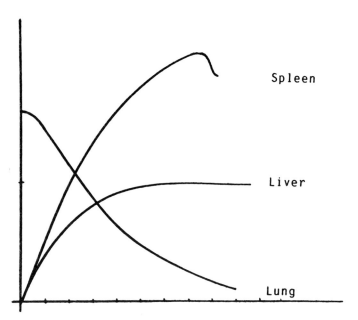

Fig. 2.   After injection of 100 uCi of In-oxinate granulocytes.

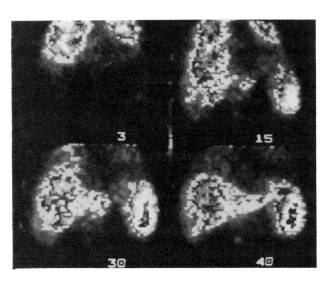

Fig. 3.   Anterior view 0-40 mn

10 CLINICAL APPLICATIONS OF 111-In-LABELLED GRANULOCYTES

D.A. GOODWIN, I.R. McDOUGALL, C. CHILES,

J.H. PALDI, D. KRIEVES AND M. GAINEY

10.1 INTRODUCTION

Since its introduction six years ago (1,2), the clinical use of 111-In labelled white cells for the detection and localization of inflammatory disease has greatly increased. In the last three years, reports from several centres have confirmed its diagnostic value (3,4,5,6). The growing interest in imaging of labelled white blood cells is due in part to the increasing availability of 111-In-oxinate and the ease of its use. Some commercial sources now have the capacity to carry out the entire white cell labelling procedure (Pharmatopes, Inc., 2944 Corvin Drive, Santa Clara, CA 95051). Nevertheless, white cell labelling with 111-In-oxinate is a relatively easy technique similar in complexity to the red cell labelling with 51-Cr needed for the determination of mass and halflife which is routinely performed in most Nuclear Medicine laboratories. Normally, autologous white cells are used and it has been shown conclusively that the 111-In labelled white cells retain their viability and chemotactic properties, and concentrate specifically in areas of inflammation and abscess following reinjection (7,8,9).

While 111-In or 67-Ga injected as the citrate or chloride will accumulate in abscesses, probably due to an increased permeability of the capillaries, the concentrations reached are not as high as with 111-In labelled white cells (10) and, more importantly, the uptake is totally non-specific. It has now been well documented in the literature that these 67-Ga and 111-In radiopharmaceuticals concentrate in various normal organs such as the colon as well as in a large variety of tumours (11). Since 111-In white cells do not normally accumulate in the gut, the examination is usually completed in 24 hours, avoiding the two or three day delay often necessary with 67-Ga-citrate.

This communication reports the results of 111-In white cell imaging in 542 patients referred over the past 5 years for investigation of acute inflammatory disease.

10.2 MATERIALS AND METHODS

The patients were selected from a total of 1138 patients (on whom 1310 scans were performed) because confirmation of the presence or absence of inflammatory disease or abscess was available either from surgery, post mortem, X-ray or the clinical course. The final study group was comprised of 542 patients on whom this follow-up information was available. Repeat white cell scans were performed on approximately 15% of the patients and were usually done to assess the treatment of a patient with a positive scan. These were counted only once, and classified as "true positive".

Autologous leucocytes were labelled with 111-In oxinate using a modification of the method of Thakur (4,6). The patients ranged in age from 1 to 88 years (mean 51), and 138 (25%) were female, the rest male. The main clinical groups investigated were suspected abscess, suspected osteomyelitis, inflammatory gastrointestinal or renal disease, and patients with an elevated white count and fever of unknown origin, especially in para- or quadriplegics in whom localizing symptoms were frequently absent.

Whole body scans were made using a Searle "Pho-Con" tomographic scanner, or an Ohio Nuclear large-field-of-view scintillation camera with a moving table 18-24 hours after the intravenous injection of 0.5-1.0 mCi 111-In labelled white cells. Cell labelling took approximately 2 hours (1 hour of which does not require technician time) and the whole body scans took 50 minutes (anterior and posterior). Spot views were made of suspicious areas seen in the whole body scan as well as of symptomatic areas: these took 5-10 minutes each. The patients spent an average of 1 1/2 to 2 1/2 hours in the Nuclear Medicine Service on the day of the study.

10.3 RESULTS

The correlation of the results of the white blood cell scan
with the final diagnosis is shown in Table 1. The statistics
calculated from the results are shown in Table 2.

Table 1.   Final Clinical Diagnosis

	+	−	
WBC-Scan +	243	24	267
−	20	255	275
	263	279	542

Table 2.

Sensitivity	92%
Specificity	91%
Positive predictive value	91%
Negative predictive value	93%
Accuracy	92%

The sensitivity, dependent on the true positive and false
negative rates (the fraction of patients with proven inflammatory
disease who had a positive scan, e.g.   243/263) was 92%.   The
specificity, dependent on the   true negative and false positive
rates (the fraction of patients proven not to have inflammatory
disease who had negative scans; 255/279) was 91%. The positive
predictive value, dependent on the true positive and false
positive rates (the fraction of patients with positive scans who
were proven to have inflammatory disease; 243/267) was 91%.   The
negative predictive value, dependent on the true negative and
false negative rates (the fraction of patients with a negative

scan who were proven not to have inflammatory disease; 255/275) was 93%. The overall accuracy, dependent on both the true positive and true negative rates (the fraction of all the patients with proven presence or absence of disease who had a scan that correctly predicted this 498/542) was 92%. These results are not significantly different from those we reported in a similar series of 312 patients in 1979 (6). Other investigators have reported similar clinical results (12). A surprising finding in view of the fact that the labelling procedure was shared by all the technical staff who had no special previous training, was the exceptionally low number of technically inadequate studies, approximately 1-2%. Figures 1-4 illustrate the clinical usefulness.

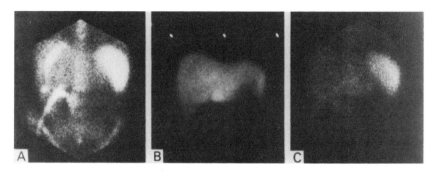

Fig. 1. 54 year old male, post cholecystectomy; fever and abdominal pain.
A: 111-In WBC scan of the anterior abdomen shows intense linear white cell concentration within the liver. A second linear concentration is seen lower on the right side where an abdominal drain is present.
B: Anterior Tc-99m sulphur colloid liver scan (10 mCi) done immediately following the white blood cell scan shows a faint linear decrease in activity in the same area in the right lobe (arrow).
C: Repeat anterior 111-In white blood cell scan done following surgical removal of a common duct stone with drainage of a large amount of pus shows clearing of liver activity.
Diagnosis: Ascending cholangitis.

190

Fig. 2. 59 year old white male with long standing polycystic disease of the liver. No change in the colloid liver scan (seen on the right), with multiple "filling" defects and a slightly enlarged liver. The HIDA Tc-99m scan showed normal liver function and gallbladder visualization. In view of the patient's fever, a white cell scan was done (shown on the left). Marked uptake of leukocytes in the large cyst in the dome of the right lobe indicating an abscess. The white cell scan became negative on antibiotic therapy.

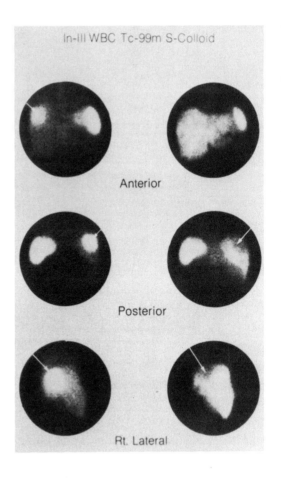

Fig. 3. 53 year old, male. T-7 paraplegic since 1954. Non-functioning left kidney secondary to chronic pyelonephritis. White cell scanning (September 80) disclosed left pyelonephritis which was treated with antibiotics. Readmission in August 81 with complaints of fever and malaise. Renal ultrasound and contrast

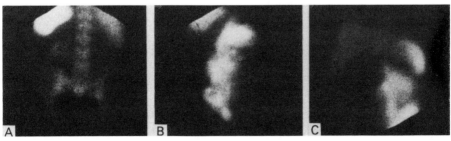

intravenous urography were unchanged since 1979. However, a repeat white blood cell scan showed an extensive collection of radiolabelled white blood cells extending from the region of the left kidney down the retroperitoneal space to the pelvis. At surgery there was a necrotic left kidney and an adjacent 15 cm abscess extending down the retroperitoneal space. Post operatively the patient's course was uneventful and he was discharged.

A: Posterior, B: Left lateral, C: Anterior

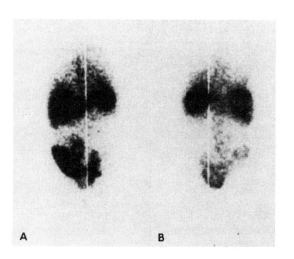

Fig. 4. This 64 year old man developed abdominal pain, fever and loose bowels 5 days post appendectomy. His temperature was 101 deg.F, his abdomen was tender with lower quadrant guarding and rebound. Abdominal films were unremarkable. The white count was 8 100. A white blood cell scan disclosed a large circumscribed collection in the right lower quadrant. At re-exploration, a large right lower quadrant abscess was drained. Post-operative healing was unremarkable and the patient was discharged the 8th post-operative day.

A: Anterior, B: Posterior

10.4 DISCUSSION

The distribution of activity seen on the 24 hour whole body white cell image reflects the distribution of the 111-In labelled leucocytes, and by virtue of the tracer principle, also the migration of all the leucocytes present in the circulation at the time of injection. Even minor increases in activity over background are important and it is necessary to obtain careful spot views of suspicious areas seen on the whole body scans as well as of areas suggested by signs and symptoms. In this way, the white cell scan provides biological information not obtainable by any other test, and this is the key to its clinical usefulness.

There is a spectrum of inflammatory diseases in which the white cell scan is clearly extremely useful and others in which it is less useful. In the first category are abdominal abscesses, either presenting initially with an acute abdominal disease such as apendicitis or pancreatitis with abscess formation, or occurring post-operatively (13,14). Incision and drainage is often lifesaving in these patients and it is crucial to know if an abscess is present and where the abscess is located. The scans are dramatic in that there is intense uptake of activity in the abscess. We have measured as much as 6% of the dose in a 5 cm diameter liver abscess within 24 hours (15). Occult abscesses outside the abdomen are often revealed by the whole body scan and discovery of these often solves a perplexing clinical problem.

Another area in which we have found the white cell scan helpful is in renal inflammatory disease (16). Perinephric abscesses take up large amounts of activity and are very easily identified in the scan. On the other hand, pyelonephritis usually shows only a faint outline of activity in the kidney parenchyma. However, we have found that even low uptake in the kidney areas is highly significant as normally no activity is seen here.

In patients with acute colitis from either Crohn's disease or ulcerative colitis, there is intense uptake in the gut and the test is very useful in acutely ill patients in whom invasive diagnostic procedures may be dangerous (17). The test cannot distinguish Crohn's disease from ulcerative colitis.

The most commonly used nuclear medical procedure for abscess detection is currently 67-Ga citrate imaging. Its major drawback is the lack of specificity, although it can be valuable in the diagnosis of chronic osteomyelitis where the white cell scan is negative. Used in conjunction with white cell imaging, the 67-Ga study remains positive, whilst the white cell scan becomes negative with adequate treatment of the acute osteomyelitis. The white cell scan becomes positive again when there is another acute flare-up of the disease.

We have found the use of sonography complementary to the white cell scan (18) in abdominal inflammatory disease, especially in patients with focal symptoms. When focal symptoms were absent, we frequently identified extra abdominal sources of sepsis using the white cell scan. Combining the two imaging modalities provided a highly accurate and sensitive means of intra-abdominal abscess detection. Computer-tomography, which shows fluid collections with exquisite resolution as well as gas within fluid collections, varies considerably in its diagnostic accuracy in abdominal inflammatory disease.

False negative 111-In-WBC studies occurred with an incidence of 8% in our series. Spleen and liver activity which is normally seen may obscure an inflammatory focus within or near either of these organs. For this reason, we advise the performance of a technetium colloid scan immediately following the white cell study should there be any question of an abscess in these areas (19). We have seen several instances of abscesses that would have been missed had not a cold defect in the technetium colloid study been visualized. We now perform the colloid scan routinely in addition to the white cell study if we are looking for a liver or spleen abscess.

In our experience, subacute bacterial endocarditis and myocardial infarction are negative in the 111-In-white cell study. Fungal or parasitic abscesses that may have a very low concentration of neutrophils may also be negative. Amoebic abscesses of the liver may appear with a "doughnut sign"; a ring of low grade uptake of cells around a cold centre (20). A well walled off abscess with a compromised blood supply may be another cause of a false negative scan.

Since a large proportion of our patients are on antibiotics at the time the scan is performed, we find it difficult to attribute false negative scans to antibiotic therapy. Similarly, patients undergoing dialysis and patients on steroids have had positive white cell scans, although these may rarely be a potential cause of false negatives.

An important cause of false positive 111-In-white cell studies is gut activity which has been spread from upper respiratory tract infections (21). This can produce quite an intense intestinal 111-In-WBC-activity, and in such cases, one should investigate the head, neck and chest for uptake of leucocytes. Frequently, the source is maxillary sinusitis. If one is still in doubt, it is important to repeat the scan 24 hours later to determine if the activity in the bowel has moved.

Clumping of the leucocytes during the labelling procedure may introduce serious artefacts of focal 111-In-WBC-activity within the lung. Normally, there is a small amount of diffuse lung activity more marked with donor cells immediately following injection, but this usually washes out by the 24 hour image. If the main area of interest is the thorax, it is useful to make a single posterior lung view shortly after the injection of the cells to check for artificial hot spots.

Ischaemia of the intestinal tract can produce an intense uptake in the small and large bowel. We have seen two patients who have gone to surgery and in both the gut activity had returned to normal by the time of the operation. We consider this as a transient phenomenon which should not be used to diagnose irreversible bowel ischaemia. Abnormal 111-In-WBC-uptake in the descending colon has been attributed to the inflammatory response from enemas (22).

Accessory spleens are another source of false positive uptake that can mimic exactly a left upper quadrant abscess. In this situation, a technetium colloid scan provides the answer. Brain infarction has been observed to accumulate leucocytes producing a positive uptake (22), which is "false positive" within the context of abscess diagnosis.

Disadvantages of the indium white cell imaging technique include the relatively large radiation dose to the liver, spleen and bone marrow: 1.3 rads, 8.5 rads and 22 rads per 500 uCi respectively (15). The 111-In-oxinate is a non-specific label for all cells, necessitating separation of the desired cell type prior to labelling. This required approximately two hours of cell preparation and labelling prior to reinjection.

SUMMARY

We studied 542 patients in detail who were referred over the past five years to the Nuclear Medicine Departments of either Stanford University or the VA Medical Center, Palo Alto, CA, for investigation of acute inflammatory disease. The results of the radionuclide imaging procedure (using 111-In-oxinate labelled granulocytes) were correlated to the clinical findings, X-ray studies, surgical procedures or other relevant evidence.

The sensitivity of 111-In-granulocyte imaging was 92%, the specificity 91%, the positive predictive value 91%, and the negative predictive value 93%. The overall accuracy was 92%. The number of technically inadequate studies was approximately 1-2%. The procedure was extremely valuable in assessing abdominal abscesses, either primary or secondary post surgical. These are usually intensely positive containing as much as 6% of the injected dose at 24 hours. Normally, there was no excretion of radioactivity in the gut or in the kidneys making interpretation much easier than with the 67-Ga-citrate scan. The application of the 111-In-oxinate white cell scan in Nuclear Medicine has proved to be highly sensitive, specific and accurate.

REFERENCES

1. McAfee J.G., M.L. Thakur: Survey of radioactive agents for in vitro labeling of phagocytic leukocytes. I. Soluble agents. J. Nucl. Med. 17:480, 1976.
2. Thakur M.L., R.E. Coleman, C.G. Mayhall, et al: Preparation and evaluation of 111-In-labeled leukocytes as an abscess imaging agent in dogs. Radiology 119:731, 1976.
3. Coleman R.E., R.E. Black, D.M. Welch, et al: Indium-111 labeled leukocytes in the evaluation of suspected abdominal abscess. Am. J. Surg. 139:99, 1980.
4. McDougall I.R., J.E. Baumert and R.L. Lantieri: Evaluation of 111-In leukocyte whole body scanning. Amer. J. Radiology 133:849, 1979.
5. Forstrom L., B. Weiblen, L. Gomez et al: Indium-111 oxine labeled leukocytes in the diagnosis of occult inflammatory disease. In: Indium-111 Labeled Neutrophils, Platelets, and Lymphocytes, Proceedings of the Yale Symposium: Radiolabeled Cellular Blood Elements, edited by M.L. Thakur and A. Gottschalk. Trivirum Publishing Company, New York, NY, Chapter 13, 123, 1981.
6. Goodwin D.A., P.W. Doherty and I.R. McDougall: Clinical use of indium-111 labeled white cells - an analysis of 312 cases. In: Indium-111 Labeled Neutrophils, Platelets, and Lymphocytes, Proceedings of the Yale Symposium: Radiolabeled Cellular Blood Elements, edited by M.L. Thakur and A. Gottschalk. Trivirum Publishing Company, New York, NY, Chapter 14, 131, 1981.
7. Zakhireh B., M.L. Thakur, H.L. Malech, et al: Indium-111 labeled human polymorphonuclear leukocytes: viability, random migration, chemotaxis, bactericidal capacity, and ultrastructure. J. Nucl. Med. 20: 741, 1979.
8. Weiblen B., L. Forstrom and J. McCullough: Studies of the kinetics of indium-111 labeled granulocytes. J. Lab. Clin. Med. 94: 246, 1978.
9. Anstall H.B. and R.E. Coleman: Donor-leukocyte imaging in granulocytopenic patients with suspected abscesses: concise communication. J. Nucl. Med. 23:319, 1982.
10. Thakur M.L., R.E. Coleman and M.J. Welch: Indium-111-labeled leukocytes for the localization of abscesses: preparation, analysis, tissue distribution, and comparison with gallium-67 citrate in dogs. J. Lab. Clin. Med. 89:217, 1977.
11. Teates C.D., S.T. Bray and B.R.J. Williamson: Tumor detection with 67-Ga-citrate: a literature survey (1970-1978). Clin. Nucl. Med. 3:456, 1978.
12. Loken M.K., L.A. Forstrom, A. Cook, et al: 111-Indium labeled leukocytes for diagnosing inflammatory diseases of the abdomen retroperitoneum. In: Proceedings of Symposium on 111-Indium Labeled Blood Elements. Mayo Clinic, 1981.
13. Fawcett H.D., M.S. Lin and D.A. Goodwin: Indium-111-labeled leukocyte imaging in acute pancreatitis with suspected complicating abscess. Dig. Dis. Sci. 24: 872, 1979.

198

14. Bicknell T.A., S. Kohatsu and D.A. Goodwin: Use of indium-111 labeled autologous leukocytes in differentiating pancreatic abscess from pseudocyst. Amer. J. Surg. 142: 312, 1981.
15. Goodwin D.A., R. Finston and S. Smith: The distribution and dosimetry of 111-In labeled leukocytes and platelets in humans. Third International Radiopharmaceutical Dosimetry Symposium, Oak Ridge, Tennessee, FDA 81-8166, 88, 1980.
16. Fawcett H.D., D.A. Goodwin, and R.L. Lantieri: 111-In leukocyte scanning in inflammatory renal disease. Clin. Nucl. Med. 6:237, 1981.
17. Stein D.T., G.M. Gray, M. Anderson, et al: Location and activity of ulcerative and Crohn's colitis by 111-indium leukocyte scan: A prospective comparison study. Submitted to Gastroenterology.
18. Carroll B., P.M. Silverman, D.A. Goodwin, et al: Ultrasonography and indium-111 white blood cell scanning for the detection of intraabdominal abscesses. Radiology 140:155, 1981.
19. Fawcett H.D., R.L. Lantieri, A. Frankel, et al: Differentiating hepatic abscess from tumor: combined 111-In white blood cell and 99m-Tc liver scans. Amer. J. Radiology 135:53, 1980.
20. McDougall I.R.: The appearance of amebic abscess of liver on 111-In-leukocyte scan. Clin. Nucl. Med. 6:67, 1981.
21. Crass J.R., P. L'Heureux and M.K. Loken: False-positive 111-In-labeled leukocyte scan in cystic fibrosis. Clin. Nucl. Med. 4:291, 1979.
22. Coleman R.E. and D. Welch: Possible pitfals with clinical imaging of indium-111 leukocytes: concise communication. J. Nucl. Med. 21:122, 1980.

11 PHAGOCYTOTIC LABELLING OF MIGRATORY BLOOD CELLS AND ITS CLINICAL APPLICATIONS

E. OBERHAUSEN AND H.J. SCHROTH

11.1 INTRODUCTION

Radioactively labelled monocytes and granulocytes may be looked upon as specific radiodiagnostic agents for the evaluation of foci of inflammation (1,2,3,4). The aim of this study was to develop and evaluate a method of white blood cell labelling which was as simple as possible and which required no sophisticated equipment.

There are at least two general ways to achieve cell labelling. The first is to separate the desired fraction of cells and subsequently label them, for instance with 111-In-oxinate. An alternative way is to use a labelling method which is selective for specific cells mixed among all the other blood cells. This is possible for granulocytes and monocytes by using colloidal substances which will be phagocytosed by these cells. The separation of the labelled cells from any unbound tracer activity can be achieved by simple centrifugation provided soluble substances are used for the labelling procedures. If colloidal or particulate substances are used as tracers, the separation is done conventionally by differential centrifugation, making use of the different densities of the cells and the colloid or particles; alternatively, as was done here, solubilizing the colloid into a soluble non-centrifugable form achieves the same purpose in an easier and more elegant way.

11.2 METHODOLOGY OF CELL LABELLING WITH 99m-Tc-Sn-COLLOID

11.2.1 Principle

Tin-II-chloride reduces 99m-Tc-pertechnetate. Reduced 99m-Tc combines with unbound tin-II-chloride to form a colloid which, on intravenous injection, will be phagocytosed by reticulo-endothelial cells, and thus may be used for the scintigraphy of the liver and spleen. This colloid will be similarly phagocytosed by monocytes and granulocytes if it is added to whole blood.

The blood cells (labelled and unlabelled) can be separated effectively and easily from the non-phagocytosed colloid, i.e. the extra-cellular unbound tracer activity by centrifugation if sodium citrate is added to the whole blood. Citrate changes the unbound colloid into a state in which it cannot be precipitated by centrifugation at 3000 g.

The relative amounts of activity taken up by monocytes or granulocytes, respectively, differ considerably depending on the experimental conditions, particularly the amount of agitation, the time and temperature of the incubation of the mixture of tin-II-chloride and 99m-Tc-pertechnetate.

11.2.2 Preparation of 99m-Tc-Sn-colloid for phagocytosis

The starting material was a lyophilized labelling kit manu-factured by RCC Amersham for the preparation of 99m-Tc-Sn-colloid for the scintigraphy of the liver and spleen. To it, a volume of 3-5 ml 99m-Tc-eluate containing about 100 mCi of pertechnetate was added. The development of the "right" colloid was facilitated by mechanical treatment, i.e. gentle shaking of the solution within the original vial on an agitating device (e.g. rotation) for 30-60 minutes. The precise period of time for agitation needed to be determined individually for each batch of tin-chloride and the device used for agitation (see below). Criterion for this optimization was a labelling efficiency in excess of 85%.

11.2.3 Labelling of white blood cells by phagocytosis

Since it was to be expected that overloading of the cells by offering too much colloid could alter their biological function, only 1/10 to 1/5 of the chemical amount of the commercial labelling kit was used for the labelling of the phagocytic cells of 10 ml whole blood.

Accordingly 1/5 to 1/10 of the volume containing the agitated 99m-Tc-Sn-colloid was removed and added to 10 ml heparinized whole blood into a vacutainer. The labelling of the phagocytic cells, i.e. the engulfment of the colloid into the cells was facilitated by gentle agitation of the mixture of heparinized blood and 99m-Tc-Sn-colloid for 30-60 minutes. The precise period of time was determined experimentally as described below. Thereafter there were two options: one was the injection of the entire mixture containing labelled cells and unbound 99m-Tc-Sn-colloid (which should not exceed 15% of the total tracer activity), the other was the separation of the labelled cells from the unbound colloid.

11.2.4 Separation of labelled cells from unbound colloid

The separation of the labelled cells from the non-phagocytosed colloid was desirable in order to avoid injection of non-cell-bound tracer activity and in order to quantify the efficiency of the cell labelling. Using 99m-Tc-Sn-colloid this was possible by simply adding 3.1% sodium citrate to the blood sample after its incubation period with the tracer colloid. So after rotation of the mixture of heparinized whole blood and 99m-Tc-Sn-colloid for 30 to 60 minutes a quantity of 1 ml 3.1%

sodium citrate was added to the vacutainer and the rotation was
continued for one more hour. Thereafter cell separation was
accomplished by centrifugation for 10 minutes at 3000 g. The
supernatant was separated from the precipitated cells, and the
cells were resuspended in 0.9% sodium chloride. The activities of
the plasma and the cells were measured in an ionisation chamber.
The resuspended cells were now ready for intravenous injection.

Table 1. Routine Procedure of Phagocytotic Labelling

The following procedure evolved after experimental evaluation:

1. Add approximately 100 mCi 99m-Tc-pertechnetate in 3-5 ml
   eluate to one vial of tin-II-chloride (RCC Amersham).

2. Rotate gently at room temperature for 30 to 60 minutes
   (see text for determination of precise time).

3. Draw 10 ml heparinized whole blood into a 20 ml
   disposable syringe, transfer into a sterile, pyrogenfree
   vacutainer.

4. Remove a volume containing 10 mCi from the pre-rotated
   99m-Tc-Sn-colloid solution and add this volume to the
   heparinized blood.

5. Rotate gently for another 30-60 minutes (see text for
   determination of precise time).

Option A: Inject whole blood (without removing unbound colloid).
Option B: Check efficiency of labelling prior to injection:
    B1: Add 1 ml sterile, pyrogenfree sodium citrate 3.1%.
    B2: Continue rotation for one more hour.
    B3: Centrifuge (3000 g, 10 minutes), remove supernatant
    B4: Assay activity in cells and supernatant.
    B5: Resuspend cells with normal saline and reinject.
    B6: Calculate efficiency of labelling.

11.3 EVALUATION OF THE 99m-Tc-Sn-COLLOID-LABELLING METHOD

11.3.1 Mechanical treatment of the 99m-Tc-Sn-colloid

The uptake of the colloid by the white blood cells greatly depended on the conditions under which the colloid was formed, and particularly the mechanical treatment of the solution during the formation of the colloid (5).

The uptake by the cells of the colloid increased with agitation and incubation time. A comparison was made between the extremes of no treatment and agitation of the vial for 0.5 hrs, and the results are shown in Table 2.

Table 2. Dependence of Labelling Efficiency on Agitation and Incubation Time of the Colloidal Solution

No treatment	6%
2 min shaking	33%
0.5 hrs standing (within vial)	78%
0.5 hrs rotation (within vial)	87%

The values indicated were measured for one specific batch of the Amersham colloid kit. There were, however, considerable differences in phagocytosis between the colloids from different batches of kits even from the same manufacturer, and the ratio of uptake between monocytes and granulocytes was very different, too. We think that the mechanical treatment of the colloidal solution influences the size of the particles, and that size is an important parameter in phagocytosis. In addition, there have been indications that, besides colloidal size, phagocytosis is also influenced by the structure of the surface of the particles.

11.3.2 Citrate effect on 99m-Tc-Sn-colloid

Citrate changed the 99m-Tc-Sn-colloid in such a way that centrifugation for 10 minutes at 3000 g did not spin it down. It evidently remained a colloid, since it accumulated in the liver and spleen like a normal colloid when it was injected into an animal, but it was probably one of much smaller size. The modification of the 99m-Tc-Sn-colloid by citrate was a time dependent process: at 20 deg.C it took from 30 to 60 minutes until all of the activity was in a non-centrifugable form. The required time depended on how long the colloid was agitated during its formation. Both times were about proportional. Before using a new batch for labelling purposes, the time was determined which was required to render 99m-Tc-colloid non-centrifugable by adding citrate to the colloid in cell free plasma. This time was determined by finding the point at which activity was no longer precipitated by centrifugation. For the evaluation of the total labelling efficiency the labelled blood sample was centrifuged at 3000 g for 10 minutes, and the activity of an aliquot of the supernatant fluid was related to the activity of a comparable volume of the cell suspension. Labelling efficiency was expressed as the percentage of the total activity bound by the cells.

11.3.3 Extent of phagocytosis

The time required for the phagocytosis during incubation of the colloid with whole blood differed individually. In extreme cases the maximum labelling efficiency was reached within 15 minutes. On average it took about 45 minutes to reach a global labelling efficiency of better than 85% for monocytes and granulocytes together. The speed and the amount of phagocytosis could be changed by adding different substances to the blood. Adding coryne bacterium parvi or PHA enhanced the phagocytosis, depending on their concentrations. The same effect was obtained with prostaglandin. The addition of bilirubine diminished phagocytosis.

11.3.4 Temperature dependence

The labelling efficiency at three different temperatures is shown in Table 3:

Table 3.   Temperature Dependence of Labelling Efficiency

Temperatures	8 deg.C	20 deg.C	37 deg.C
Labelling efficiency	41.0	87.6	58.7

The results given in Table 3 are the mean results of 10 determinations. At present we have no explanation as to why the labelling efficiency at 20 deg.C was higher than that at 37 deg.C.

11.3.5 Relative uptake by monocytes and granulocytes

To differentiate between the activities in granulocytes, monocytes and in the supernatant fluid, a separation by means of a density gradient was necessary. A discontinous Percoll gradient was used with densities of 1.06, 1.08 and 1.12 g/cu.cm. After centrifugation with 3000 g for 30 minutes, the activity profile was measured along the test tube. Figure 1 shows such an activity profile together with the separation of the different cellular fractions according to their density. With this procedure the efficiency of labelling with 99m-Tc-Sn-colloid by phagocytosis could be evaluated totally and separately for monocytes and granulocytes. As can be seen from the activity profile, there was much more activity in the monocytes than in the granulocytes. Therefore, with the colloid that was used, an almost specific labelling of the monocytes was obtained.

206

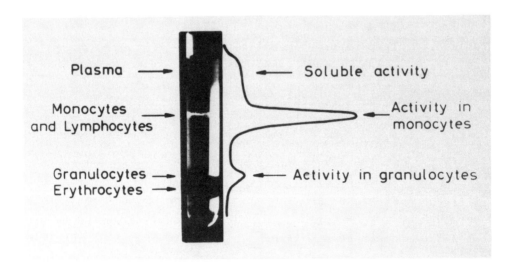

Fig. 1. Separation of different cell fractions and their activity
       profile.

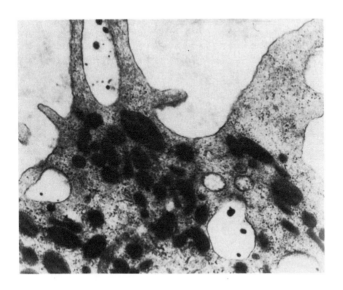

Fig. 2. Electron microscopic picture of a monocyte with phago-
       cytosed colloid.

11.3.6 Cell labelling by phagocytosis - discussion

The results of the labelling procedure showed that the labelling of monocytes and granulocytes with 99m-Tc-Sn-colloid by phagocytosis was principally possible, although considerable differences in the overall labelling efficiency occurred.

Since phagocytosis is a vital function of the cells, individual differences were to be expected. Secondly, the labelling efficiency depended very much on the treatment of the colloid solution. With a normal kit, manufactured for liver and spleen scintigraphy, some effort was necessary to obtain a standardization of the labelling procedure. It was the aim of the experiments to obtain labelled monocytes and granulocytes with as nearly normal behaviour in-vivo as possible.

Since it was to be expected that too much colloid in the cells would change their function, only 1/10 or 1/5 of a commercial kit was used for labelling 10 ml of blood. Figure 2 shows the electronmicroscopic picture of a monocyte with colloidal particles in a vacuole.

11.4 VIABILITY TESTING OF THE 99m-Tc-Sn-COLLOID-LABELLED CELLS

11.4.1 Adsorption onto glass-surfaces

According to several authors (6) the viability of monocytes and granulocytes can be tested by their ability to adsorb onto glass-surfaces. As a test system we used silicon tubing (60 cm length and 0.3 cm diameter) filled with glass beads of 0.2 mm diameter. The surface of the glass beads in this system was sufficiently large to absorb all the monocytes and granulocytes from the 10 ml samples of whole blood, with which these tubes were filled. The blood samples tested contained varying chemical amounts of tin colloid labelled with varying activities of 99m-Tc.

The amount of colloid present in 10 ml of whole blood was varied between 40 ug and 0.125 ug, and the activities of 99m-Tc ranged from 10 to 100 uCi. The incubation time of the labelled cells within the tubes was 1 hr at 37 deg.C. After the incubation period the non-adsorbed cells were eluted with 20 ml of RPMI 1640. Independent from the amount of colloid and the used activities, only about 25% of the labelled cells could be eluted. About 75% of the cells were fixed onto the glass-surface.

11.4.2 Repeat of the phagocytotic cell labelling after 24 hours

As a second criterion of the viability of the cells, we tested their ability for phagocytosis by repeating the cell labelling after 24 hrs. Ten ml of whole blood were labelled in the usual way with 12.5 ug 99m-Tc-Sn-colloid. The labelling efficiency was 84%. Then the blood sample was kept under slight rotation for 24 hrs at 37 deg.C. After this time a second labelling procedure was performed which again yielded an efficiency of 86%. This showed that even 24 hrs after the first labelling the cells with 99m-Tc-Sn-colloid were in a condition which allowed a second labelling with an almost identical efficiency. This appeared to be only possible if the cells were in a viable state and capable of phagocytosis. If it was assumed that a 10 ml sample of whole blood contained a total of 5.0 x 10E07 leucocytes and 1.0 x 10E06 monocytes, then the monocytes with their diameter of about 10 um had a mass of about 500 ug. This had to be related to 25 ug 99m-Tc-Sn-colloid which was added to the 10 ml sample of whole blood for phagocytosis. Since the mass of the monocytes was 20 times larger than that of the colloid, it appeared reasonable that the second labelling of the cells should have had the same efficiency as the first; particularly if it was considered that one monocyte was able to phagocytose several erythrocytes.

11.4.3 Discussion of the viability testing

The two in-vitro tests described above show that there is a high probability that after labelling with 99m-Tc-Sn-colloid the cells remained in a viable state with a normal function. The ultimate assessment of their function was only assessable from their in-vivo behaviour.

11.5 STUDIES OF 99m-Tc-Sn-COLLOID-LABELLED CELLS IN RATS

11.5.1 Activity distribution in the liver and spleen of the rat

For this investigation Sprague-Dawley rats were used. From one animal 6 ml of blood were taken and divided into 6 samples of 1 ml each. To three of the samples equal chemical amounts of colloid were added, but the activity was changed by a factor of ten from sample to sample. In the other three samples the activity was kept constant, but the chemical amount of colloid was changed by a factor of ten from sample to sample. After cell-labelling, rats were injected, each one with 0.5 ml of labelled blood from one sample. The injection was performed into a tail-vein. Thirty minutes after the injection the animals were sacrificed and the activities of tissue specimens of the liver and spleen, and of 1 ml of whole blood were measured. The measurements showed that the activity accumulation in the liver and spleen was independent of the amount of colloid and the activity used for the cell labelling.

Table 4.   Accumulated Activities in Different Organs

Organ	Activity-accumulation (%)	Standard deviation
Liver	51.2	2.5
Spleen	8.0	0.4
Blood (%-dose/ml)	0.88	0.08

This experiment was in good agreement with our findings in patients, but gave no solution to the phenomenon of the accumulation of cell bound ativity in the liver and spleen.

11.5.2 Biological filtration of 99m-Tc-Sn-colloid-labelled cells

Removal of labelled cells from one animal and reinjection into another animal can be considered as biological filtration. Accordingly, labelled cells were injected via a tail-vein into one rat. Blood was then drawn from this animal after 30 minutes and injected into a second rat. In the first rat the activity concentration in the blood was 0.9% of the injected activity and it was 4.4% in the second. If a total blood volume of 10 ml was assumed, then about 9% of the total activity was in the blood of the first rat, and about 44% of the transferred activity in that of the second. Since it is known that more than half of the blood monocytes are confined to the vessels (10), then one may conclude that almost all the labelled cells were within the circulating system of the second rat. The scintigram of the first rat showed the maximum activity in the liver and spleen, but in the second rat the activity distribution was intravascular, similar to that observable after the injection of 99m-Tc-labelled albumin.

11.5.3 Discussion of the animal studies

The two animal experiments described yielded no definitive result with respect to questions as to the nature of the uptake of cellbound activity in liver and spleen. There still remained two possibilities:
1) In contradiction to the in-vitro tests described a large proportion of the cells might have been damaged by the labelling procedure, and the damaged cells might be sequestered in the reticulo-endothelial system.
2) The functional state of the cells might have changed by the labelling procedure, and a large fraction of them might have left the circulating system. The biological filtration, as applied in our second experiment, could have separated the two fractions of cells. At any rate the findings in rats again confirm the old finding of a recovery of about 50% in the circulating blood of the activity of the reinjected labelled white blood cells.

11.6 BIODISTRIBUTION OF 99m-Tc-COLLOID-LABELLED CELLS IN HUMANS

After reinjection of the labelled autologous monocytes and granulocytes, accumulation of the activity in the liver and spleen was observed in all cases, yet the extent was variable.

Figure 3 shows the time activity curve for the activity in both organs. The curve gives the mean values from measurements in 14 patients. For these measurements the labelled cells were not separated from the activity in the supernatant fluid. Since there was a labelling efficiency of about 85%, there was also non-phagocytosed colloid present for accumulation in the liver and spleen. Therefore, the percentage of activity attributable to labelled cells needed reduction by a factor of 0.85, as indicated in Figure 3.

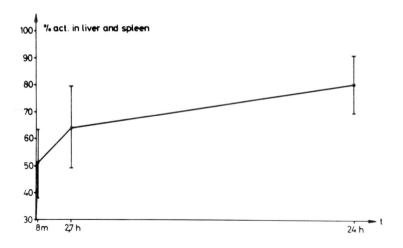

Fig. 3. Time activity curve of liver and spleen.

Accumulation in the liver and spleen has also been reported for cells which were labelled with 111-In-oxinate (7,9). The following probable reasons for the activity accumulation in liver and spleen after 111-In-oxinate-labelling have been discussed: chemical damage by the oxinate, or damage by the radiation of the 111-In-oxinate. For lymphocytes labelled with 111-In-oxinate a change in their in-vivo behaviour has been shown (9): With increasing activities in the lymphocytes, the accumulation of activity rose in the spleen and fell in the lymphocytes.

In our own experiments it was found that the in-vitro transformation of lymphocytes to lymphoblasts under stimulation with PHA did not appear to be associated with an increasing concentration in the activity of 111-In-oxinate.

Knowing these results from the labelling with 111-In-oxinate, it was obvious that the accumulation of the activity in the liver and spleen with colloid labelled cells could have also been caused by cell damage. If this were so, it would have to be some kind of cell damage which was not detectable in our in-vitro tests. If we assumed that cell damage occurred from cell labelling with 99m-Tc, two parameters had to be taken into consideration: the amount of colloid and its activity. The cells were therefore labelled with amounts of colloid and Tc-99m, which were shown to be innocuous by the studies of the activity distribution in rats (section 11.5.1).

11.7   CLINICAL STUDIES - PROCEDURE AND RESULTS

Independent of the more theoretical considerations concerning the general distribution of the labelled cells in the body, a labelling procedure is only of value provided it is clinically relevant.   In this part of our study the labelled cells were used in the scintigraphic evaluation of abdominal abscesses and inflammations of the skeleton.

11.7.1   Patient procedure

The method of 99m-Tc-Sn-colloid-labelling of white blood cells (monocytes and granulocytes) was used as described above (section 11.2.5):   10 ml whole blood, 1/5 to 1/10 of the Amersham Sn-colloid kit, 99m-Tc-activity between 10 and 15 mCi.   The first scintigraphies were made 15 minutes after the reinjection of the labelled cells.   In acute inflammations with a high blood flow accumulation of activity could be seen even after that short period of time.   The final scintigraphic pictures were taken 3-4 hrs after the reinjection of the cells.

11.7.2   Abdominal abscesses

For the past three years we have used 99m-Tc-colloid-labelled leucocytes for the scintigraphic evaluation of abdominal abscesses and inflammations in over 250 cases.

214

11.7.2.1 Illustrative cases - abdominal suppuration -

Our clinical results are illustrated by the following cases:

Case I: This 20 year old patient was appendectomized for a purulent appendicitis. Five days after operation she developed fever again and leucocytosis. The scintigraphy with labelled cells demonstrated a perityphlitic abscess (Figure 4 shows the ventral scintigraphy).

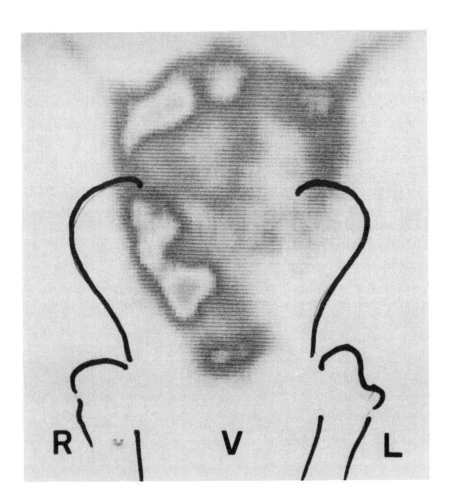

Fig. 4. Ventral scintigraphy of a perityphlitic abscess

Case II: Figure 5 shows the ventral scintigraphy of the abdomen of a 53 year old patient. Because of an endocarditis she had been under antibiotic therapy for 3 months. Under this therapy she had had diffuse pain in the total abdomen with a varying amount of diarrhoea for 4 weeks. In the scintigraphy we found an activity accumulation in the colon ascendens and transversum. The diagnosis of a colitis was confirmed by the further diagnostic procedures.

Fig. 5

Ventral
scintigraphy
of a colitis.

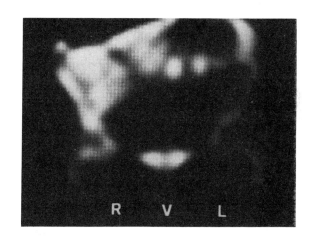

Case III: In a 64 year old patient with a history of a previous hemicolectomy the clinical signs suggested the possibility of a subphrenic abscess (Figure 6).

216

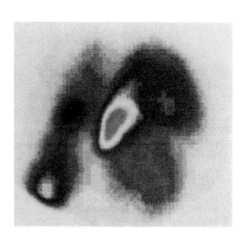

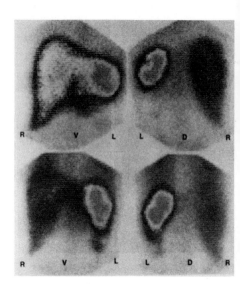

Fig. 6. Right lateral scintigraphy of a subphrenic abscess

Fig. 7. Liver-spleen-scintigraphy
(upper part) and scintigraphy with
labelled cells of a septic infarct
of the spleen

The scintigraphy in the right lateral view, obtained
32 minutes after the injection of the labelled cells showed
accumulation of activity on both sides subphrenically.

Case IV: A 42 year old patient was nephrectomized on both
sides because of a malignant hypertension. After a prolonged
convalescent period she developed septic temperatures. The liver
and spleen scintigraphy with 99m-Tc-Sn-colloid showed a high
activity accumulation in the spleen and, in the dorsal view, some
irregularity of the uptake in the middle of the organ (Figure 7).
With the labelled cells the uptake in the spleen was much more
accentuated and the organ was larger. On the same day the
cardiologists diagnosed an endocarditis. Therefore a septic
infarct in the spleen was probable. This diagnosis was confirmed
at autopsy.

11.7.2.2 Clinical results of WBC imaging in abdominal abscesses –

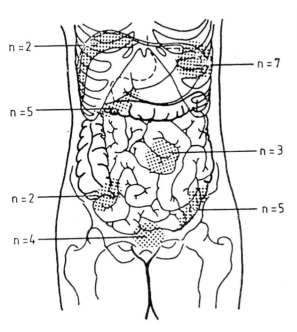

n = 2
n = 7
n = 5
n = 3
n = 2
n = 5
n = 4

Fig. 8. Distribution of diagnosed inflammations in the abdomen

Together with our Department of General Surgery we have evaluated our results in 57 cases (11). In 23 cases no pathological activity accumulation was found, which was in complete agreement with the results of other diagnostic methods or the course of the disease. In 5 cases an extra-abdominal activity accumulation was found which could be confirmed with other diagnostic means or by surgery. In 28 patients activity accumulation was found in the abdomen. The distribution of the various accumulations is shown in Figure 8.

All the above positive findings were confirmed by surgery or at autopsy. Only in one case there was one focus of questionable accumulation which could not be confirmed.

11.7.3 Inflammation of the skeleton

In a cooperative study with the Departments of Orthopedics and Traumatological Surgery over 300 patients with the tentative diagnosis of osseous suppuration were examined.

11.7.3.1 Illustrative cases - osseous suppuration -

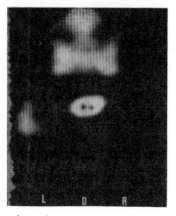

Fig. 9. Dorsal scintigraphy of a septic loosening of an endo-prothesis

Case V: Figure 9 shows the dorsal view of the pelvis of a 65 year old patient. The endoprothesis of the hip joint had been implanted 3 years ago; the patient has had increasing complaints in the left hip for 6 months prior to our investigation. The scintigram (2 hrs after reinjection) showed a clearly increased activity accumulation in the lateral part of the left hip.

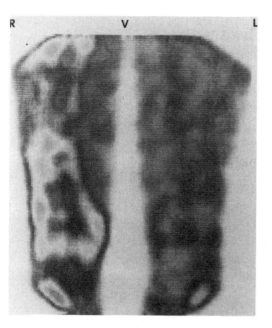

Case VI: Figure 10 shows the ventral view of the femur of a 42 year old patient who had had an open fracture of the right femur two years ago, and in the last 3 months he had had increasing complaints. The scintigraphy with the labelled cells showed a large area of pathological uptake in the right femur representing osteomyelitis. In several cases it is helpful to take not only static scintigrams but to also take sequential scintigrams immediately after the injection of the labelled cells.

Fig. 10. Ventral scintigraphy of the femurs with an osteomyelitis of the right one

Case VII: A 10 year old girl had pain in the right thigh. The sequential scintigrams (Figure 11) showed a higher blood flow in the right thigh. In the static scintigram (3 hrs after reinjection) one could see (Figure 12) a high accumulation of activity in the middle of the femur. Surgery revealed a phlegmon of the bone marrow.

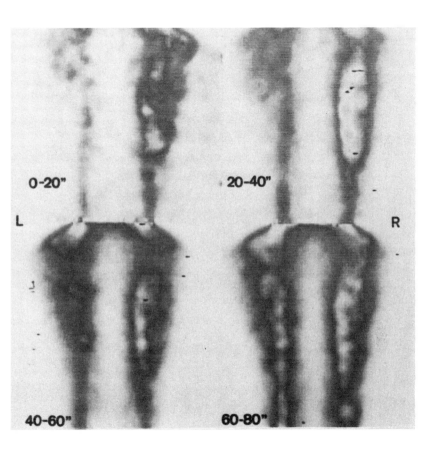

Fig. 11.
Sequential scintigraphy with higher blood flow in the right thigh

220

Fig. 12.

Scintigraphy
of the bone
marrow

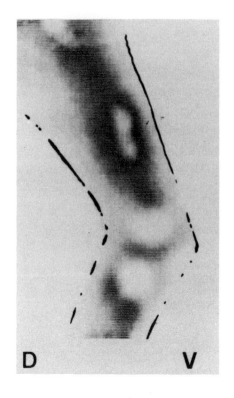

11.7.3.2 Clinical results of WBC imaging in skeletal pathology –
    The main question in the orthopedic patients was how to
distinguish between septic and aseptic loosening of an
endoprothesis. Of the patients we have examined, more than a
hundred have been reoperated in order to renew the prothesis.
Bacteriological and histological specimens had been taken in
83 patients during the operation, so that the results of the
scintigraphy could be compared with the bacteriological and
histological findings. In 36 patients (43%) an accumulation of
the labelled cells was found and there were also other positive
findings. In 28 (34%) patients there was no activity accumulation
and no positive finding. That means the correct diagnosis was
established in at least 77%. Two scintigraphies (2.5%) were false
positives and 12 (14%) were false negatives. In 5 cases (5%) the
scintigraphy and the bacteriological findings were negative, but
the histological finding was questionably positive. These results
do not look as promising as those from abscesses in the abdomen,

but it has to be taken into account that the differentiation between septic and aseptic loosening is much more difficult, and that the bacteriological and histological findings are also questionable in many cases. Some of the difficulties in scintigraphy with labelled cells in orthopedic cases are that many of the inflammations are chronic, that one has to distinguish between bone marrow and inflammation, and that infiltrations of macrophages may exist around an endoprothesis without bacteriological inflammation.

11.8 CONCLUSIONS

The method presented for labelling monocytes and granulocytes has to be compared with the 111-In-oxinate method. With 111-In-oxinate all the blood cells are labelled, therefore a separation of the leucocytes before labelling is necessary. In the method described here, only the phagocytosing cells are labelled, therefore the labelling procedure can be done in samples of whole blood, and a separation is not necessary if the labelling efficiency is greater than 80%. Another advantage of the method is the use of 99m-Tc-Sn-colloid which is always available, and activities in the range of 10-15 mCi can easily be used. The energy of the 99m-Tc together with activities used allow a successful scintigraphy to detect the accumulation of monocytes and granulocytes. Compared with 111-In-oxinate, labelling with 99m-Tc-Sn-colloid is much cheaper, especially if one takes into account the radioactive decay of 111-In. Both methods have the disadvantage that a large part of the activity is accumulated in the liver and spleen. Therefore further work has to be done to find the real reason for this accumulation, and, if possible, to avoid it. This disadvantage, however, should not hinder the use of the method successfully in the diagnosis of foci of septic inflammation.

SUMMARY

A method for the labelling of monocytes and granulocytes with 99m-Tc-Sn-colloid in whole blood is described. The basis of the method is the phagocytosis of the Sn-colloid by the monocytes and granulocytes. After an incubation period of 30-40 minutes the fraction of the colloid (10-20%) which is not phagocytosed can be transformed into a non-centrifugable form by adding sodium citrate. After this the separation of the labelled cells from the non-phagocytosed activity is possible by simple centrifugation. The main advantage of the method is that labelling can be done in whole blood. Like the other methods so far described for white blood cell labelling, there is the disadvantage that more than half of the activity is accumulated in the liver and spleen after the reinjection of labelled cells. Experiments in rats have revealed that about 90% of the administered cell bound activity were removed from the circulation and were taken up in the liver and spleen. By venipuncture of such a rat it was possible to remove circulating labelled cells of which, on reinjection into a second rat, about one half remained in the circulation. This evidence indicated that phagocytotic tagging of white blood cells with 99m-Tc-Sn-colloid yielded viable, labelled cells.

The main evidence regarding the viability of a sufficient fraction of the labelled cells were the results of the clinical studies in over 250 patients in whom the labelled cells were localized in foci of suppurative inflammation.

REFERENCES

1. Segal A.W., R.N. Arnot, M.L. Thakur, and J.P. Lavender: Indium-111 labelled leucocytes for localization of abscesses. Lancet 13:1056, 1976.
2. Schroth H.-J., R. Berberich, and E. Oberhausen: Der Nachweis entzuendlicher Veraenderungen mit Tc-99m-markierten Leukozyten. Der Nuklearmediziner 4,2:209, 1981.
3. Thakur M.L., R.E. Colunan, and M.J. Welch: Indium-111 labelled leucocytes for the localization of abscesses: preparation, analysis, tissue distribution, and comparison with gallium-67 citrate in dogs. J. Lab. Clin. Med. 89:217, 1977.
4. Schroth H.-J., K.P. Mueller, E. Oberhausen, and R. Berberich: Cell labelling with colloidal substances in whole blood. Eur. J. Nucl. Med. 6:469, 1981.
5. Schroth H.J., E. Oberhausen, R. Berberich: Cell labelling with colloidal substances in whole blood. Eur. J. Nucl. Med. 6:469, 1981.
6. Van Furth R.: Mononuclear phagocytes in immunity, infection and pathology. Blackwell Scientific Publications, England, 1975.
7. Lavender J.P., and A.M. Peters: Indium-111 labelled leucocytes for localization of abscesses. Proc. Brit. Inst. Radiol. 53:926, 1980.
8. Ducassou D., J.P. Nouel, and A. Brendel: Le marquage des elements figures du sang pur l'indium radioactif - Methodologie - Resultats - Indications. In: Radioaktive Isotope in Klinik und Forschung, Vol. 13, part 1, p. 91, 1978.
9. Chisholm P.M.: Recirculation of Indium-111 labelled lymphocytes in the rat and man. Proc. Brit. Inst. Radiol. 53:929, 1980.
10. Meuret G., and G. Hoffmann: Monocyte kinetic studies in normal and disease states. Br. J. Haematology 24:275, 1973.
11. Koch B., N. Wolf, Ch. Schwaiger, E.H. Farthmann, H.-J. Schroth, R. Berberich, H. Wilhelm, and E. Oberhausen: Lokalisationsdiagnostik und Differentialdiagnose postoperativer intraperitonealer Abscesse mit 99m-Technetium-Zinn-Kolloid-markierten Granulocyten. Chirurg 53:149, 1982.

12 MICRODOSIMETRY OF LABELLED CELLS

K.G. HOFER

12.1 INTRODUCTION

The diagnostic use of radipharmaceuticals is based on the principle of maximizing medical benefits while minimizing patient risk from radiation exposure. To establish a rational basis for designing nuclear medical procedures, modern dosimetric models take into consideration not only obvious factors such as the type and amount of radionuclide administered, the decay characteristic and radiation spectrum of the nuclide, the physical and biological halflives, etc., but also more subtle factors such as the biokinetics of the radiopharmaceutical, the residence time of the radionuclide in various body compartments, and variations in the intrinsic radiosensitivity of different tissues (1).

However, most of the dosimetric models developed so far are based on the assumption that the biological hazards of internal radiation emitters can be predicted on the basis of the random distribution of radiation energy around the site of radionuclide decay. This assumption may be justified for high energy beta or gamma emitters, but can lead to grossly misleading results when applied to low energy beta emitters or nuclides which decay by electron capture and/or internal conversion, followed by emission of a burst of low energy electrons (Auger electrons, Coster-Kronig electrons). Examples of this type of radioactive decay include the low energy beta emitter 3-H and numerous Auger emitters such as 51-Cr, 55-Fe, 57-Co, 64-Cu, 67-Ga, 75-Se, 77-Br, 99m-Tc, 111-In, 113m-In, 123-I, 125-I, 201-Tl, and many other radionuclides currently employed in Nuclear Medicine.

A common feature of these radionuclides is the fact that they emit extreme low energy radiations with ranges less than or comparable to cellular dimensions. Therefore, the damage produced by these radionuclides depends to a large extent on the geometrical relationship between the pattern of radiation energy deposition and the radiosensitive cellular structures. In other words, the cytotoxicity of the low energy emitters depends on whether the radionuclide decay occurs within the cell nucleus, in the cytoplasm, or outside the cells. Due to the strong dependence of the damage on the microscopic distribution of the energy, an accurate determination of the inhomogeneity in intracellular dose distribution is required to assess the biological hazards of such low energy emitting radionuclides.

Moreover, radioactive decay within cells may cause additional damage due to atomic transmutation and associated effects such as recoil of the daughter nuclide, chemical consequences of isotope change, excitation and ionizations of the daughter species, or molecular disruption caused by charge imbalances associated with atomic transmutation. Damage from such transmutation events is related not only to the absorbed radiation dose, but to the number of disintegrations per unit mass, that is, to the specific activity of the radionuclide within the biological system. Although atomic transmutation effects are highly localized perturbations which most likely are not important for decay events occurring outside cells, these effects can become significant if the decay takes place in direct association with important biological molecules such as the DNA (2-4). Thus, both radiation and non-radiation effects need to be considered in evaluating the potential risks resulting from the diagnostic or therapeutic administration of unsealed radionuclides.

This article will examine the biological effects of low energy electron emitters, in particular Auger emitters in relation to the microdistribution of the radiation dose within different subcellular compartments. In addition, an attempt will be made to assess the significance of basic microdosimetry and cytotoxicity concepts to Nuclear Medicine.

226

12.2   RADIOACTIVE DECAY WITHIN THE CELL NUCLEUS

Previous studies have indicated that a given number of radioactive decays within the cell nucleus usually produces significantly greater cytotoxic effects than the same number of decays occurring at extranuclear sites. This is true both for low energy beta emitters such as 3-H (5-7) and for Auger emitters (8-11).

Figure 1 demonstrates the extreme radiotoxicity of the Auger emitter 125-I when incorporated as 125-I-iododeoxyuridine (125-IUdR) into the DNA of L1210 lymphoid leukemia cells (12). For comparison, Figure 1 also shows the dose survival curve for I-131 (administered as 131-IUdR) and 3-H (administered as 3-H-TdR).

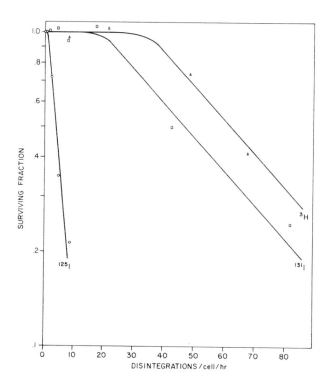

Fig. 1.   Fractional survival of murine L1210 lymphoid leukemia cells labelled in-vivo with various doses of 125-IUdR, 131-IUdR, or 3-H-TdR. The surviving fraction is plotted as a function of disintegrations/cell/hr at the time of labelling (12).

From the data it is apparent that the toxic effects obtained with DNA associated 125-I greatly exceed those observed in cells whose DNA was labelled with either 3-H or 131-I. Expressed in terms of disintegrations per cell, the D(o) (that is the dose required to reduce cell survival along the exponential portion of the curve to 37%) was 4 disintegrations/cell x hr for 125-I, 43 for 131-I, and 43 for 3-H.

In the experiments shown in Figure 1 the radionuclide was administered to exponentially proliferating cells growing in-vivo in the peritoneal cavity of mice. As a result, it was not possible to accurately calculate the cumulative number of decays/cell or the cumulative dose/cell. Subsequent in-vitro studies on several different mammalian cell lines indicated that, even when expressed in terms of cumulative decay and dose values per cell, DNA associated 125-I remained extremely cytotoxic (8,9,12-19).

Figure 2 shows the 125-I survival data for 3 different cell lines, Chinese hamster ovary cells [D(o): 100 decays/cell; 74 rad], Chinese hamster V79 cells [D(o): 39 decays/cell; 50 rad], and mouse L5178Y leukemia cells [D(o): 46 decays/cell; 78 rad]. By comparison, the D(o) values for 3-H and external X-rays in the same experiments ranged from 230-250 rad (data not shown).

More recent studies have shown that other Auger emitters, such as 77-Br administered as 77-BrUdR, are also highly toxic to mammalian cells (20). Moreover, the decay of Auger emitters within cell nuclei remains highly cytotoxic even if the radionuclides are not covalently bound to DNA. For example, 125-I introduced into bone marrow cells in the form of 125-I labelled iodoantipyrine yields a D(o) value of 64 rad (10), which is virtually identical to the 46-74 rad values shown in Figure 2 for 125-IUdR. It should be stressed that iodoantipyrine is a molecule which diffuses freely through cells and does not become directly linked to DNA. It appears, therefore, that the decay of intranuclear Auger emitters is extremely cytotoxic whether or not these radionuclides are covalently attached to DNA.

228

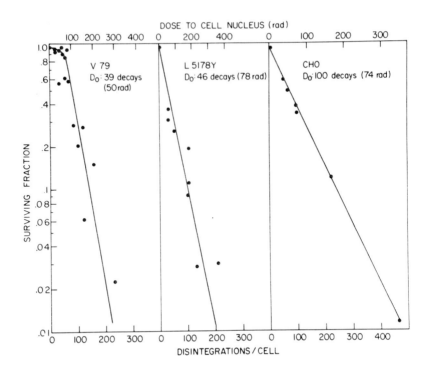

Fig. 2. Fractional survival of Chinese hamster V79 cells, murine L5178 leukemia cells, and Chinese hamster ovary cells, plotted as a function of the cumulative 125-I disintegrations/cell and cumulative rad doses to the cell nucleus (9,15).

Expressed differently, the toxic effects of intranuclear Auger emitters resemble those observed with high linear energy transfer (LET) radiations such as alpha particles, even though Auger emitters do not actually produce any high LET radiations. The resemblance is expressed not only in the shape of the dose survival curve [narrow shoulder or no shoulder, small D(o)], but also in the fact that the oxygen enhancement ratio for intranuclear Auger emitters is very small (21). It is now generally accepted that biological systems irradiated in the presence of molecular oxygen are much more sensitive to ionizing radiations than systems irradiated at low levels of oxygen

229

(hypoxia or anoxia). This effect is known as the oxygen effect, and it is particularly pronounced with low LET radiations such as X-rays, gamma-rays, electrons, and beta particles. With high LET radiations such as neutrons, protons, and alpha particles the oxygen effect gradually diminishes and finally disappears (22,23). It is of considerable interest, therefore, that the oxygen enhancement ratio (OER) for 125-IUdR is only 1.4, whereas the OER for intranuclear 3-H is about 2.8-3.0 (Figure 3). This confirms the notion that although 125-I emits only low LET electrons, the intranuclear decay of this radionuclide induces effects which are comparable to those achieved with high LET radiations.

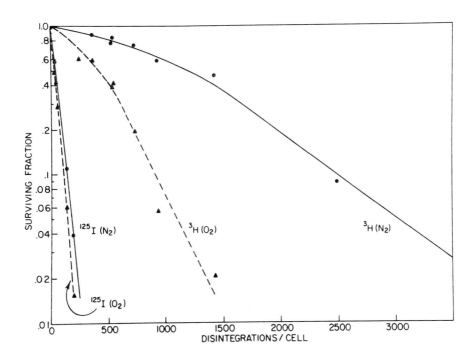

Fig. 3. Fractional survival of Chinese hamster V79 cells subjected to 125-I or 3-H decays either under oxygenated (dashed lines) or hypoxic (solid lines) conditions (21).

The actual mechanisms responsible for the unusual radiotoxicity of intranuclear 125-I remain unclear. It appears likely that the excessive cytotoxicity results from the fact that decay by electron capture and/or internal conversion is usually accompanied by emission of a burst of low energy electrons (Auger electrons, sometimes also Coster-Kronig electrons) due to the vacancy cascade occurring in the perturbed parent atom. In the case of 125-I the initial electron capture process results in a 125-tellurium nucleus and 35.5 keV excess energy. In 7% of the disintegrations, a 35.5 keV photon is emitted. In the remaining 93% of disintegrations, this energy ejects another electron from the inner shell by internal conversion. The electron vacancies created by the initial electron capture event and by the internal conversion event lead to the emission of two showers of Auger electrons. The number of electrons emitted during 125-I decay in the condensed phase ranges from 1-56 with a mean of 21.2 (24). The great majority of these electrons have energies of less than 1 keV, i.e. their range in unit density material is only about 25 nm. Emission of such dense showers of low energy electrons results in a highly charged daughter atom and in a high density of electron irradiation in the immediate vicinity of the disintegrating radionuclide (8,11,18,24).

Based on these decay features two different hypotheses have been advanced to explain the extreme radiotoxic consequences of intranuclear Auger emitters: (1) high local concentrations of radiation energy at the DNA from low energy Auger electrons; (2) charge induced molecular fragmentation at the site of decay in the DNA. Microdosimetry calculations (8,11,18,24) show that at least in small target regions (diameter 50 nm or less) more radiation energy is deposited on average by the electron shower from decaying 125-I than by the passage of a high LET alpha particle traversing an identical target sphere (Figure 4). In other words, the radiation energy deposited in the immediate vicinity of the decaying 125-I atoms appears sufficient to produce high LET-like biological damage.

Although microdosimetric calculations alone cannot fully prove the electron irradiation hypothesis, experiments with 125-I administered to cells in the form of radioactive iodoantipyrine tend to support this hypothesis (10). As discussed above, these experiments involved the introduction of 125-I into bone marrow cells via a method which does not lead to covalent attachment of the radionuclide to DNA. Yet, 125-I administered in this fashion remained as cytotoxic as in its DNA associated form.

Equally high cytotoxicity was observed in experiments when 125-I was administered to mammalian cells in the form of iodinated Synkavit. Again, although Synkavit is not incorporated into the DNA, 125-I administered in this form induces the typical high LET-like pattern of cell mortality characteristic for intranuclear 125-I (25). Moreover, the results of a limited number of experiments involving the administration of iodinated Synkavit to hypoxic cells suggest a low OER of about 1.4, identical to the OER observed with 125-IUdR.

Fig. 4.

Average radiation energy deposited in spheres of various diameters by decaying 125-I and 3-H (solid lines), or by a 5 MeV alpha-particle traversing the sphere (dashed line).

For mathematical details on these calculations as well as other types of microdosimetry calculations see references 8,11,18, 20,24.

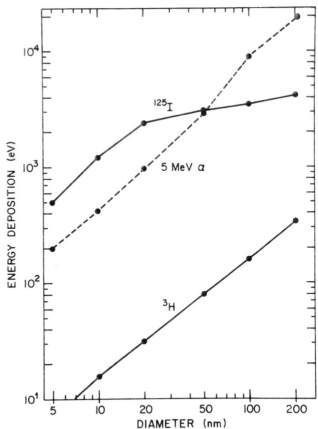

These results have important implications concerning the mechanism of cell damage by Auger emitters. As pointed out above, transmutation effects have a very short range and are effective only in the immediate vicinity of the decay event. Since 125-I administered via iodoantipyrine or Synkavit is not attached to the DNA, the high cytotoxocity observed in cells subjected to these agents supports the notion that the highly localized deposition of radiation energy from Auger electrons is responsible for the toxic manifestations of intranuclear 125-I decay (8,10,18).

Nevertheless, discussion on possible alternate mechanisms for 125-I toxicity continues. Several studies have conclusively shown that the charge instabilities associated with electron capture decay can result in the molecular disruption of organic molecules (26,27), so the possibility cannot be excluded that both charge effects and radiation effects contribute to the cytotoxic consequences of intranuclear electron capture decay (24).

12.3 RADIOACTIVE DECAY IN THE CYTOPLASM

Although the extreme cytotoxicity of intranuclear radioactive decay has attracted considerable interest, so far only two studies have been undertaken to evaluate the radiotoxocity of Auger emitters located in the cytoplasm of the cells (8,11). Figure 5 presents the result of these studies, one involving 67-Ga, the other 75-Se.

The nuclide 67-Ga is now widely used clinically for the detection of malignancies (28,29) and to an even greater extent for the confirmation of suspected inflammatory processes (30). When administered in the form of 67-Ga-citrate, most of the intracellular 67-Ga appears to be located in the cellular cytoplasm, particularly in lysosomes (8,29,31). As a result, the intracellular decay of 67-Ga primarily irradiates the cytoplasm (8).

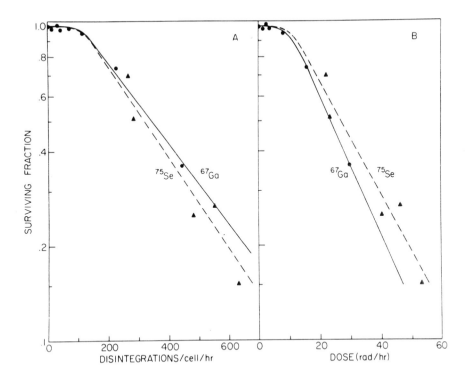

Fig. 5. Fractional survival of murine L1210 lymphoid leukemia
cells labelled in-vivo with 67-Ga-citrate (solid lines) and
Chinese hamster V79 cells labelled in-vitro with 75-Se-seleno-
methionine (dashed lines). The surviving fraction is plotted as a
function of disintegrations/cell/hr (Panel A) or rad dose to the
cell nucleus (Panel B) at the time of labelling (8,11).

The solid lines in Figure 5 show the results of an experiment
on L1210 lymphoid leukemia cells labelled with various doses of
67-Ga-citrate. The data are presented as surviving fraction
plotted against disintegrations/cell x hr at the time of labelling
(estimates on cumulative disintegrations x cells are almost
impossible to obtain for exponentially growing tumour
populations). From the data it is apparent that although 67-Ga is
an Auger emitter, the cytoplasmic decay of this radionuclide does
not produce excessive cell lethality. In fact, the D(o) (the

number of disintegrations required to reduce the surviving fraction to 37% along the exponential portion of the curve) is astonishingly high, 340 disintegrations/cell x hr. This value is 85 times higher than the D(o) value for intranuclear 125-I decays (4 disintegrations/cell x hr) obtained on the same cell line under identical treatment conditions (Figure 1).

A similar lack of radiotoxicity from cytoplasmic electron capture decays was noted with 75-Se (Figure 5, dashed lines). In these experiments Chinese hamster V79 cells were labelled with 75-Se-selenomethionine, a compound which is mainly incorporated into cytoplasmic proteins (11). Like 67-Ga, cytoplasmically located 75-Se proved surprisingly non-toxic to mammalian cells [D(o) about 270 disintegrations/cell x hr].

Microdosimetry calculations indicated that most of the radiation energy liberated from the cytoplasmic decays of 67-Ga and 75-Se was deposited in the cytoplasmic region of the cell (8,11). Only a very small fraction of the total decay energy reached the cell nucleus. To test the hypothesis that cell killing is a function of radiation dose to the cell nucleus (rather than dose to the entire cell), the dose-survival values for the two radionuclides were recalculated as a function of dose rate per nucleus. Using this procedure, the dose survival curves for 67-Ga and 75-Se became virtually superimposed (Figure 5b). In terms of dose rate to the cell nucleus, the D(o) value was 20.9 rad/hr for 67-Ga and 24 rad for 75-Se. Interestingly, this is very similar to the 21 rad/hr D(o) value observed in L1210 cells subjected to chronic irradiation from intranuclear 3-H decays (12). These results suggest that with cytoplasmically located Auger emitters the high LET-like local burst of radiation energy is "wasted" on the radio-resistant cytoplasm. However, a small component of the electrons emitted during the vacancy cascade are high energy electrons. These electrons manage to penetrate into the cell nucleus but (since such electrons have low LET radiations) they produce a typical low LET survival curve with a wide shoulder and a large D(o).

12.4 RADIOACTIVE DECAY ON THE CELL SURFACE

Some types of radiopharmaceuticals are known to become attached to the outer membrane of cells. For example, "tumour-specific" antibodies can be radioactively labelled and used either for the radioimmunodetection of cancers (32) or as "homing carriers" for radionuclide therapy (33,34). As with cytoplasmically located radionuclides, so far only sporadic attempts have been made to evaluate the microdosimetric and cytotoxic consequences of radionuclide decay at the cell surface.

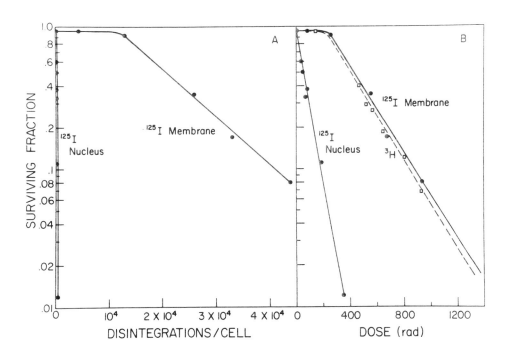

Fig. 6. Fractional survival of Chinese hamster ovary (CHO) cells subjected to various doses of 125-I either in the form of 125-IUdR (125-I Nucleus) or as 125-I labelled concanavalin A (125-I Membrane). The survival data are plotted as a function of cumulative disintegrations/cell (Panel A) or as a function of rad dose to the cell nucleus (Panel B). For comparison, Panel B also shows a radiation survival curve for CHO cells subjected to various doses of 3-H-TdR (9).

Figure 6 shows the results of one such study where 125-I was attached to the plasma membrane of CHO cells in the form of 125-I labelled concanavalin A (9).

For comparison, Figure 6 also contains the 125-IUdR data previously shown for CHO cells in Figure 2. As discussed above 125-I bound to DNA of CHO cells is extremely cytotoxic [D(o): 100 decays/cell]. In contrast, the membrane associated 125-I was very non-toxic with a D(o) of 12 500 decays/cell, or more than 120 times the D(o) value observed for intranuclear 125-I (Figure 6a). Even when expressed in terms of cumulative radiation dose to the cell nucleus (Figure 6b), intranuclear 125-I [D(o): 74 rad] was much more toxic than membrane associated 125-I [D(o): 265 rad]. However, there was a close agreement between 125-I-membrane and 3-H-DNA dose survival curves. These results confirm the conclusion that 125-I decays outside the cell nucleus exert their toxic effects via the longdistance irradiation of the cell nucleus. As pointed out above, only a small fraction of the electrons emitted are energetic enough to reach the cell nucleus, i.e., very large numbers of 125-I decays at the cell membrane are required to produce a cytotoxic radiation dose in the nucleus.

12.5 RADIOACTIVE DECAY IN THE EXTRACELLULAR SPACE

Since many of the radiopharmaceuticals used in Nuclear Medicine remain completely outside the cells, precise information on the potentially lethal effects of Auger emitters in the extracellular space would be of considerable interest. However, only a single well controlled study is available on this subject (10). This study compares the cytotoxicity of two extracellular Auger emitters (125-I administered in the form of 125-I-albumin, and 55-Fe in the form of 55-Fe-transferrin) to that of an intracellular Auger emitter (125-I administered is 125-I-iodo-antipyrine). In these experiments, suspensions of murine bone marrow cells were exposed for various times to extracellular 125-I and 55-Fe and intracellular 125-I, and the survival of the bone marrow stem cells was evaluated with the spleen colony assay.

The results shown in Figure 7 are expressed in rather unusual dose units, namely surviving fraction as a function of accumulated radioactive disintegrations per cu.um frozen cell suspension. This makes it somewhat difficult to compare the results with standard dose-survival parameters in other investigations.

Fig. 7.
Fractional survival of murine bone marrow stem cells suspended in solutions containing either 125-I-iodoanti-pyrine, 125-I-albumin, or 55-Fe-transferrin (10).

Nevertheless, from the data shown in Figure 7 it is immediately apparent that once again intranuclear 125-I is very radio-toxic, whereas extra-cellular 125-I and in particular extra-cellular 55-Fe are very non-toxic to bone marrow cells. In terms of disintegration per cu.um of cell suspen-sion, the $D(o)$ for 125-I-iodoantipyrine (intracellular) is 0.17 disintegrations per cu.um, whereas the $D(o)$ for extracellular Auger emitters is much higher, 1.74 disintegrations per cu.um for 125-I-albumin and 11.36 disintegrations per cu.um for 55-Fe-transferrin. Expressed in standard dose units (radiation to the cell nucleus), the $D(o)$ is 64 rad for 125-I-iodoantipyrine, 362 rad for 125-I-albumin, and 277 rad for 55-Fe-transferrin (10).

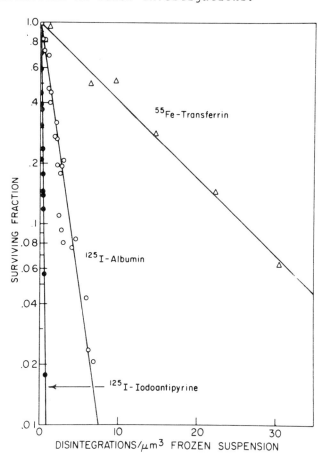

12.6   CYTOTOXICITY OF RADIONUCLIDES

The data presented in the foregoing sections of this article appear to possess serious implication for cell labelling and Nuclear Medicine. Although additional studies on the biological hazards of Auger emitters are urgently needed, the findings reviewed above appear to support the following general conclusions:

(1) Decay by electron capture within the cell nucleus is highly destructive to mammalian cells.

(2) Identical electron capture decays occurring in the cytoplasm, the outer cell membrane, or in the extracellular space appear to be relatively inefficient in killing mammalian cells.

(3) Microdosimetric analysis of the data suggests that regardless of the point of decay, the cytocidal effects of Auger emitters result exclusively from deposition of radiation energy in the cell nucleus.

(4) Absorption of radiation energy in the cytoplasm or at the plasma membrane appears to contribute little, if anything, to the cell-damaging effects of radionuclides.

It is evident that the rational use of Auger emitters in Nuclear Medicine requires detailed information on the intracellular distribution of the radionuclides. Auger emitters are very well suited for diagnostic applications in situations where the radiopharmaceutical remains outside the cell nucleus. Conversely, Auger emitters should not be used for diagnostic purposes in conjunction with radiopharmaceuticals which can penetrate into the cell nucleus, because even small numbers of Auger decays within the cell nucleus can cause devastating cytocidal effects.

Unfortunately, with few exceptions, our current knowledge on the intracellular distribution pattern of most radio-pharmaceuticals is too limited to permit a rational decision as to whether or not a particular agent is a suitable carrier for Auger emitters. Several examples where the intracellular distribution of radiopharmaceuticals has been established have been reviewed in previous papers (25,35). These examples include iododeoxyuridine (cell nucleus), iodinated Synkavit (cell nucleus), radioactive antibodies (cell membrane and/or cytoplasm), 67-Ga-citrate (cytoplasm), 111-In-oxine (cytoplasm), 111-In-bleomycin (cytoplasm), 57-Co-bleomycin (cell nucleus), and various radionuclides such as 99m-Tc, 123-I, 125-I and 131-I used for the diagnosis of thyroid disease (extracellular space and cytoplasm). For most other radiopharmaceuticals the information on their cellular uptake and intracellular radionuclide distribution is insufficient to permit a meaningful radiobiological evaluation.

In conclusion, the data reviewed here suggest that the biological toxicity of Auger emitters is largely a function of subcellular radionuclide distribution. As demonstrated most dramatically by the more than 100-fold cytotoxicity differential between DNA associated and membrane associated 125-I [D(o) of 100 vs. 12 000 decays/cell], even minor differences in intracellular radionuclide distribution can drastically alter the biological consequences of radionuclide decay. In spite of the obvious importance of these findings to Nuclear Medicine, very little attention has been devoted to this subject so far. This is surprising since many investigators have expressed concern about the adequacy of currently available dosimetric procedures which yield dose estimates that may be in error by a factor as high as 2 or 3 (1). If this margin of error is perceived to be uncomfortably high, a phenomenon which suggests error factors in excess of 100 should be seriously investigated.

SUMMARY

Many radionuclides commonly employed in Nuclear Medicine decay by electron capture and/or internal conversion. This type of decay is frequently accompanied by emission of bursts of low energy electrons (Auger electrons, Coster-Kronig electrons). Due to the short range of these electrons, most of their radiation energy is deposited in the immediate vicinity of the site of decay. As a result, the biological damage produced by Auger emitters depends largely on the intracellular location of the radionuclides at the time of decay: Auger emitters decaying within the cell nucleus are extremely radiotoxic, but the same type of decay event occurring outside the cell nucleus in the cytoplasm, at the plasma membranes, or in the extracellular space is surprisingly non-toxic. For example, if the Auger emitter 125-I is attached to different subcellular sites, the toxicity differential may be as high as 100-fold or higher, with D(o) values for cell killing ranging from less than 100 decays/cell to more than 12 000 decays/cell.

Microdosimetry calculations suggest that this phenomenal toxicity differential results from inhomogeneities in the intracellular dose distribution. Most of the radiation energy from low energy Auger electrons is deposited within 25 nm from the point of decay, resulting in extremely high concentrations of radiation energy in the immediate vicinity of the decay event, with only minor overlap irradiation of distant cell compartments. These findings suggest that conventional dosimetry calculations based on the assumption of uniform dose distribution are inadequate for estimating the radiation hazards from Auger emitters. Depending on the radiopharmaceutical used, one and the same Auger emitter may exhibit either a much higher or much lower radiotoxicity than predicted by classical radiation dosimetry. In other words, Auger emitters are exceedingly dangerous when used in conjunction with radiopharmaceuticals which accumulate within the cell nucleus, whilst only minor biological damage will result if the same Auger emitter is attached to a carrier compound which remains localized outside the cells or at least outside the cell nucleus.

REFERENCES

1. Watson E.E., A.T. Schlafke-Stelson, J.L. Coffey and R.J. Cloutier (Eds): Third International Radiopharmaceutical Dosimetry Symposium. HHS Publication (FDA) 81-8166, Oak Ridge, Tennessee, 1981.
2. Krisch R.E. and M.R. Zelle: Biological effects of radioactive decay. The role of transmutation effect. Advanc. Radiat. Biol. 3:177-213, 1969.
3. Halpern A. and G. Stoecklin: Chemical and biological consequences of beta-decay. Radiat. and Environm. Biophys. 14:167-183, 257-274, 1977.
4. Apelgot S. and J.P. Adloff: Transmutation effects of P-32 and P-33 incorporated in DNA. Curr. Top. Radiat. Res. 13:61-95, 1978.
5. Marin G. and M.A. Bender: A comparison of mammalian cell killing by incorporated 3-H-thymidine and 3-H-uridine. Int. J. Radiat. Biol. 7:235-244, 1963.
6. Burki H.J. and S. Okada: A comparison of killing of cultured mammalian cells induced by decay of incorporated tritiated molecules at -196 deg.C. Biophys. J. 8:445-456, 1968.
7. Burki H.J., S. Bunker, M. Ritter and J.E. Cleaver: DNA damage from incorporated radioisotopes: Influence of the 3-H location in the cell. Radiat. Res. 62:299-312, 1975.
8. Hofer K.G., C.R. Harris and J.M. Smith: Radiotoxicity of intracellular 67-Ga, 125-I and 3-H: Nuclear versus cytoplasmic radiation effects in murine L1210 leukemia. Int. J. Radiat. Biol. 28: 225-241, 1975.
9. Warters R.L., K.G. Hofer, C.R. Harris and J.M. Smith: Radionuclide toxicity in cultured mammalian cells: Elucidation of the primary site of radiation damage. Curr. Top. Radiat. Res. Q. 12:389-407, 1977.
10. Commerford S.L., V.P. Bond, E.P. Cronkite, and U. Reincke: Radiotoxicity of intranuclear 125-I atoms not bound to DNA. Int. J. Radiat. Biol. 37:347-554, 1980.
11. Kassis A.I. and S.J. Adelstein: Radiotoxicity of 75-Se and S-35: Theory and application to a cellular model. Radiat. Res. 84:407-425, 1980.
12. Hofer K.G. and W.L. Hughes: Radiotoxicity of intranuclear tritium, 125-iodine and 131-iodine. Radiat. Res. 47:94-109, 1971.
13. Feinendegen L.E., H.H. Ertl and V.P. Bond: Biologica toxicity associated with the Auger effect. In: Proceedings of the Symposium on Biophysical Aspects of Radiation Quality (Vienna: IAEA), p. 419, 1971.
14. Roots R., L.E. Feinendegen and V.P. Bond: Comparative radiotoxicity of 3-H-IUR and 125-IUdR after incorporation into DNA of cultured mammalian cells. In: Proceedings of the Third Symposium on Microdosimetry, edited by H.G. Ebert, p.371. Euratom, 1971.
15. Burki H.J., R. Roots, L.E. Feinendegen and V.P. Bond: Inactivation of mammalian cells after disintegration of 3-H or 125-I in cell DNA at -196 deg.C. Int. J. Radiat. Biol. 24:363-375, 1973.

16. Bradley E.W., P.C. Chan and S.J. Adelstein: The radiotoxicity of iodine-125 in mammalian cells. I. Effects on the survival curve of radioiodine incorporated into DNA. Radiat. Res. 63:555-563, 1975.
17. Chan P.C., E. Lisco, H. Lisco and S.J. Adelstein: The radiotoxicity of iodine-125 in mammalian cells. II. A comparative study on cell survival and cytogenetic responses to 125-IUdR, 131-IUdR, and 3-HTdR. Radiat. Res. 67:332-343, 1976.
18. Hofer K.G., G. Keough and J.M. Smith: Biological toxicity of Auger emitters: Molecular fragmentation versus electron irradiation. Curr. Top. Radiat. Res. Q. 12:335-354, 1977.
19. Warters R.L. and K.G. Hofer: Radionuclide toxicity in cultured mammalian cells: Elucidation of the primary site for radiation-induced division delay. Radiat. Res. 69:348-358, 1977.
20. Kassis A.I., S.J. Adelstein, C. Haydock, K.S.R. Haydock, K.D. McElvany and M.J. Welch: Lethality of Auger electrons from the decay of bromine-77 in the DNA of mammalian cells. Radiat. Res. 901:362-373, 1982.
21. Koch C.J. and H.J. Burki: The oxygen enhancement ratio for reproductive death induced by 3-H or 125-I damage in mammalian cells. Int. J. Radiat. Biol. 28:417-425, 1975.
22. Munson R.J., G.J. Neary, B.A. Bridges and R.J. Preston: The sensitivity of Escherichia coli to ionizing particles of different LETs. Int. J. Radiat. Biol. 13:205-224, 1967.
23. Berry R.J.: Growing points in mammalian radiobiology and their implications for radiotherapy. Radiol. Clinics N. Amer. 7:281-292, 1969.
24. Charlton E.E., J. Booz, J. Fidorra, Th. Smit and L.E. Feinendegen: Microdosimetry of radioactive nuclides incorporated into the DNA of mammalian cells. In: Sixth Symposium on Microdosimetry, edited by J. Booz and H.G. Ebert, p.91. London, Harwood Academic Publishers Ltd, 1978.
25. Hofer K.G.: Toxicity of radionuclides as a function of subcellular dose distribution. In: Third International Radiopharmaceutical Dosimetry Symposium, edited by E.E. Watson, A.T. Schlafke-Stelson, J.L. Coffey and R.J. Cloutier, p.371. HHS Publication (FDA) 81-8166, 1981.
26. Carlson T.R. and R.M. White: Formation of fragment ions from CH3 Te-125 and C2H2 Te-125 following nuclear decays of CH3 125-I and C2H2 125-I. J. Chem. Phys. 38:2930-2934, 1963.
27. Stoecklin G.: Chemical and biological effects of beta-decay and inner shell ionization of biomolecules: A new approach to radiation biology. In: Proceedings Sixth Int. Congress Radiat. Res., edited by S. Okada, M. Imamura, T. Terasima, and H. Yamaguchi, p.382. Toppan Printing Co., Ltd., 1979.
28. Andrews G.A. and C.L. Edwards: Tumor scanning with gallium-67. JAMA 233:1100-1103, 1975.
29. Hayes R.L.: Factors affecting uptake of radioactive agents by tumor and other tissues, In: Tumor Localization with Radioactive Agents, p.29. IAEA-MG 50/14, 1976.

30. Staab E.V.   and W.H. McCartney: Role of gallium-67   in
    inflammatory disease. Semin. Nucl. Med. 8:219-234, 1978.
31. Glickson J.D.,   R.B. Ryel,   M.M. Bordenca,   K.H. Kim   and
    R.A. Gams: In vitro binding of 67-Ga to L1210 cells. Cancer
    Res.   33:2706-2713, 1973.
32. Goldenberg D.M. (Ed.):   Radioimmunodetection   of   Cancer,
    p.2957. AUICC Workshop, In: Cancer Res. 40, 1980.
33. Smith R.T.: Tumor-specific immune mechanisms. N.E.J.   Med.
    278:1207-1214, 1268-1275, 1311-1326, 1968.
34. Ghose T.   and A. Guclu: Cure of mouse lymphoma with
    radio-iodinated antibody. Eur. J. Cancer 10:787-792, 1974.
35. Hofer K.G.:   Radiation biology and potential therapeutic
    applications of radionuclides.   Bull.   Cancer 67:343-353,
    1980.

13 CONJUGATE COUNTING APPLIED TO THE SCINTIGRAPHIC QUANTIFICATION OF RADIONUCLIDE DISTRIBUTIONS (SCINTIMETRY)

R. NICOLETTI AND G.F. FUEGER

13.1 INTRODUCTION

This paper describes the application of the technique of conjugate counting to numerical radionuclide images of emitted and transmitted activity for the quantification of radionuclide distribution in the human body. This task represented a methodological difficulty since the inception of radionuclides for diagnostic studies. It is illustrated by the great effort in the past to standardize the radio-iodine uptake test (1,2), and the similarly great effort nowadays directed at the quantitative estimation of cardiac work in ECG-gated radionuclide ventriculography (3).

Thyroid radio-iodine content has traditionally been c o u n t e d (and was estimated by comparison with a phantom yielding percentage of the administered dose). Sacral radioiron content likewise was counted and related to a comparable value of counts/min resulting in a value of relative uptake. Correlation of such values to a body region was accomplished by the correct anatomical positioning of the probe. With the arrival of imaging devices, such as scanners or scintillation cameras, the regional distribution of a tracer was recognizable as an analog image. In order to obtain digital information, the surface radiation from the radiostrontium content of the knee joints (4), for instance, was detected by rectilinear scanning with a focussed collimator and the counts per unit distance were transformed in a digital value which was printed out (5,6). The quantification of radionuclide distributions in the body by means of a scintigraphic device, e.g. scanner or scintillation camera, was termed "scintimetry". The true activity content of the body regions under study was not measureable by simple surface counting or imaging, of course. On the other hand, the measurement of

activity of the one lateral and its counterpart other lateral
(opposing) surface of the body was used a long time ago for the
estimation of the 226-Ra content (7). From such measurements an
arithmetic as well as a geometric mean could be derived, of which
the latter was shown to be more useful. To compensate for self
absorption, an additional measurement of transmitted activity was
related to the activity of the unattenuated source (all under
standardized conditions of geometry). Sorenson (8) studied
systematically this type of measurement, the conjugation of
transmission and emission measurements, and its methodological
errors, not only for point sources and uptake probes, but also for
volume sources to be detected by profile scanners and
scintillation cameras.

Quantification in Nuclear Medicine by the application of
conjugate counting as developed by Evans (7) and Sorenson (8) to
radionuclide imaging of opposing body surfaces may be termed
"conjugate scintimetry". This approach was applied by Wicks (9)
to the biodistribution of 99m-Tc-MAA in humans and by Mostbeck
(10) to the quantitative estimation of activity in lymph nodes.
In the present paper this work was extended. The main problems of
geometry and attenuation were analyzed; phantom measurements were
carried out to establish the magnitude of the error of conjugate
scintimetry and a computer program for the analysis of patient
data was developed.

13.2 BASIC CONSIDERATIONS

13.2.1 Relationship between true activity and measured counts

The object to be measured is a distribution of radioactivity
which varies in time and space. The following considerations
assume that variations with time during one measurement are neg-

ligible so that the activity varies in spatial coordinates only:

> object: activity a(x,y,z)

The recorded image consists of a two-dimensional distribution of count rates:

> result: count rate r(u,v)

As the three-dimensional activity-distribution is projected onto a two-dimensional image, the count rate in each image element is related to the activity in the field of view by the equation

$$r(u,v) = K \int_V a(x,y,z) \cdot \eta(x,y,z) \cdot s(x,y,z) \, dV \qquad \ldots [1]$$

K is an efficiency factor which contains photon efficiency of isotope, crystal-efficiency and efficiency of instrument electronics (including discriminator setting), $\eta(x,y,z)$ is the tissue attenuation factor, s(x,y,z) is the point source sensitivity of the collimator. (6,11,12,13)

13.2.2   Relative and absolute quantification

Relative quantification is the comparison between the activity content in one region of a given subject and another region of the same subject expressed as a percentage of the sum of activity in all regions under study. In many cases the knowledge of relative quantitative data is sufficient and absolute measurements are not necessary.

Absolute quantification is the measurement of true activity content in a given tissue region, expressed in Becquerel (Curie) or in percent of the administered activity in Becquerel (Curie).

In either case it is necessary that in equation 1
1) the efficiency factor K is kept constant
2) an appropriate attenuation correction is performed

3) the collimator sensitivity function is taken into account

For absolute quantification a calibration procedure has to be performed additionally, which relates the count rate (counts per minute) to activity (Becquerel, Curie).

An essential condition for all kinds of quantitative measurements is precise control of instrument performance. Linearity and stability of electronics, uniformity, spatial and temporal resolution and spatial linearity of imaging systems are the parameters which have to be controlled not only regularly, but also before and after conjugate imaging for quantification purposes to assure the proper operation of the instruments and to obtain valid data. (14,15)

13.2.3 Collimator sensitivity and spatial resolution

The point source sensitivity function s (equation 1) describes the response of the collimator to a point source. An ideal sensitivity function would be independent of z, that is the distance of the source to the collimator, whereas the dependence on x and y would look like a single impulse. That means maximum sensitivity for all sources on the collimator axis and zero sensitivity for all sources off the axis.

In practice these conditions are never satisfied. The dependence on z is very high with flat field and focussed collimators. Fortunately it can be kept reasonably small with certain dual detector arrangements and with the Anger scintillation camera (see section 13.3.2).

The dependence on x and y is a bell shaped function which is responsible for the limited spatial resolution of scintigrams. This problem is treated by the linear system theory which states that the true activity-distribution can be restored by deconvolution of the measured count rate distribution with the impulse response function of the recording instrument. Because of the distance dependence of the impulse response function this deconvolution is a very difficult task. Many attempts have been made to improve scintigrams by various kinds of filters, but no important clinical value of this type of image processing has been established until now. (16,17)

Fortunately, with conjugate scintimetry image processing is not the major problem, because in most cases the interest is not directed at small details but at the activity content of larger regions. Therefore, equation 1 can be simplified to the following equation:

$$r_{\Delta F} = K. \int_Z a_{\Delta V}(z).\eta(z).s(z)\,dz \qquad \qquad \dots[2]$$

$r_{\Delta F}$ is the count rate in a small image region ΔF. Working with a computer it is convenient to set ΔF equal to one picture element (pixel) of the image matrix, so $r_{\Delta F}$ is the count rate of one pixel. $a_{\Delta V}$ is the activity in the corresponding volume element (voxel) ΔV. As in equation 1, η and s are tissue attenuation and collimator sensitivity respectively but dependent on distance only. K is the same efficiency constant as in equation 1.

Equation 2 is much easier to handle. Errors due to count rate distributions from neighbouring voxels (so-called cross-talk) cancel within one region. Certain problems arise at the boundaries of regions. If the organ or region of interest can easily be defined and the surrounding tissue has very low activity, the error can be kept small by selecting the boundaries of the region a certain distance away from the organ edges. But near high activity differences region boundaries have to be selected with care and results judged with criticism. (6,14)

13.2.4   Sources of errors

Simplification is a necessary tool in managing such problems as to measure the activity content in an organ. But it is also necessary always to be aware of error possibilities introduced by those simplifications. Another source of errors is the not-ideal performance of measuring instrumentation.

With quantitative determination of activity by means of scintigrams possible sources of errors are (8,14):

1) Dependence of attenuation and collimator sensitivity on distance: On the one hand there has not yet been found a method to completely remove the distance dependence. On the other hand we cannot correct for distance dependence, because the distribution of the activity source is unknown. So distance dependence of attenuation and collimator sensitivity are major problems.

2) Finite spatial resolution of instrument: This problem has already been discussed above (section 13.2.3): cross-talk from surrounding tissue alters the value of measured counts. Another consequence of finite spatial resolution is the fact that organ boundaries never can be determined exactly.

3) Scattered radiation: Another kind of cross-talk from surrounding tissue is scattered radiation, which cannot be eliminated by discriminator setting. Scattered radiation also originates in the collimator and in other materials near the detector crystal.

4) Attenuation effects: For simplification a constant linear attenuation factor is assumed (see section 13.3.3). This does not hold true in practice with tissues of various densities.

5) Tissue background: Because of the projection of a three-dimensional volume onto a two-dimensional image, separation of activity in a z-direction is not possible. When the activity content of an organ is to be determined, activity of overlying and underlying tissue has to be subtracted. This is done by background subtraction whereby background activity is estimated from surrounding tissue activity. Activity contents of overlying organs cannot be separately determined. An approach to solve these problems is emission computed tomography.

250

13.3 THE METHOD OF CONJUGATE SCINTIMETRY

13.3.1 Approaches to quantification

It is clear from equation 2 that if a constant relationship is to be preserved between measured count rate and amount of activity, either of two conditions must be satisfied:
1) Of all three functions, $a(z)$, $\eta(z)$ and $s(z)$ the distribution with z has to be known.
2) If the distribution of $a(z)$ is unknown then η and s have to be constant and independent of distance.

Two approaches to quantitative measurement have been discussed:
1) Spectro-analytic techniques: From the attenuation ratio of two different gamma-ray energies the depth of activity can be determined. After this, corrections for $\eta(z)$ and $s(z)$ can be made (8,18).
2) Conjugate scintimetry which will be discussed in the following.

13.3.2 Collimator sensitivity

As stated above in cases of unknown activity distribution $a(z)$, the attenuation η and the collimator sensitivity s have to be kept constant. Let us consider collimator sensitivity first:

The distance dependence of collimator sensitivity (frequently referred to as geometry effects) can be reduced to a minimum if appropriate arrangement of detectors and appropriate collimation is used. This holds true for whole body counters, scanners and for scintillation cameras (8,16,19,20). Unfortunately there is one serious restriction. The imaged area (region of interest) has to be large in comparison to the area of activity, otherwise errors due to limited spatial resolution occur (see section 13.2.3

and 13.2.4). However, these errors are accepted in today's practice because until now no method to remove them has been developed (the same problems arise in emission tomography). As mentioned above, if one is aware of these problems, by properly judging the results valid data are available.

13.3.3 Attenuation

If one measures a source which is embedded in attenuating tissue, the value of attenuation is dependent on the depth of the source. Correction of attenuation is possible only if the source depth is known.

The concept of conjugate scintimetry replaces attenuation dependence on depth by dependence on total body thickness (8,16). This is done by simultaneously counting the activity from two opposite directions and combining the results by the geometric mean:

$$N_o = \sqrt{N_a \cdot N_p} \cdot \exp(\mu T/2) \qquad \ldots [3]$$

N_a ... anterior counts
N_p ... posterior counts
μ ... tissue attenuation coefficient
T ... total body thickness

Body thickness can be measured or determined experimentally by transmission measurement:

$$T = (1/\mu_t) \cdot \ln (I_o/I) \qquad \ldots [4]$$

μ_t ... tissue attenuation coefficient for transmission measurement
I_o ... unattenuated counts from transmission source
I ... attenuated transmission counts

If we combine equations 3 and 4 we get:

$$N_o = \sqrt{N_\alpha \cdot N_p} \; (I_o /I)^{\mu/2\mu_t} \qquad \qquad \ldots [5]$$

Because of scattering effects μ is not equal to μ_t (8). The quotient μ/μ_t has to be determined experimentally with phantom measurements.

13.3.4 Influence of source thickness and distribution

So far we have dealt with point sources only. Usually we have volume sources of variable thickness and distribution. Genna (21), Sorenson (8) and Thomas (22) analysed the influences of thickness and distribution and described methods for correction.

13.3.5 Calibration factor

To get the absolute activity from count-measurements the calibration-factor C [cpm/MBq] has to be determined. This is done by measuring a known activity, contained in a syringe or a phantom.
The complete formula is therefore:

$$A = (F/C) \cdot \sqrt{N_\alpha \cdot N_p} \cdot (I_o /I)^{\mu/2\mu_t} \qquad \qquad \ldots [6]$$

with

$$F = (f\mu T/2)/\sinh (f\mu T/2) \qquad \qquad \ldots [6a]$$

A ... activity (MBq)

C ...   calibration factor (cpm/MBq)

F ...   correction factor for source thickness as suggested
         by Sorenson (8)

f ...   fraction of total body thickness occupied by the
         source (thus fT is source thickness)

13.4   EXPERIMENTAL DATA WITH PHANTOM MEASUREMENTS

The phantom measurements described in the following were
intended as preparatory work for studies with In-111-labelled
cells. These patient studies are discussed in the following
article of this book (23).

13.4.1   Method and instrumentation

Because of lack of a whole body scanner we had to use a
single detector large field of view scintillation camera (Picker
Dynacamera 4/15/61) which is connected to a computer system
(Informatek Simis 4).

Phantoms used were a Machlett-Alderson head phantom with
skull with two tumour-phantoms inside, and Machlett-Alderson liver
and spleen-phantoms within a body-shell. For transmission
measurements a flat flood-source of 45 cm diameter and 1 cm
thickness was used.

The isotope used was Indium-111. Activity varied with the
various measurements and ranged between 170 µCi (6.3 MBq) and
1300 µCi (48 MBq). All measurements were done with discriminator
settings for both Indium-peaks (172 keV and 247 keV) as well as
for the 247 keV peak only.

Each phantom study consisted of two steps:

1) Transmission measurement: The flood source was filled
with a known amount of activity and fixed in front of the detector
parallel to the detector surface at such a distance that the

phantom could be positioned between the detector and the flood source. Two images were acquired, one of the flood source without phantom between source and detector, and one transmission image of each phantom.

2) Emission measurement: The flood source was removed, and the phantom was filled with known amounts of activity. Two images of the phantom from opposing directions were acquired.

Counts were calculated using equation 6 and setting μ_t equal to μ. For comparison we calculated all counts with and without correction by the factor F correcting for source thickness.

For determining the calibration factor C we used two methods:

1) Counts per minute per μCi were calculated from activity, total area and imaged area of the flood source which was used for the transmission measurement.

2) Counts per minute per μCi were calculated by imaging a syringe filled with known activity.

13.4.2 Results of phantom measurements

1) Correction for organ thickness: All calculations were performed with and without correction for organ thickness. Without correction all values were larger, but the maximum deviation was $< + 4\%$.

2) Discriminator setting: All calculations were performed with discriminator setting for both Indium-111 peaks (172 keV and 247 keV) as well as for the 247 keV peak only. Using both peaks scatter effects were much more evident, resulting in larger errors than using the higher peak only (see Table 1).

Table 1.   Results of Phantom Measurements
                (see text for explanations)

---

a) Influence of organ thickness correction:

   Deviation without correction: < + 4.0%

---

b) Error in relative quantification

   using 247 keV In-111 peak only
   for fractions > 15%   + 2.3 (+/- 3.2)%

   using 247 keV In-111 peak only
   including fractions < 15%   - 2.1 (+/- 14.2)%

   using both In-111 peaks   + 1.5 (+/- 14.8)%

---

c) Error in absolute quantification
   (activities used ranged between 170 and 250 μCi)

   Calibration factor calculated by
   flood source method

        using 247 keV peak only   + 34.0 (+/- 5.0)%
        using both peaks   + 37.0 (+/- 13.0)%

   Calibration factor calculated by
   syringe method

        using 247 keV peak only   + 6.0 (+/- 4.0)%
        using both peaks   + 8.0 (+/- 10.0)%

Table 2.   Computer Program for Conjugate Scintimetry
With a Single Detector Scintillation Camera.
(see text for explanations)

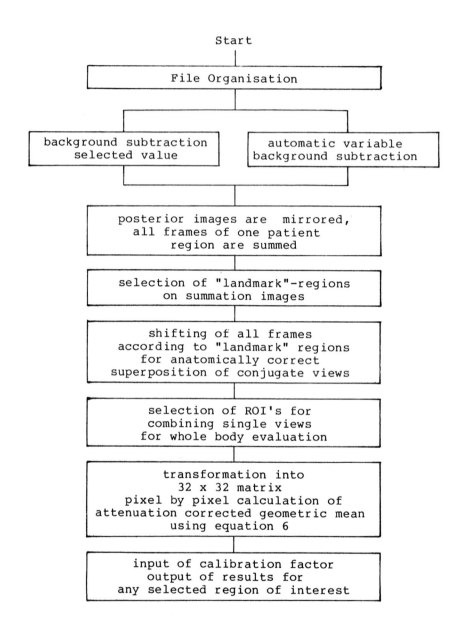

3) Error in relative quantification: Relative quantification measurements delivered the following results: The difference between calculated and true activity fractions was + 2.3 (+/- 3.2)% for fractions larger that 15%. Measurements of smaller fractions (< 15%) were associated with larger errors: - 2.1 (+/- 14.2)%.

4) Error in absolute quantification: For calculation of activity both calibration methods described above were used. With calculating the calibration factor by the flood source method, activity was overestimated by + 34 (+/- 5)%. Using the syringe method the error was + 6 (+/- 4)%.

An overview of the results is given in Table 1.

13.4.3 Discussion of the results

The results of our phantom measurements confirm that conjugate counting delivers reasonably good results in the quantification of activity contents in organs. The error proves to be smaller than +/- 10% if an appropriate calibration procedure is used.

An appropriate calibration procedure is the measurement of a syringe with known activity content. Using the transmission source for calibration procedures seems not to be reliable. The reason for this fact is to be investigated.

If isotopes with two or more peaks such as 111-Indium are used, for quantification purposes only one peak is to be used. Otherwise scatter effects increase the error in quantification. A slight but not essential decrease in the quantification error is obtained by correcting for organ thickness.

13.5 COMPUTER PROGRAM

The following section describes our computer program for conjugate scintimetry with a single detector scintillation camera. Two major problems in using a single detector scintillation camera for conjugate scintimetry proved to be

1) Anatomically correct superpositioning of separately acquired anterior and posterior views.

2) Assembling multiple single views into a whole body image if whole body data were desired.

Managing these problems was facilitated by the use of a computer macro program which was written at our Institute. A simplified flow chart of this program is shown in Table 2.

The single steps of the program are:

1) File organisation: The program is able to accept up to 21 images for one whole body study: opposing views of four regions (usually head, chest, upper abdomen and lower abdomen) at two points in time, four transmission images (one for each patient region) and one image of the unattenuated disc phantom. These images have to be presented to the program in a certain order.

2) Background subtraction: For determination of organ activity background subtraction is necessary. Two modes are available in the program: subtraction of a user selectable constant value (no background subtraction is possible by an input of zero) or an automatic background subtraction using a special program developed at our Institute. This program substracts a variable background value depending on surrounding background above and below the organ.

3) Superposition of anterior, posterior and transmission images: Anterior and posterior images of the same patient region are summed after mirroring of posterior images. On these summation images rough "landmark"-regions around anatomical structures are selected. Then these regions are superimposed on the single anterior, posterior and transmission images; the user has to shift the single images until they fit into the regions.

4) Assembling the single views to a whole body image: All views are shown simultaneously on the display. Rectangular

regions are selected which - assembled together - would provide a whole body image (neglecting the extremities).

5) Calculation of attenuation corrected geometric mean: To keep errors due to the finite spatial resolution of the system and due to poor superposition of the anterior and posterior views small, the 64x64 matrices are transferred to 32x32 matrices. After this a pixel by pixel calculation of attenuation corrected geometric mean using equation 6 is performed. Results are stored in separate frames representing images of attenuation corrected geometric mean.

6) After user input of the calibration factor the activity content in any user defined region is calculated and printed out.

This program has been used for patient studies described in the following article in this book (23).

13.6 CONJUGATE SCINTIMETRY VERSUS EMISSION TOMOGRAPHY

The main problem with conjugate scintimetry is the superposition of activity from organs which lie on top of each other, caused by the fact that a three-dimensional distribution is projected onto a two-dimensional image.

This problem is basically removed by emission computed tomography, so tomography appears to provide a new and accurate means of getting quantitative data. However there are numerous other problems which result in severe limitation of the accuracy of quantitative measurements. Not all of these problems have been solved in a satisfactory way until now. These problems are (24,25):

1) Statistical uncertainty is increased by noise propagation due to the image reconstruction process, therefore instrument sensitivity has to be further improved to satisfy statistical requirements.

2) Attenuation correction is a problem which arises particularly with single photon emission computed tomography.

3) Errors are introduced by the decrease in resolution with

distance from a parallel hole collimator as used with single photon emission computed tomography.

4) Scattered radiation and - in positron emission computed tomography - accidental coincidences are further sources of errors.

5) The partial volume error occurs if only part of the volume described by the region of interest and the transverse section thickness is occupied by the organ of interest.

From these facts must be deduced that the single photon emission tomography has a high likelihood for success in studies of the brain but not in quantification of activity distributions of the body regions (24). With positron emission computed tomography quantification problems are less severe but this technique requires a cyclotron close to the Nuclear Medicine Department which is a considerable financial restriction.

13.7 CONCLUSION

Theoretically, emission computed tomography is the method of choice for getting quantitative data. However, considering all the physical and technical problems which arise with this method, the method of conjugate scintimetry, too, is a valid technique for in-vivo-quantification of human tracer distributions and has a justified existence, since it is a technique which requires no special instrumentation, is easy to perform and provides data of reasonable accuracy as our phantom measurements have confirmed.

SUMMARY

A quantitative description of radioisotope distribution is
essential for metabolic studies and for dosimetry. One approach
to get quantitative data is conjugate counting, i.e. the counting
of opposing body surface activities in order to obtain the
activity content of the underlying body region:
Regional attenuation corrected mean counts are obtained from
the numerical radionuclide transmission and emission images of
opposing surface areas, and are related either to the administered
tracer activity or the attenuation corrected mean surface counts
of the whole body.
Two main problems of this method are geometric effects and
tissue attenuation. These problems can be overcome to a great
extent by appropriate selection of detector arrangement,
measurement technique and algorithm. We have performed conjugate
counting on phantoms with a single detector scintillation camera.
The results of these phantom studies are presented in this paper.
They show that absolute quantification is possible with an error
smaller than +/-10 %. Further on a computer program is described
which performs all the image handling and data processing. Of
course, conjugate counting is restricted to two-dimensional
imaging. True three-dimensional data can only be achieved by
emission computed tomography. But considering all physical and
technical problems arising with emission tomography, conjugate
counting remains a valuable and valid technique which requires no
special instrumentation, is easy to perform and provides data of
reasonable accuracy.

262

REFERENCES

1. Hine G.J. and J.B. Williams: Thyroid radioiodine uptake measurements. In: Instrumentation in Nuclear Medicine, Vol.1, pp.327-350. Academic Press, New York, 1967.
2. IAEA Consultants Meeting on the Calibration and Standardization of Thyroid Radioiodine Uptake Measurements. Published simultaneously in ten scientific journals, referenced in Reference No.19 of this paper.
3. Budinger T.F.: Physiology and Physics of Nuclear Cardiology. In: Nuclear Cardiology, edited by J.T. Willerson, pp.9-78. F.A. Davis Company, Philadelphia, 1980.
4. Bauer G.C.H. et al.: Sr-85 scintimetry in osteoarthritis of the knee. J. Nucl. Med. 10:109-116, 1969.
5. Kenny P.J. and E.M. Smith: Quantitative organ visualization in Nuclear Medicine. University of Miami Press, Florida, 1971.
6. Nicoletti R.: Quantitative Scintigraphie. Thesis. Technische Universitaet Graz, 1980.
7. Evans R.D.: Radium poisoning. II. The quantitative determination of the radium concent and radium elimination rate of living persons. Am. J. Roentgenol. 37:368-378, 1937.
8. Sorenson J.A.: Methods for Quantitating Radioactivity in vivo by External Counting Measurements. Thesis. University of Wisconsin, 1971.
9. Wicks R., K. Rosenspire, R. Ackerhalt, M. Langan, J.J. Steinbach and Monte Blau: Distribution of Tc-99m administered as labeled Microspheres for lung imaging. Radiopharmaceutical Dosimetry Symposium, Oak Ridge, Tenn., 1981.
10. Mostbeck : Personal communication, 1983.
11. Beck .R.N., L.T. Zimmer, D.B. Charleston, P.V. Harper and P.B. Hoffer: Advances in Fundamental Aspects of Imaging Systems and Techniques. In: Medical Radioisotope Scintigraphy 1972, Vol. I. International Atomic Energy Agency, Vienna, 1973.
12. Kenny P.J.: What is Quantitative Organ Visualization in Nuclear Medicine? In: Quantitative Organ Visualization in Nuclear Medicine. P.J. Kenny and E.M. Smith (Eds.), University of Miami Press, Coral Gables, 1971.
13. MacIntyre W.J., S.O.Fedoruk, C.C. Harris, D.E. Kuhl and J.R. Mallard: Sensitivity and Resolution in Radioisotope Scanning. A report to the International Commission on Radiation Units and Measurements. In: Medical Radioisotope Scintigraphy, Vol. I. International Atomic Energy Agency, Vienna, 1969.
14. Johnston R.E.: Objectives and Problems in Calibration Procedures for Making Quantitative Measurements. In: Quantitative Organ Visualization in Nuclear Medicine. P.J. Kenny and E.M. Smith (Eds), University of Miami Press, Coral Gables, 1971.

15. Nicoletti R.: Qualitaetskontrolle nuklearmedizinischer Untersuchungsgeraete. In: Wissenschaftliche Berichte der 6. Jahrestagung der Oesterreichischen Gesellschaft fuer Biomedizinische Technik, Graz, 1981.
16. Budinger T.F.: Quantitative Nuclear Medicine Imaging: Application of Computers to the Gamma Camera and Whole-Body-Scanner. In: Recent Advances in Nuclear Medicine. Progress in Atomic Medicine, Vol. 4. J.H. Lawrence (Ed), Grune and Stratton, New York-London, 1974.
17. Todd-Pokropek A.: Image Processing in Nuclear Medicine. IEEE Transactions on Nuclear Science, Vol. NS-27, No.3, June 1980.
18. Johnston R.E. and A.B. Brill: Inherent Problems in the Quantitation of Isotope Scan Data. In: Medical Radioisotope Scintigraphy, Vol. I. International Atomic Energy Agency, Vienna, 1969.
19. Williams E.D., H.I. Glass, R.N. Arnot and A.C. de Garreta: A Dual Detector Scanner for Quantitative Uptake and Organ Volume Studies. In: Medical Radioisotope Scintigraphy. Vol. I. International Atomic Energy Agency, Vienna, 1969.
20. Arimizu N. and H. Kakehi: Area Scanning for Quantitative Measurement of Radioactivity in Internal Organs. In: Medical Radioisotope Scintigraphy, Vol. I, International Atomic Energy Agency, Vienna, 1969.
21. Genna S.: Analytical methods in whole-body counting. In: Clinical Uses of Whole-Body Counting. International Atomic Energy Agency, Vienna, 1966.
22. Thomas S.R., Maxon H.R. and J.G.Kereiakes: In vivo quantitation of lesion radioactivity using external counting methods. Medical physics 3:253-255, 1976.
23. Fueger G.F. and R. Nicoletti: 111-In labelled white blood cells: biodistribution and techniques of in-vivo-quantification. In: This book.
24. Budinger T.F.: Physical Attributes of Single-Photon Tomography. J. Nucl. Med. 21:579-592, 1980.
25. Budinger T.F., S.E. Derenzo and R.H. Huesman: Role of Tomography in Providing Radionuclide Distribution and Kinetic Data. In: Third International Radiopharmaceutical Dosimetry Symposium. U.S. Department of Health and Human Services, Rockville, 1981.

14 111-In-LABELLED WHITE BLOOD CELLS:
BIODISTRIBUTION AND TECHNIQUES OF IN-VIVO QUANTIFICATION

G.F. FUEGER AND R. NICOLETTI

14.1 INTRODUCTION

The normal organ and tissue distribution of neutrophil leucocytes is still largely unknown (1). Although the organ and tissue localization of 111-In observed with a scintillation camera may be due not only to viable neutrophils, but to damaged cells, protein bound 111-In-oxinate or 111-In-transferrin, or a combination of these (1), the quantification of the biological distribution of the 111-In activity appears desirable if for no other reason but dosimetric considerations. This work analyzes the activity distribution after injection of 111-In labelled mixed white cell preparations in humans using a scintillation camera and an associated computer. Such equipment is widely available, and it appears better to obtain quantitative approximations now than to wait until equipment of theoretical superiority might become available at some later time. Conjugate scintimetry was used as the method of quantification, as described in the preceding chapter.

14.2   METHOD

Table M.1   Patients

Name   Id./Nr.   Age   Weight   Sex
Code   (y)   (kg)

                  OXIN I

JNDL   76781   16   62   m
NEUB   76848   54   75   m
ERKG   75404   22   52   f
ALTB   76423   32   82   m

                  OXIN II

TTSL   79726   45   74   m
RCHL   79048   58   70   m
WLBR   79537   29   63   f

                  TROP

MSSR   33985   54   75   m
BRGR   63165   38   95   m
BRTR   79110   65   67   m

14.2.1   Patients, studies, chelating agents

The study concerned ten patients of which two were female and eight male. The patients' ages ranged between 16 and 65. Blood concentration measurements and conjugate scintimetry were carried out in each patient. 111-In-oxinate was used in seven patients, 111-In-tropolonate in three patients. Autologous plasma was not added to the last rinse of the labelled cells with normal saline

in four of the seven patients studied with 111-In-oxinate.
Accordingly, "OXIN I" refers to the four patients whose cells were
labelled without addition of autologous platelet poor plasma (PPP)
to the last rinse; "OXIN II" refers to the three patients whose
cells were rinsed with normal saline and autologous PPP. "TROP"
refers to the three patients whose cells were labelled with
111-In-tropolonate. PPP was used for resuspension of the labelled
cells prior to injection in each case.

14.2.2   Patient procedure

Blood was drawn for cell separation and labelling, if
possible on the ward, in order to avoid having the patient wait in
the Department of Nuclear Medicine during the procedure. The
suspension of 111-In labelled cells in PPP was injected
intravenously in the Department of Nuclear Medicine. Blood
samples were drawn at 15,30,45,90 and 180 minutes, 22 and 48 hrs
following injection. The imaging procedure was carried out
nominally at 3 hrs and 22 hrs following injection with variations
depending on patient transport. The true time interval between
the starts of each imaging procedure was noted. Imaging at each
time point consisted of one set of transmission images and two
sets (3 hrs and 22 hrs) of emission images of opposing aspects of
the skull, the chest, the upper and the lower abdomen (see section
14.2.5). All images were fed into the computer. Additionally
24-hr urine collections were carried out. For the technical
details of the scintillation camera and computer used see
section 14.2.5 and the preceding chapter of this book by Nicoletti
and Fueger.

14.2.3 Cell separation

The separation of white blood cells from whole blood was carried out by the following procedure: Three 30 ml syringes were filled each with 5.0 ml Macrodex, 0.1 ml Heparin. Twenty ml blood was drawn directly into each of these syringes. Macrodex contained 6 g Dextran-60 per 100 ml of 0.9% sodium chloride. The syringes were placed with their tips upwards into beakers, and were kept standing at 37 deg.C for 45-60 minutes in order to achieve sedimentation of most of the erythrocytes and suspension in the supernatant of most of the white cells. The supernatant leucocyte and platelet rich plasma (LRPR-P) was centrifuged at 100 g and 20 deg.C for 10 minutes in order to obtain granulocytes and lymphocytes in the precipitate. This pellet was resuspended in phosphate buffered saline for labelling with one of the 111-In-chelates (see below). The supernatant platelet rich plasma (PRP) was decanted and spun a second time at 1000 g and 20 deg.C for 10 minutes to yield platelet poor plasma (PPP). The cell separation was modified in order to avoid the addition of colloidal polycarbohydrates to the whole blood for sedimentation purposes, since microscopic slides of the concentrates of the white blood cells showed the cells to have engulfed considerable quantities of colloidal Macrodex. It is hypothesized that this might impair the subsequent biological activity of the granulocytes; it has further been stated that phagocytosis "activates" the granulocytes and that this activation starts the "clock" of the granulocyte survival (Egger, Chapter 5). Therefore the following modification was adopted:

The three syringes were filled with 4.5 ml ACD instead of 5.0 ml Macrodex. Heparin (0.1 ml) was still used in order to forestall later fibrin formation by changes in the calcium ion concentration, particularly in order to enhance resuspendability of the granulocytes; 24.5 ml whole blood was drawn up with ACD instead of the 20 ml for Macrodex. This modification had in some patients the disadvantage that the sedimentation of the red and emission images of each of the regions.

14.2.4 Labelling procedure

The pellet of granulocytes and lymphocytes obtained from the centrifugation of the leucocyte and platelet rich plasma was resuspended in 2.0 ml heparinized phosphate buffered saline (PBS), pH = 7.4. To this resuspension 0.5 to 1.5 mCi 111-In-oxinate or tropolonate plus 1.0-2.0 mCi 111-In-chloride was added. 111-In-oxinate was buffered with 0.35 ml TRIS buffer per 1 ml in order to buffer the solution to pH = 7 just prior to its addition to the cell suspension in PBS for labelling. The mixture was incubated at 37 deg.C for 30 minutes and intermittantly gently agitated. At the end of the incubation time 5 ml PPP was added, (excepting four cases designated "Oxinate I"; see below). Thereafter the cell suspension was centrifuged at 100 g and 20 deg.C for 10 minutes. The supernatant was decanted and kept for activity measurement, the pellet was resuspended in 5.0 ml PPP, the activity was assayed, a drop was inspected microscopically [Boehringer Test simplets H(E)], and, if satisfactory, intravenous injection followed without any extended or intentioned waiting period. This procedure was carried out initially without reinjection of the labelled cells many times for practice purposes and is now used routinely. A labelling efficiency of better than 85% was consistantly obtained. The procedure is referred to in the text below as "Oxinate II". It was modified as follows:

Oxinate I: In four patients the addition of 5 ml PPP to the suspension of cells in PBS containing 111-In-oxinate was omitted at the end of the labelling incubation. This was described as "no addition of plasma to the last wash of the labelled cells" in the text below, and was designated "Oxinate I".

Tropolonate: In three patients 111-In-tropolonate was used for the labelling of the cells. The pellet of cells obtained from the first 100 g centrifugation was resuspended in 3.0 ml Hepes buffer rather than 2.0 ml phosphate buffered saline. To this was added 100 ul tropolonate in a concentration of 4.4 x 10E-04 and 150 ul 111-In-chloride according to the procedure elaborated by Danpure et al. (2). For the constitution of Hepes buffer stock solution and further details, see Danpure, Chapter 8.

Table M.2

WHITE CELL SEPARATION

3 SYRINGES (30 ml)

5 ml Macrodex, 0.1 ml Heparin, 20 ml blood
or alternatively
4.5 ml ACD, 0.1 ml Heparin, 24.5 ml blood

SEDIMENTATION
37 deg.C/45-60 min

CELL RICH SUPERNATANT (PRLRP)
transfer into plastic centrifuge tubes

ERYTHROCYTE SEDIMENT
may be discarded or reinjected

CENTRIFUGE CELL RICH PLASMA
100 g/10 min/20 deg.C

SUPERNATANT (PRP)   WBC PELLET

CENTRIFUGE   RESUSPEND

1400 g/10 min/20 deg.C   a) 2.0 ml PBS or
                                     b) 3.0 m Hepes buffer

PLATELET POOR PLASMA   INCUBATE WITH 111-IN

Table M.3

111-IN LABELLING OF WBC's

WBC SUSPENSION
2.0 ml PBS or 3.0 ml Hepes buffer

ADDITION OF 111-In
add 0.5-1.5 mCi 111-In-oxinate,   pH = 2.4
0.35 ml TRIS buffer per ml 111-In, pH = 7

or

add 100 ul tropolonate (4.4 x 10E-04 M)
+ 150 ul 111-In-chloride

INCUBATION WITH 111-In
Oxin: 37 deg.C/30 min
Trop: 20 deg.C/10 min

PLASMA WASH *)
add 5.0 ml platelet poor plasma

CENTRIFUGE
100 g/10 min/20 deg.C

SUPERNATANT   PELLET
assay for free 111-In   resuspend in PPP
                               assay for bound 111-In
                               inspect microscopically
                               if satisfactory, inject

*) not with OX I

14.2.5 In-vivo quantification of organ radioactivity

The method of conjugate scintimetry was applied as described in the preceding chapter. The disc phantom was made from lucite; it had a circular chamber, 45 cm in diameter and 1 cm thick. It was filled with 111-In-EDTA in order to avoid a low pH, and precipitation of hydroxides. Radioactivities of about 1-2 mCi were usually added to the chamber. The phantom was inserted underneath the top of the examining table into a custom built holder, so as to not to impair positioning of the patient, and the unattenuated disc phantom was imaged and stored. Likewise transmission images were fed into the computer for the following regions: Lateral skull, chest, upper abdomen, lower abdomen. The distance was fixed at 35 cm between collimator face and table top. This was followed by the injection of the labelled cells. Numerical emission images were acquired into the system between 2-3 and 21-22 hrs after the injection of the labelled cells, and the following views were obtained: right and left lateral views of the skull, anterior and posterior aspects of the chest, the upper and the lower abdomen. The patient was positioned supine for the anterior images, and prone for the posterior views. A total of 21 images was obtained (Table M.4):

Table M.4   Patient Procedure: Images

	- 0.5 hrs	2 - 3 hrs		22 - 23 hrs	
unatt. disc.	PHANT				
Skull	TRANS	RLAT	LLAT	RLAT	LLAT
Chest	TRANS	ANT	POST	ANT	POST
Upper abd.	TRANS	ANT	POST	ANT	POST
Lower abd.	TRANS	ANT	POST	ANT	POST

Acquisition time for each individual frame was 5 minutes.

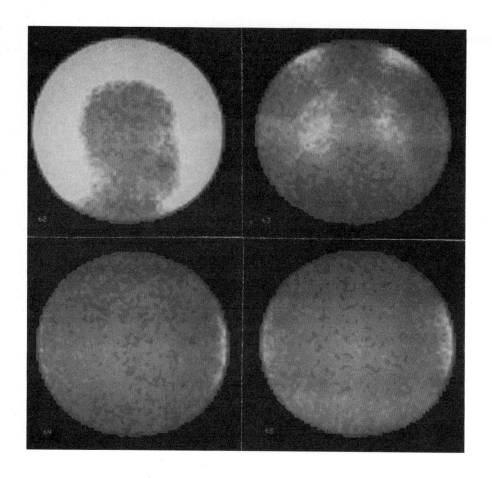

Fig. M.1. Transmission images of skull, chest, upper and lower abdomen. Unattenuated activity surrounds the imaged body structures. Variable attenuation is recognizable in the chest and the upper abdomen due to the lungs.

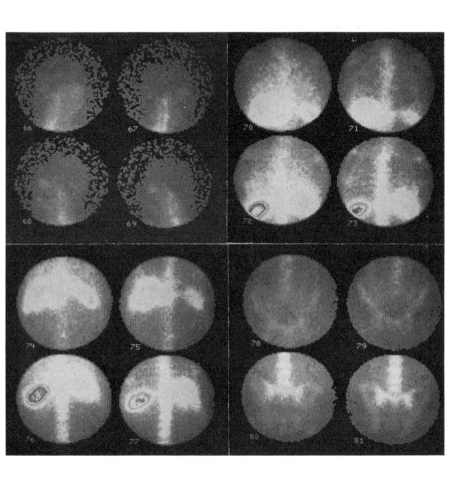

Fig. M.2. Emission images, obtained at 3 and 22 hrs following
injection: right and left lateral views of the skull, anterior
and posterior of the chest, of the upper and lower abdomen.

The frames were processed to achieve the following:

a) anatomically correct superposition of all images of each region

b) calculation of attenuation corrected geometric mean cts./t x area

c) summation of the attenuation corrected mean counts of all four imaged parts of the body to obtain a sum value of the entire imaged body at 3 and 22 hrs following injection.

d) quantification of the localized uptake of the 111-In-activity within the spleen, liver, lungs or other selected body regions (see below) at 3 and 22 hrs following injection.

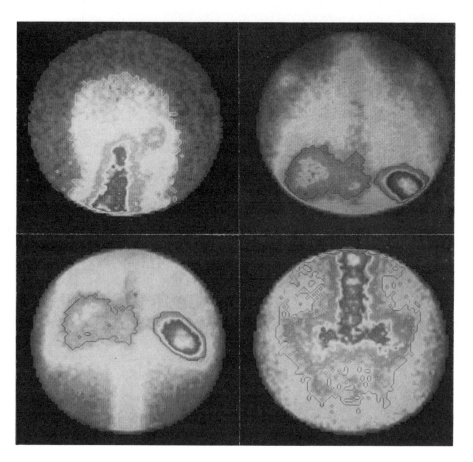

Fig. M.3. Landmark regions. Such regions were used to achieve as accurately as possible a superposition of all transmission and emission images of each of the regions.

These aims were arrived at by the following steps: Summation of all four emission frames of each region after appropriate mirroring in order to obtain a coarse summation image. (The considerable skill of the technicians allowed such a gross summation since they were able to position the patients repeatedly in a quite comparable way. This resulted in individual images of a given body region such that no exaggerated shift occurred in the body structures relative to each other within one set of four frames of each body region). Four coarse summation images were obtained: one each for the skull, the chest, the upper and lower abdomen. Using these summation images the next step was to create a "landmark" region for each of the four sets of frames. The landmark ROI's served as reference areas in order to allow anatomically accurate superposition by shifting each single image. So, as an example, the mirrored posterior 2-hr-image of the upper abdomen was superimposed on its counterpart anterior 2-hr-image and on its (precedingly likewise shifted) transmission image. Then the 64x64 matrices were transferred into 32x32 matrices to keep errors due to cross-talk and due to the inevitable small inaccuracies of superposition minimal. After this a pixel by pixel calculation of the attenuation corrected geometric mean counts/t x area was performed on the corresponding views of the skull, the chest, the upper and the lower abdomen forming a new numerical image of each imaged part of the body. The geometric mean was calculated from the opposing emission images. The attenuation correction was calculated from the corresponding transmission image in order to correct for self absorption and distance losses. This resulted in four numerical images containing the attenuation corrected geometric mean cts/t x area in 32x32 matrices, one each for the skull, the chest, the upper and the lower abdomen. Quantification of the attenuation corrected geometric mean counts was carried out with two aims to be achieved: one was to arrive at a quantification of localized accumulations of the 111-In-activity, the other was the summation of the total attenuation corrected activity included in the conjugated imaging procedure. Two further sets of regions of interest were created: One set was aimed at quantifying localized accumulations ("organ ROI's"), it consisted of the following regions: Skull and cervical spine, right lung, left lung, heart, thoracic spine, liver, spleen, lumbar spine and pelvis.

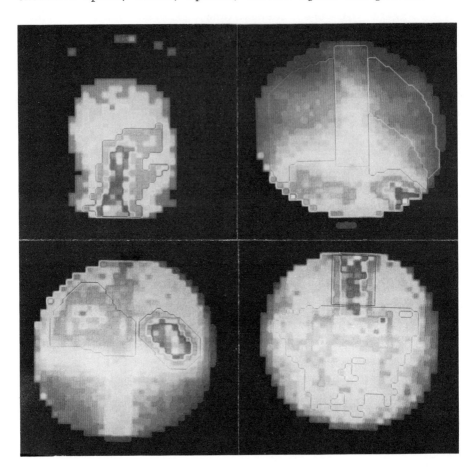

Fig. M.4. Organ regions. These regions were used to quantify the activity content of various organs respectively body regions from the numerical image representing attenuation corrected, geometric mean counts.

The other set was aimed at summation of the total attenuation corrected activity; it consisted of four all encompassing regions ("body ROI's"): one each for the skull and neck, chest, upper and lower abdomen.

Fig. M.5.

Summation regions. Such regions were used to sum the 111-In-activity content of the skull, chest and abdomen without overlap.

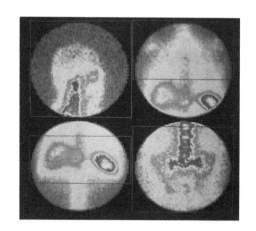

Great care was taken to avoid overlap between these regions of each part of the body.

The procedure described above was facilitated and greatly eased by a computer program described in the preceding chapter (Nicoletti and Fueger).

14.2.6 Activity in blood, blood cells, plasma and urine

The percentages of the administered activity in the blood at various times were calculated in classical fashion from the measured activity concentrations of the samples and the comparison standard. Blood volume was taken as 7.5% of body weight, haematocrit as 50%. The percentage of the administered activity in the red blood cell volume was considered to represent the intravascular cell bound activity. The amounts of tracer found in the total volumes of whole blood, blood cells and plasma are listed in Table R.2.

The percentage of the administered activity excreted in urine

was determined from 24-hr-collections of urine. The urinary
excretion was given in Table R.13.

14.2.7 Halftimes

The halftimes of 111-In in the blood were calculated between
the time points 0,3,22 and 48 hrs. The amount of tracer present
in the blood at t=0 was assumed to be 100%; the amounts present
at 3 hrs, 22 hrs and 48 hrs were determined experimentally. The
analysis of the fractions with different halftimes was done
graphically. The halftimes were listed in Table R.14.

14.2.8 Whole body activity

As described above, conjugate scintimetry yielded attenuation
corrected geometric mean counts/t x area for several organ
regions, and for the imaged total of head and trunk at two
different time points (3 hrs and 22 hrs). The whole body activity
was constituted by the tracer content of the head and trunk, which
had been measured, and that of the arms and legs, which, for
reasons of expediency had not been included in the conjugate
imaging procedure. A certain percentage of the administered dose
had been "lost" in the arms and legs (see section 14.2.11); The
tracer content of the extremities was estimated on the basis of
the 111-In-percentage in blood at 3 hrs and 22 hrs. The blood
activity, as a representative and reliable value, was allocated on
the basis of the masses to the head and trunk (65%) and to the
arms and legs (35%). Multiplication of the blood activity by
0.35 yielded the 111-In-activity of the arms and legs. The whole
body activity was summed by adding the calculated activity of arms
and legs to the measured activity of head and trunk. See also
below, section 14.2.11.

14.2.9 In-vivo distribution of 111-In

The counts/t x area of the organ regions were related to the whole body counts/t x area and expressed as percentage. The regions containing predominately skeletal structures were summed to yield a measure of bone marrow uptake. The region of the heart and left lung were added to account for the inevitable overlap. Thus the percentages of the administered activity were calculated for the liver, the spleen, the right lung, the heart and left lung, the bones and bone marrow of skull, spine and pelvis. The percentage of the administered activity within a certain body region was obtained by the following equation:

% = (organ activity) x 100/(whole body activity)

14.2.10 Balancing of the organ activities

The percentages of the administered dose in the body regions are listed in Tables R.4a,b.

In order to balance the percentages of the administered activity found by in-vivo conjugate counting in the various body regions with those found by in-vitro counting of whole blood, the blood content of the organs (contained within the organ regions of interest) needed to be estimated. Based on reference man, the anthropomorphic model (3), the blood content of the heart, the lungs, the liver, the spleen, and the bones of the torso was estimated. The estimates (as listed in Table M.5) total 1490 ml respectively 28.4%. This amount of blood was included in the organ ROI's, whereas about 72% of the tracer concentration present in whole blood at the time of conjugate counting (2-3 hrs, 21-22 hrs) was not "seen" within the organ regions of interest. For balancing the fractions, therefore, only 72% of the 111-In amount present in whole blood at 3 hrs, or 22 hrs respectively, needed to be added to the fractions found within the organ regions from conjugate counting.

| Table M.5 | | | Masses | and | Blood | Content | of | Body | Regions |

Structure	Mass (g)	Mass (%)	Blood Content (ml)	Content (%)	Reference
Total body	70000	100	5250	100	(3)

Included   in   Conjugate   Counting

Structure	Mass (g)	Mass (%)	Blood Content (ml)	Content (%)	Reference
Head	5100	7.3	-	-	Approx.by author
Torso	40100	57.3	-	-	
Subtotal HT	45200	64.6	3090	58.8	
Heart-wall	299	-	-	-	
-contents	431	-	431	-	(7)
Lungs	1000	-	525	-	10% of TBV (3)
Liver	1800	-	270	-	15% of liver (3)
Spleen	180	-	90	-	60 - 125 ml (3)
Bones	5000	-	175	-	35 ml/kg (3)
Subt. Organs	8710	12.4	1490	28.4	

Excluded from Conjugate Counting

Structure	Mass (g)	Mass (%)	Blood Content (ml)	Content (%)	Reference
Arms	6100	-	-	-	Approx.by author
Legs	18700	-	-	-	
Soft tissues	19800	-	495	9.5	25 ml/kg (3)
Bones	5000	-	175	3.3	35 ml/kg (3)
Subtotal extremities	24800	35.4	670	12.8	

14.2.11 111-In-activity in arms and legs

The extremities contained significant tracer amounts, and not negligible quantities as was thought initially. This became apparent when the measured 22-hr-activities of the head and trunk were corrected for decay so that they could be compared to the 3-hr-activities. Decay was corrected for the time interval between the two procedures of conjugate imaging of each individual patient, whose data were being analyzed. This decay correction yielded head and trunk activities at 22 hrs that were constantly greater by a few percent than the comparable values at 3 hrs. This difference was not due to different counting losses at the two time points, as was established by phantom measurements. This seeming increase was due to the exclusion of the arms and legs from the measurements. The tracer content of the arms and legs lost from the conjugate measurement was greater at 3 hrs than at 22 hrs, so that the head and trunk activities did not represent 100%, but a lesser percentage which was lower at 3 hrs than at 22 hrs.

The observation that the decay corrected values of the 22-hr-activities of the head and trunk exceeded the 3-hr-value by a few percent, was complemented by two findings: The ratio of the organ activity to the non-organ activity did not change significantly between the two measurements (3 hrs and 22 hrs). The organ activity showed no significant increase relative to the head and trunk activities between 3 and 22 hrs. The following Table M.6 lists the fractional activities of the organ and the non-organ regions. The second observation was the lack of correlation between the non-organ activity and the activity content of whole blood. It had been conceivable that high blood activities might have caused high non-organ activities, i.e. body background, but this was not the case.

Table M.6   Fractional Activities of Organ and Non-Organ Regions
(Trunk only, arms and legs excluded)

	3 hrs		22 hrs	
	Organ counts	Non-Organ counts	Organ counts	Non-Organ counts
JNDL	0.83	0.27	0.80	0.20
ERKG	0.80	0.20	0.78	0.22
ALTB	0.60	0.40	0.58	0.42
NEUB	0.80	0.20	0.79	0.21
TTSL	0.84	0.26	0.85	0.25
RCHL	0.70	0.30	0.71	0.29
WLBR	0.84	0.26	0.83	0.27
MSSR	0.66	0.34	0.67	0.33
BRTR	0.78	0.22	0.77	0.23
BRGR	0.74	0.26	0.73	0.27

The correlation coefficients between the non-organ activities and the tracer amounts in the total blood volume for the ten 111-In patients were 0.244 (3 hrs) and 0.268 (22 hrs) indicating no correlation. Extrapolation of the non-organ activity of the head and trunk to that of the arms and legs therefore appeared unreasonable and, when tried, on the basis of their relative masses (Table M.5) yielded no balance in the activity distribution, yet, consideration of the tracer contents in the arms and legs was necessary. The activity in legs and arms was in large measure due to the tracer content of the blood; perhaps also due to extravascular labelled cells which might have migrated into tissues, yet a differentiation between intravascular and extravascular labelled cells was impossible by planar conjugate counting. A certain amount of tracer activity had to be expected in the active bone marrow of the heads of humerus (and femur) and the bordering proximal parts of the bone shafts.

The percentage presumably present in arms and legs could be estimated on the basis of the blood activity. The arms and legs constituted about 35% of the body mass and contained about 12.5% of the blood volume (Table M.5).

Multiplying the 111-In content in the total blood volume at 3 and 22 hrs by the factors 0.35, 0.25 and 0.128 yielded a percentage of the administered activity which presumably could have been present in the extremities, and therefore would have escaped detection. Since the blood activity was higher at 3 hrs than at 22 hrs the "lost" percentage was greater at 3 hrs than at 22 hrs. The three sets of presumably lost percentages (blood activity times 0.35 or 0.25 or 0.128) were added to the 3-hr and 22-hr activities of the head and trunk. Only those correction factors could have been correct which in individual patients would yield identical whole body activities at 3 and 22 hrs (decay taken into consideration). This was, indeed, found when a fraction of 0.35 of the indium activity in whole blood was considered to be present in arms and legs: This correction revealed a ratio of 0.992 +/- 0.016 between the 22-hr and 3-hr values of the whole body activities. Using a fraction of 0.25 or 0.128 of the blood activity rendered too low (0.975 +/- 0.023) or too high (1.007 +/- 0.016) a ratio considering that the mean cumulated 22-hr urinary excretion was found at 0.34 +/- 0.3% of the administered activity.

This proved that the head and trunk activities did not represent the total administered activity, but a lesser amount, and that the diminuition was different at 3 and 22 hrs, and that the blood activity could be used as a correcting parameter. This was taken into account individually for each patient studied.

14.3   RESULTS

14.3.1   Cell labelling

The labelling efficiencies and the liver to spleen ratios are listed in Table R.1. Relatively increased hepatic uptake was considered a sign of hypotonic change of the labelled granulocytes (6). The efficiencies were related to essential features of the labelling technique (Table R.1.).

Table R.1   Labelling Efficiency and Uptake Ratios Liver/Spleen

Name Code	Id. Number	Labelling Eff.	Uptake Ratio Liver/Spleen	Chelating Agent
JNDL	76781	88	0.80	OX I
NEUB	76848	89	1.96	OX I
ERKG	75404	91	0.86	OX I
ALTB	76423	86	0.77	OX I
TTSL	79726	85	1.26	OX II
RCHL	79048	77	1.13	OX II
WLBR	79537	84	0.98	OX II
MSSR	33985	81	0.49	TROP
BRGR	63165	74	0.72	TROP
BRTR	79110	77	0.84	TROP

Table R.2   Mean 111-In-Activities in Whole Blood, Blood Cells
                   and Plasma Volumes   (% Administered Activity)

I   OXIN I
           Whole Blood   Blood Cells   Plasma

	Whole Blood	Blood Cells	Plasma
15 min	48.6 +/- 3.7	39.1 +/- 7.9	9.7 +/- 6.6
45 min	39.4 +/- 3.5	28.8 +/- 5.4	9.2 +/- 2.8
90 min	35.4 +/- 5.0	25.2 +/- 4.5	9.6 +/- 1.7
180 min	28.7 +/- 6.0	20.2 +/- 4.9	8.5 +/- 1.4
22 hrs	16.2 +/- 7.2	9.7 +/- 4.9	6.6 +/- 2.4
48 hrs	14.9 +/- 8.0	9.6 +/- 5.6	5.2 +/- 2.4

II   OXIN II
           Whole Blood   Blood Cells   Plasma

	Whole Blood	Blood Cells	Plasma
15 min	35.8 +/- 16.6	28.5 +/- 15.7	7.2 +/- 1.5
45 min	33.8 +/- 15.8	27.5 +/- 16.4	6.4 +/- 1.0
90 min	29.8 +/- 16.1	24.5 +/- 16.5	5.2 +/- 1.5
180 min	24.9 +/- 15.2	19.7 +/- 14.9	5.2 +/- 0.7
22 hrs	10.9 +/- 4.1	7.9 +/- 3.7	3.1 +/- 0.9
48 hrs	6.7 +/- 2.2	3.8 +/- 1.9	2.9 +/- 0.3

III   TROP
           Whole Blood   Blood Cells   Plasma

	Whole Blood	Blood Cells	Plasma
15 min	55.2 +/- 1.0	42.4 +/- 5.7	12.7 +/- 5.8
45 min	51.9 +/- 5.2	43.6 +/- 6.4	7.9 +/- 5.3
90 min	50.2 +/- 4.9	42.8 +/- 7.7	7.5 +/- 5.2
180 min	46.0 +/- 2.0	37.0 +/- 5.1	8.9 +/- 6.9
22 hrs	33.1 +/- 2.9	25.5 +/- 0.2	7.6 +/- 3.1
48 hrs	31.5 +/- 0.85	21.6 +/- 5.0	9.8 +/- 4.2

14.3.2 111-In activity in whole blood

The percentages of the administered activity found in the total volumes of whole blood at the time points 15,45,90,180 minutes and 22 and 48 hrs following injection are listed in Table R.2. (averages) and R.3 (individual patient data).

Table R.3   Percentage of administered In-111-activity in whole blood volume (data of individual patients)

I	OXIN I					
	15 min	45 min	90 min	180 min	22 hrs	48 hrs
JNDL	45.0	42.5	42.4	35.2	24.4	20.4
ERKG	53.2	34.3	35.0	28.8	19.6	18.5
ALTB	46.3	40.4	32.9	30.2	13.2	-
NEUB	50.0	40.3	31.1	20.7	7.8	5.7
II	OXIN II					
	15 min	45 min	90 min	180 min	22 hrs	48 hrs
TTSL	34.8	31.1	25.6	20.7	13.6	9.2
RCHL	52.8	50.8	47.5	41.7	13.1	4.9
WLBR	19.7	19.6	16.2	12.2	6.2	6.0
III	TROP					
	15 min	45 min	90 min	180 min	22 hrs	48 hrs
MSSR	56.0	56.9	55.7	45.9	31.1	31.8
BRTR	54.0	46.4	46.4	44.0	31.7	32.1
BRGR	55.5	51.2	48.5	48.1	36.4	30.5

There was no case in whom the 15 minute concentration of
111-In in whole blood amounted to 100% or at least nearly that
much, so that the calculation of the total blood volume based on
the dilution method and the 15 minute labelled cell concentration
would have been possible. Among ten cases the 15 minute
concentrations of 111-In in whole blood ranged between a low of
19.7 and a high of 56%. Similarly, there were between 12.2 and
48.1% in blood at 3 hrs, and 6.2% - 36.4% at 22 hrs following
injection (for the halftimes see below, section 14.3.8,
Table R.14.

14.3.3   111-In in-vivo distribution

In-vivo imaging and quantification by means of conjugate
scintimetry and region of interest analysis revealed that on
average the liver, the spleen and the bone marrow accumulated
about equal percentages of approximately 20% each. The percentage
seen in the lungs and the heart was about 10% of the administered
dose at 3 hrs, and it declined to slightly over 8% at 22 hrs.

The averages were listed in Tables R.4a and R.4b, the data
from the individual patients in Tables R.5 and R.6.

The one patient in the series (RCHL) who had an abscess and
leucocytosis had the lowest uptake of all the patients in the
spleen, and a particularly high accumulation in the bone marrow.
Tropolonate revealed a tendency toward higher bone marrow uptake,
and lower accumulation in the liver than oxinate. The addition of
autologous plasma to the last rinse of the labelled cells revealed
no significant influence on the in-vivo distribution, but there
was a tendency toward increased liver uptake.

288

Fig. R.1.   Assembly of multiple posterior scintigraphic images demonstrating 22-hr-distribution of 111-In-labelled mixed white cells, as they can be easily prepared for routine clinical use. Note uptake in regions of active bone marrow as well as liver and spleen. (Left petrous pyramid is missing because of surgical resection.)

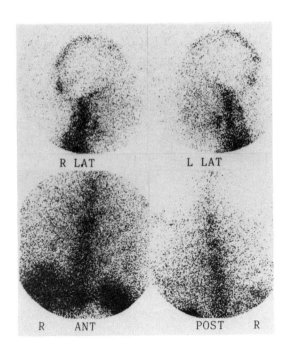

Fig. R.2. Additional views of the same patient as in Figure R.1., complementing the visualization of the 22-hr-distributionjected labelled cel.s into the marginated leucocyte pool.

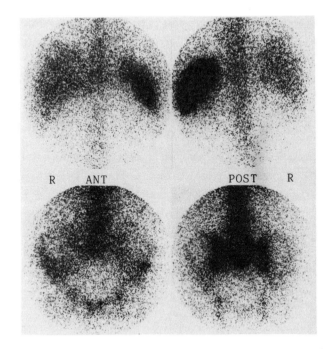

Table R.4a.   Mean Organ Distribution of 111-In-WBC at 3 and 22 hrs p.i. (Percentage of Administered Activity)

	MEAN		OXIN I	
	3 hrs p.i.	22 hrs p.i.	3 hrs p.i.	22 hrs p.i.
Spleen	19.8 +/- 5.3	19.0 +/- 5.7	19.9 +/- 2.6	20.0 +/- 3.3
Liver	19.4 +/- 8.8	21.2 +/- 9.0	20.9 +/- 7.8	23.1 +/- 8.4
Rt.Lung	4.6 +/- 1.4	3.9 +/- 0.8	5.0 +/- 1.8	3.6 +/- 1.0
Lt.Lung, heart	5.3 +/- 1.5	4.5 +/- 0.8	6.0 +/- 2.1	4.4 +/- 0.9
Skull, Spine, Chest, Pelvis	18.2 +/- 4.6	21.3 +/- 6.0	16.3 +/- 3.9	18.4 +/- 3.9
Subt.org.	67.3 +/- 9.6	69.9 +/- 8.8	68.0 +/-10.0	69.3 +/- 9.7
Non-org. cts."body backgd."	21.9 +/- 6.9	23.1 +/- 7.6	22.4 +/- 9.2	24.8 +/-10.1
Cell-bound activity	8.8 +/- 4.0	4.8 +/- 3.0	7.1 +/- 1.7	3.4 +/- 1.7
Plasma-bd. activity	2.7 +/- 1.3	2.0 +/- 1.0	3.0 +/- 0.5	2.3 +/- 0.8
Total	100.6 +/- 1.5	99.9 +/- 0.2	100.5 +/- 1.2	99.8 +/- 0.2
	N = 10		N = 4	

p.i. = post injection

Table R.4b   Mean Organ Distribution of 111-In-WBC at
3 and 22 hrs p.i. (Percentage of Administered Activity)

| | OXIN II | | TROP | |
	3 hrs p.i.	22 hrs p.i.	3 hrs p.i.	22 hrs p.i.
Spleen	22.4 +/- 9.5	21.3 +/- 9.9	17.0 +/- 1.7	15.5 +/- 1.7
Liver	25.1 +/-10.0	27.4 +/- 8.4	11.9 +/- 4.1	12.6 +/- 4.0
Rt.Lung	3.8 +/- 1.1	3.8 +/- 0.8	4.9 +/- 0.9	4.4 +/- 0.6
Lt.Lung, heart	4.4 +/- 0.8	4.0 +/- 0.6	5.2 +/- 0.4	5.3 +/- 0.6
Skull, Spine, Chest, Pelvis	17.0 +/- 6.0	20.2 +/- 8.7	21.8 +/- 3.0	26.2 +/- 3.3
Subt.org.	72.7 +/-11.4	76.7 +/- 8.1	60.9 +/- 5.2	63.9 +/- 4.2
Non-org. cts."body backgd."	18.6 +/- 6.3	19.4 +/- 7.6	24.5 +/- 5.0	24.5 +/- 4.4
Cell-bound activity	6.9 +/- 5.2	2.8 +/- 1.3	13.0 +/- 1.8	8.9 +/-0.05
Plasma-bd. activity	1.8 +/- 0.3	1.1 +/- 0.3	3.1 +/- 2.4	2.7 +/- 1.0
Total	99.9 +/- 0.1	99.9 +/- 0.1	101.4 +/- 2.5	100.1 +/- 0.1
	N = 3		N = 3	

Table R.5   Individual Organ Distribution
                   of 111-In-WBC   at 3 hrs p.i.

	JNDL	ERKG	ALTB	NEUB	TTSL	RCHL	WLBR	MSSR	BRTR	BRGR
		OXIN I				OXIN II			TROP	
Spleen	22.7	20.4	19.8	16.5	25.1	11.9	30.3	15.1	17.5	18.5
Liver	18.2	17.6	15.2	32.4	31.8	13.5	29.9	7.5	12.6	15.6
Rt.L.	6.8	5.8	2.5	4.7	3.3	5.1	3.1	4.7	5.8	4.1
Lt.L. heart	8.0	7.7	4.7	3.8	3.7	5.2	4.2	5.6	5.4	4.8
Skull, Spine, Chest, Pelvis	17.3	20.1	10.9	17.0	13.8	23.9	13.2	22.5	24.4	18.5
Subt. organs	73.0	71.6	53.1	74.4	77.7	59.6	80.7	55.4	65.7	61.5
Non- org.cts. "body backgd."	15.0	20.5	35.9	18.3	15.0	23.8	14.9	28.5	18.9	26.0
Cell- bd.act.	8.9	7.5	7.1	4.8	5.2	12.7	2.7	14.1	13.9	10.9
Plasma bd.act.	3.4	2.6	3.4	2.5	2.0	1.9	1.5	2.0	1.5	5.9
Total	100.3	102.2	99.5	100.0	99.9	100.0	99.8	100.0	100.0	104.3

Table R.6   Individual Organ Distribution
                   of 111-In-WBC at 22 hrs p.i.

	JNDL	ERKG	ALTB	NEUB	TTSL	RCHL	WLBR	MSSR	BRTR	BRGR
		OXIN I				OXIN II			TROP	
Spleen	24.0	20.9	18.6	16.3	25.3	10.0	28.5	14.1	15.1	17.4
Liver	19.8	20.2	16.8	35.5	32.9	17.7	31.6	8.1	14.2	15.6
Rt.L.	3.6	4.0	2.2	4.4	3.6	4.7	3.1	4.5	4.9	3.7
Lt.L. heart	4.3	5.5	4.2	3.4	3.6	4.7	3.8	5.8	5.4	4.6
Skull, Spine, Chest, Pelvis	20.7	22.1	13.3	17.3	15.9	30.2	14.5	27.4	28.7	22.4
Subt. organs	72.4	72.7	55.1	76.9	81.3	67.3	81.5	59.9	68.3	63.7
Non-org.cts. "body backgd."	18.6	20.4	40.0	20.4	13.8	28.0	16.4	29.3	20.6	23.6
Cell-bd.act.	5.2	4.4	2.5	1.4	3.3	3.7	1.3	9.0	8.9	8.9
Plasma-bd. act.	3.3	2.5	2.1	1.3	1.4	0.9	0.9	2.0	2.2	3.9
Total	99.5	100.0	99.7	100.0	99.8	99.9	100.1	100.2	100.0	100.1

14.3.4 Correlation of 111-In blood clearance to organ uptake

The activities not found in the blood, of course, were the difference between the administered activity (100%) and its percentage found in the blood. These differences are a measure of cumulated removal from the blood:

Table R.7 Cumulated Percentages of 111-In Removed from Whole Blood

	Overall range	Average		
		OXIN I	OXIN II	TROP
0 - 0.25 hrs:	44 - 80%	64%	51%	45%
0 - 3.00 hrs:	52 - 88%	75%	71%	64%
0 - 22.00 hrs:	64 - 94%	90%	84%	77%
0 - 48.00 hrs:	68 - 95%	93%	85%	78%
	N = 10	N = 4	N = 3	N = 3

The calculated cumulated removal of 111-In from the blood indicates that considerable amounts of the administered activity were either trapped in the lungs or accumulated in the spleen, liver or bone marrow, and were thereby prevented from appearing in the peripheral blood. There were only slight differences among the three variations in the labelling technique in that respect. This consideration led to the question what fraction of the tracer activities removed from the blood could be found in the organs.

The activities found in the organs could have come from the blood content of the organs only. Yet, the total of the organ activities could not exceed the cumulated removal from the blood. Table R.8 lists the percentage of 111-In removed from the blood between 0 and 3 hrs following injection and the sum of the percentages found within the organ regions.

294

The percentage of 111-In which disappeared from the blood
between 0 and 3 hrs was correlated to the percentages found within
the organ regions at 3 hrs following injection, i.e. a
correlation between the elimination from the blood and the uptake
in the organ. An average of 67.25% of the administered activity
disappeared from the circulating blood and an average of 67.27%
was found within the organ regions. The correlation coefficient
was 0.741, the mean uniformity amounted to 1.0003. (Figure R.1,
Table R.8) It was found that the organ activities at 3 hrs
corresponded well to the activities removed from the blood up to
this time point.

Table R.8   Elimination from Blood Compared to
                   Uptake in Organ Regions 0-3 hrs

	Diff. (%) Whole blood	Diff. (%) Organ regions
JNDL	64.8	73.0
ERKG	71.2	71.6
ALTB	69.8	53.1
NEUB	79.3	74.4
TTSL	79.3	77.7
RCHL	58.3	59.6
WLBR	87.8	80.7
MSSR	54.1	55.4
BRTR	56.1	65.7
BRGR	51.9	61.5
Mean	67.25	67.27
S	12.3	9.6
Mean uniformity		1.00029
Corr.coeff.		0.741

Between 3 to 22 hrs there was an average decrease of about 13% in the whole blood activity divided in about 11% leaving the cell fraction and about 2% leaving the plasma-bound fraction. The uptake in the organ region reflected in no way this disappearance. It was probably caused by migration of labelled cells into tissues since there was no change in the relative tracer content of the non-organ region, and it is, of course, impossible to differentiate between intra- and extravascular radioactivity.

Table R.9   Elimination from Blood Compared to Uptake
                   in Organ or Non-Organ Regions 3-22 hrs

	Diff.(%) Blood Cells	Diff.(%) Plasma Volume	Diff.(%) Subt. Org.	Diff.(%) Non-Org.
JNDL	- 10.6	- 0.2	- 0.6	+ 3.6
ERKG	- 8.8	- 0.5	+ 1.1	- 0.1
ALTB	- 13.3	- 3.7	+ 2.0	+ 4.1
NEUB	- 9.5	- 3.4	+ 2.5	+ 2.1
TTSL	- 5.4	- 1.7	+ 3.6	- 1.2
RCHL	- 25.9	- 2.6	+ 7.7	+ 2.2
WLBR	- 4.1	- 1.8	+ 0.8	+ 1.5
MSSR	- 14.5	- 0.3	+ 4.5	+ 0.8
BRTR	- 14.2	+ 1.9	+ 2.6	+ 1.7
BRGR	- 5.9	- 5.8	+ 2.2	- 2.4
Mean	- 11.2	- 2.15	+ 2.6	+ 1.97

14.3.5 Cell-bound 111-In-activity

The tracer activities found within centrifuged blood cells
were considered to be predominantly bound to leucocytes. The
cell-bound activities ranged between a low of 14.1% and a high of
approximately 19% of the administered activity at 15 minutes
following injection, between about 8% and 40% at 3 hrs, and
between 4% and 25% at 22 hrs.

Table R.10   Percentage of Administered 111-In Activity in
                    Blood Cell Volume (Data from Individual Patients)

I	OXIN I					
	15 min	45 min	90 min	180 min	22 hrs	48 hrs
JNDL	41.3	34.1	31.4	25.5	14.9	13.1
ERKG	48.9	27.6	27.5	21.3	12.5	12.5
ALTB	30.4	21.7	21.8	20.4	7.1	-
NEUB	35.9	31.8	21.9	13.6	4.1	3.1
II	OXIN II					
	15 min	45 min	90 min	180 min	22 hrs	48 hrs
TTSL	26.1	23.7	18.6	14.9	9.5	6.0
RCHL	45.4	45.5	43.2	36.4	10.5	2.3
WLBR	14.1	13.2	11.7	7.8	3.7	3.2
III	TROP					
	15 min	45 min	90 min	180 min	22 hrs	48 hrs
MSSR	46.9	50.3	50.5	40.2	25.7	22.2 R
BRTR	44.4	43.0	42.6	39.7	25.5	26.4 P
BRGR	36.0	37.5	35.1	31.2	25.3	16.4 R

The average amounts of 111-In activity recoverable in blood
cells showed no significant difference from group to group. The

amounts found early showed no relationship to the subsequent time course of the activity. The individual patient values found at various time points were listed in Table R.10. For average values see Table R.2.

No appreciable, distinct increase in the cell-bound recoverable 111-In fraction could be demonstrated by two modifications in the labelling process, i.e. exchanging oxinate for tropolonate or vice versa or by carefully removing excess 111-In from the preparation of the labelled cells prior to injection. If there was any effect at all, it was a tendency to keep the cell-bound fraction stable for 1.5 hrs when tropolonate was used or when autologous platelet poor plasma was added to the final rinse of the 111-In-oxinate labelled cells.

14.3.6 Plasma-bound 111-In activity

The percentages of 111-In activity found in plasma were listed in Table R.11 (individual patients) and Table R.2 (averages). The plasma-bound 111-In activity was considered "free" indium and was thought to have been eluted or expelled from intact cells or derived from ruptured cells. An increase in the relative amount of 111-In in plasma during the observation period would have been a sign of shortened survival or damage of labelled cells, respectively.

Sizeable quantities of 111-In were recovered in plasma at 15 minutes following injection: These activities were lowest (5-9%) when 111-In-oxinate was used for labelling and when autologous plasma was added to the last rinse of the labelled cells. They were highest (10 and 15%) when oxinate was used without addition of autologous plasma. When tropolonate was used for labelling and autologous plasma was added to the last wash of the labelled cells, the fraction of unbound indium within the total plasma volume ranged between 9 and 20% of the administered activity. So it was clearly demonstrable that the addition of autologous plasma to the last wash of the labelled cells did not abolish the appearance of free 111-In in the patients' plasma. This must have been eluted from the labelled cells during the first minutes of the labelled cells within the blood stream. It could possibly also stem from an active process of expulsion from the cells or from ruptured cells. The use of tropolonate showed no improvement in this respect, i.e. no significant reduction in free indium in comparison to preparations of labelled cells in which oxinate had been used. The subsequent time course of plasma bound 111-In was analyzed with respect to the cell bound tracer activity (see following section) and with respect to the halftime.

Table R.11   Percentage of Administered 111-In Activity in Plasma Volume (Data from Individual Patients)

I	OXIN I					
	15 min	45 min	90 min	180 min	22 hrs	48 hrs
JNDL	3.7	8.4	10.9	9.7	9.5	7.2
ERKG	4.3	6.6	7.5	7.5	7.0	5.9
ALTB	15.9	13.2	11.0	9.8	6.1	-
NEUB	14.9	8.4	9.1	7.1	3.7	2.6

II	OXIN II					
	15 min	45 min	90 min	180 min	22 hrs	48 hrs
TTSL	8.7	7.4	7.0	5.8	4.1	3.2 P
RCHL	7.4	5.4	4.3	5.3	2.7	2.6 P
WLBR	5.6	6.4	4.4	4.4	2.6	2.8 R

III	TROP					
	15 min	45 min	90 min	180 min	22 hrs	48 hrs
MSSR	19.2	6.6	5.2	5.7	5.4	9.6 D
BRTR	9.6	3.4	3.8	4.3	6.2	5.7 D
BRGR	19.4	13.7	13.4	16.9	11.1	14.1 D

14.3.7 Relative amounts of cell bound and plasma bound 111-In

The mean percentages of the administered activity found in the packed red cells, and in the plasma (see Table R.2) at each time point were each divided by the amount of the administered activity in whole blood at that time to yield a ratio of the activity concentrations in blood.

Table R.12   Ratios of 111-In Activities in Packed RBC and PLASMA
              (derived from average In activities)

	15 min	90 min	180 min	22 hrs	48 hrs
I OXIN I	80/20	82/18	79/21	72/28	57/36
II OXIN II	80/20	71/29	70/30	60/40	64/36
III TROP	77/23	85/15	80/20	77/23	69/31

The total of 100 equals the percentage of the administered activity in whole blood at each time point.

The plasma bound indium remained, relative to the cell bound 111-In, at about the same level of approximately 20% for the first three hours when oxinate was used and autologous platelet-poor-plasma was added to the last wash of the labelled cells; it increased to 28% until 22 hrs following injection. When tropolonate was used to mediate cell labelling with 111-In, the plasma bound activity ranged between 15 and 23% up to 22 hrs and so remained the same relative to the the cell-bound radioactivity (see Tables R.10 and R.11). Very little difference could be observed in this respect between tropolonate and oxinate.

During the time interval between 22 and 48 hrs following injection there was a relatively larger increase in the relative plasma bound activity in comparison to the time before 22 hrs p.i. At 48 hrs about one third of the blood activity was in the plasma in each of the cell preparations.

300

14.3.8 Urinary excretion

The amounts of 111-In found in 24 hr collections of urine are listed in Table R.13. The mean value amounted to 0.34 +/- 0.3% of the administered activity. Even if the observed value were to underestimate the cumulated 24 hr urinary elimination of 111-In by a factor of 4 (i.e. three voidings missed) the urinary 24 hr excretion would be no higher than about 2%.

Table R.13

Cumulated 24 hr urinary excretion of 111-In administered as oxinate or tropolonate labelled WBCs.

JNDL	-
ERGK	1.05
ALTB	0.41
NEUB	0.25
RCHL	0.19
MSSR	0.06
WLBR	0.45
BRTR	0.10
BRGR	0.14
TTSL	0.40
Average	0.34 +/- 0.3

Table R.14   111-In-Labelled   Blood   Cells
Halftimes in Whole Blood (hrs)

	I:	0 - 3 hrs
	II:	3 - 18 hrs
	III:	18 - 48 hrs
	IV:	48 - infinity

----

			biol.	eff.
OXIN I	I	75.0%	1.5	1.5
	II	13.0%	2.5	2.4
	III	5.4%	34.5	22.8
	IV	6.6%	67.44	67.44
OXIN II	I	72.0%	1.6	1.6
	II	11.5%	3.1	3.0
	III	1.5%	246.0	52.9
	IV	15.0%	67.44	67.44
TROP	I	54.0%	2.7	2.6
	II	12.0%	3.8	3.6
	III	2.0%	240	52.6
	IV	32.0%	67.44	67.44
MEAN	I	67.0%	2.7	1.8
	II	12.1%	3.8	3.0
	III	3.0%	130 hrs	44.4
	IV	10.4%	67.44	67.44

302

14.3.9 Kinetic considerations

The outstanding observation was the seeming non-uniformity from patient to patient of the kinetic behaviour of the cell-bound and plasma-bound 111-In activity between 0.25 and 1.5 hrs following injection (see Tables R.10 and R.11). The cell-bound activity displayed three types of time course:
a) initial increase, followed by plateau
b) minimal decline or
c) distinct decline.

An initial rise of the cell-bound radioactivity was observed in two of our ten patients and the maximum of the cell bound radioactivity appeared between 45 and 90 minutes. There were three patients in whom the cell-bound radioactivity remained at a plateau between 15 and 45 minutes. In some patients this plateau like time course extended as long as 90 minutes following injection.

The patients whose cell-bound 111-In activity plateaued or rose during the initial 45 or 90 minutes respectively (MSSR, BRTR, BRGR, RCHL, WLBR) showed no systematic response in the plasma-associated 111-In activity: It descended more or less briskly in the patients MSSR, BRTR, BRGR, whereas it plateaued in RCHL and even rose in WLBR; in two further patients, JNDL and ERKG, the plasma-associated 111-In activity rose while the cell-bound activity descended briskly.

It is probably best to consider this period as a period of mixing during which at least three processes occur simultaneously:
a) trapping of labelled cells in the lungs followed by continuous release
b) transfer of 111-In from the cell-bound fraction to the plasma-bound fraction; some of this 111-In should form colloid, to be taken up by the liver, spleen and bone marrow, some of the 111-In should be bound by transferrin.
c) uptake of labelled cells into the spleen, liver and bone marrow, a process which is perhaps equivalent to the mixing of the injected labelled cells into the marginated leucocyte pool.

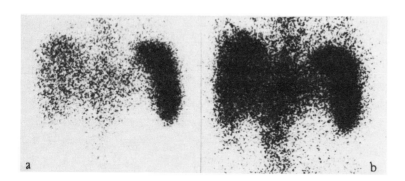

Fig. R.3. Relative increase in hepatic uptake between 3 and 20 hrs following injection. Although the degree of this relative hepatic uptake is exaggerated due to different intensity settings, the images confirm the average scintimetric data which suggest continuing uptake of slight degree between 3 and 24 hrs.

The amount of 111-In removed from whole blood by 3 hrs could be found within the spleen, liver, bone marrow, lungs and heart at 3 hrs (see section 3.4).

The uptake of 111-In activity into the accumulating organs was virtually complete by 3 hrs. There was very little change in the tracer content of the organ regions after 3 hrs. The observed differences in the average values of the percentages accumulated in the various organs are so small that no definite conclusion can be drawn other than that no significant change appears to take place (Tables R.4a and R.4b). There appears to prevail a tendency, however, for the lungs, heart and spleen to release small amounts of activity during the time period between 3 and 24 hrs, for the liver, the bones and the non-organ regions to accumulate minimal amounts.

The halftimes of the 111-In activity in the blood, blood cells and plasma are listed in Table R.14.

14.3.10   Radiation dosimetry considerations:

This study revealed the liver, the spleen, the bones with active bone marrow, the heart, the lungs, the blood and the body as a whole as significant source regions.   Virtuallly no elimination was observed up to 22 hrs and certainly no elimination from the body should be assumed beyond 22 hrs.

14.4 DISCUSSION

The method of labelling granulocytes in-vitro with 32-P labelled di-isopropyl-fluorophosphate (32-DFP), a label which is not reutilized, was used extensively to study granulocyte kinetics (4).   These studies revealed that only about one half of the injected labelled cells appeared in the circulating peripheral blood.   Since 32-P is a beta-emitter, imaging studies have not been possible with this tracer, only the time course of the labelled cells in blood was studied.

Hence, the initial trapping of the labelled cells in the lungs as well as the subsequent accumulation in the liver, spleen and bone marrow remained undetected.   The margination of leucocytes within the confines of blood vessels along capillary walls, however, was used as an explanation for the missing labelled cells: The one half of the injected labelled white blood cells, which was not recovered in the peripheral circulating blood, was postulated to mix with the marginated white blood cells, and therefore the concept of the marginated pool of leucocytes was established and was quantitatively estimated at one half of the total pool of leucocytes;   the second half of the total amount of the intravascular leucocytes was termed the circulating pool since this was found in the peripheral blood.

In the newer studies gamma emitters, particularly 111-In, were used to label leucocytes, so that the visualization of localized accumulations in the body was possible.   Thus it was learned that labelled granulocytes localize in the lungs immediately following the injection, and accumulate within the liver, spleen, and bone marrow somewhat later.

Our study has shown that the localization in the lungs is a transient phenomenon and that only about 10% of the administered activity can be found within the lungs and the heart at 3 hrs after injection. It revealed further that the blood levels may remain at about the same level between 15 minutes, and as late as 90 minutes after injection. Barbara Weiblen et al. (5) found in their patients that the concentration in blood peaked after about 2 hrs after injection. This can be explained by considering variable amounts of labelled cells being trapped in the lungs and variable rates of release from the lungs.

The amount of the activity trapped within the lungs most likely depended on the details of the labelling procedure and the handling of the cells, but perhaps also on the particular characteristics of the pulmonary microcirculation in individual patients (we have had one or two patients in whom nearly all of the injected activity was recovered in the circulating blood at 15 minutes after injection; patients, who were not studied by conjugate imaging).

At the same time, while labelled leucocytes are continuously released from the lungs there is uptake of 111-In in the liver, spleen and bone marrow. Goodwin et al. (6) have shown that the uptake in the liver will be higher if the labelled white blood cells suffer hypotonic damage during cell separation and labelling. Among our ten patients we found three patients in whom the liver uptake was in the order of 30%, whereas it was between about 7-18% in the six other patients. The uptake in the spleen ranged around 20% and deviated to the extreme values of 12% in one patient and 30% in another patient. Uptake in bone marrow ranged around 18% at 3 hrs, and deviated extremely to a low of 11% only in one patient and up to 24% in one other patient. The uptake in bone marrow was higher than was thought previously. At 3 hrs after injection the localized 111-In activity accounted for approximately 67% of the administered activity. Another 22% was diffusely distributed in the tissues of the trunk and head representing intravascular radioactivity as well as interstitial radioactivity. Another 11% accounted for the 111-In content in arms and legs at 3 hrs after injection.

There was good correlation in the total amount of radioactivity which had left the blood and the amount of radioactivity found within the regions of localized uptake. It was shown by Weiblen et al. (5) that the subcutaneous injection of epinephrine 4 hrs after the injection of autologous 111-In labelled granulocytes could again mobilize labelled granulocytes into the circulation from the marginal pool, causing a granulocytosis of 22 or 100%. The epinephrine injection had resulted in a prompt mobilization of leucocytes within 5 minutes, which became maximal at about 20 minutes and then returned towards normal. The idea of the spleen serving as an organ for the transient storage of neutrophils and perhaps other leucocytes is supported by one of our patients (RCHL) who had marked leucocytosis because of an abscess and the lowest splenic uptake of 111-In WBC's.

We found that very little change occurred in the in-vivo distribution between 3 hrs and 22 hrs following injection. There was only slight diminution of the activity in the lungs and heart: We observed a drop from about 10% to about 8%. There was a tendency for the bone marrow and liver to increase their uptake, and there was a tendency for the spleen to release some of the accumulated radioactivity between 3 and 22 hrs following injection. The ratio between the activities of the organ regions and the non-organ regions showed no significant change between 3 hrs and 22 hrs.

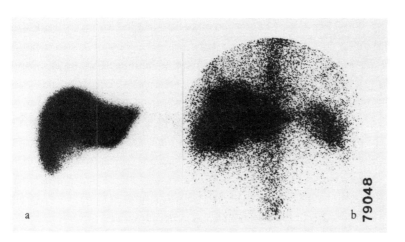

Fig. R.4. Extraordinarily low uptake of 111-In WBC's in spleen
and localized uptake in gallbladder area due to empyema
a) 99m-Tc-colloid liver scan   b) 111-In WBC scan

The kinetic behaviour of labelled leucocytes in the blood
stream could easily be explained on the basis of the data
obtained.

The time course of radioactivity in the blood between 0 and
3 hrs is the consequence of release from the lungs on one hand and
uptake in the cumulating regions of the spleen, liver and bone
marrow on the other hand. The time course between 3 hrs and
22 hrs is characterized by continued disappearance from the blood
which is not associated with any definitive increase in the uptake
of the localizing region, and which therefore should represent
migration of labelled cells into the extravascular interstitial
tissues. The true rate of leucocyte migration from blood into
tissue, i.e. disappearance from the blood stream should therefore
be measured only after 3 or 4 hrs following injection. Our study
revealed biological halftimes of 2.5 - 3.8 hrs during this period
of observation. Some radioactivity was lost from the cell-bound
fraction during the period 3 hrs to 22 hrs, not because of cell
migration out of the vascular compartment, but by leakage or
expulsion of 111-In from the cells or by rupture of cells and
transfer of 111-In into the plasma-bound fraction.

The concentration (and relative amount) of 111-In in plasma
should increase as time goes on if there were significant release

of 111-In from the labelled cells by elution, expulsion, leakage or cellular rupture. A certain increase in the plasma-bound 111-In was observed when oxinate was used as a chelating agent and when no autologous plasma was added to the final rinse of the labelled cells. It was not observed until 22 hrs following injection when tropolonate was used and it was distinctly lower with oxinate when the prefinal plasma addition was carried out. An opposite trend occurred after 22 hrs: The indium concentration in plasma increased sharply with OXIN II (oxinate-plus-plasma-wash) and with tropolonate (also plus plasma wash), whereas it dropped with OXIN I (oxinate-without-plasma-wash). This was interpreted to indicate that significant cell damage occurred with OXINATE II and tropolonate (plus plasma) only after 22 hrs, whereas the rate of cellular decay, i.e. the transfer of 111-In from the cell-bound fraction to the plasma-bound fraction occurred much earlier, namely during the first 18 hrs or so, when no autologous plasma had been added to the last rinse of the oxinate labelled cells. From this different behaviour in the transfer of 111-In from the cell-bound fraction to the plasma-bound fraction it was concluded that the addition of autologous plasma to the final rinse of the labelled cells had a protective effect on the cells which lasted for about one day, and that survival times of labelled cells within the blood stream should be estimated beginning between 3 or 4 hrs after injection, and not after 22 to 24 hrs after injection.

As much as we would have liked to find a distinctly different behaviour of tropolonate over oxinate we could find no truly significant difference in the in-vivo distribution, perhaps because of suspending and labelling the white cells in saline rather than in plasma. There can be no doubt that autologous plasma is the best environment for white blood cells.

From the view point of radiation dosimetry it is important to recognize that no significant biological elimination occurs and that the spleen, the liver, the bone marrow, the lungs, the heart, the blood and the body as a whole have to be considered significant source regions during the first 24 hrs, whereas only the spleen, liver, bone marrow and the body as a whole represent significant source regions thereafter.

SUMMARY

The distribution of 111-In-labelled leucocytes in 10 patients was quantified by conjugate scintimetric imaging using a scintillation camera and an associated computer. The in-vivo quantification was derived from numerical images representing the attenuation corrected geometric mean of radionuclide images of opposing surfaces of the skull, the thorax, the upper and lower abdomen. The leucocytes were labelled in phosphate-buffered normal saline using 111-In-oxinate or tropolonate. The following mean percentages of the administered tracer activity were found at 3 hrs (A) and at 22 hrs (B):

A: spleen 19.8, liver 19.4, chest 9.9
B: spleen 19.0, liver 21.2, chest 8.4

A: bone and marrow: 18.2, body background 21.9
B: bone and marrow: 21.3, body background 23.1

A: vasc. cell bound act.: 8.8, plasma: 2.7
B: vasc. cell bound act.: 4.8, plasma: 2.0

The ratio between the activities found within organ regions of interest (ROI) and those found within non-organ ROI's did not change significantly between 3 and 22 hrs. The disappearance of the 111-In activity from the blood revealed three components with the following percentages and halftimes:

   I: 0-3 hrs: 67.0%, 2.7 hr biol, 1.8 hr eff
  II: 3-18 hrs: 12.1%, 3.8 hr biol, 3.0 hr eff
 III: 18-48 hrs: 3.0% 130 hr biol, 44.4 hr eff
  IV: beyond 48 hrs: 10.4%, 67.44 hr physical

The addition of autologous plasma to the final rinse of the cells labelled in buffer had a protective effect which lasted about 24 hrs. Survival times of labelled cells are best estimated between 4 and 24 hrs following injection.

310

REFERENCES

1. McAfee J.G.: Importance of Cell Labelling Techniques. In: Indium-111-Labeled Neutrophils, Platelets and Lymphocytes, edited by M.L. Thakur and A. Gottschalk, pp.1-6. Trivirum Publishing Company, New York, 1980.
2. Danpure H.J., S. Osman and F. Brady: The labelling of blood cells with 111-Indium-tropolonate. Brit.J.Radiol. 55:247-429, 1982.
3. Snyder W.S., M.R. Ford and G.G. Warner: Estimates at specific absorbed fractions for photon sources uniformly distributed in various organs of heterogeneous phantom(s)? MIRD-Pamphlet No.5, edited by the Society of Nuclear Medicine, Inc., New York, 1978.
4. Kaboth W.: Kinetik der Granulozytopoese. In: Klinische Haematologie, edited by H.Begeman, 2nd ed., pp.67-70. Thieme, Stuttgart, 1975.
5. Weiblen B.J., J. McCullough, L.A. Forstrom and M.K. Loken: Kinetics of Indium-111-labeled Granulocytes. In: Indium-111 Labeled Neutrophils, Platelets and Lymphocytes, edited by M.L. Thakur and A. Gottschalk, pp.23-32. Trivirum Publishing Company, New York, 1980.
6. Goodwin D.A., P.W. Doherty and I.R. McDougall: Clinical Use of Indium-111-Labeled White Cells: An Analysis of 312 Cases. In: Indium-111 Labeled Neutrophils, Platelets and Lymphocytes, edited by M.L. Thakur and A. Gottschalk, pp. 131-146. Trivirum Publishing Company, New York, 1980.
7. Coffey J.L. and E.E. Watson: S values for selected radionuclides and organs with the heart wall and heart contents as source organs. Third International Radiopharmaceutical Dosimetry Symposium, Oak Ridge, 1981.

15 RADIATION DOSIMETRY OF LABELLED LEUCOCYTES

B. BJURMAN, L. JOHANSSON, S. MATTSSON, B. NOSSLIN,
P.I. OLSSON, B. PERSSON AND S.E. STRAND

15.1 INTRODUCTION

The most important clinical application of labelled white blood cells (WBC) is the identification and localization of abscesses and inflammatory processes by scintigraphy after the injection of 111-In labelled autologous leucocytes (1,2). Lymphocytes labelled with 111-In are now also used for studies of lymphocyte migration and distribution in man (3). 99m-Tc has also been used for leucocyte labelling (4-9). Earlier fundamental studies on blood cell kinetics were performed with the use of 32-P-DFP (10). 51-Cr has also been employed in non-imaging applications such as cell kinetic studies etc. (11).

The purpose of the present work is to review the available data on the in-vivo distribution of labelled WBC in man in order to define a model applicable to dosimetric calculations. Calculations have been performed for the radionuclides 111-In, 51-Cr and 99m-Tc as well as for 97-Ru; the latter being of potential interest.

15.2 IN-VIVO DISTRIBUTION OF LABELLED WBC

For blood cell labelling with 111-In, three chelating agents are mainly in use, namely oxinate (1,2,12) acetylacetone (13) and tropolone (14). In the cell suspension not only leucocytes are labelled but also some erythrocytes and thrombocytes. There are several methods for cell separation described in the literature, giving rise to different compositions of the reinjected cell suspensions. Furthermore, when the cells are separated, labelled and washed they may suffer from varying degrees of chemical as well as mechanical damage (15). These facts, as well as the patient's condition, will influence the in-vivo distribution of the activity.

Published data on the distribution in man of 111-In labelled WBC are scarce. Biokinetic data have so far been reported for a total number of about 30 patients (1,16,17,18).

After an intravenous injection of 111-In WBC there is an early and transient uptake in the lungs and a rapid early fall in the blood activity, mainly caused by an accumulation in the spleen, liver and bone marrow. Other organs have not been observed with such a high specific uptake. No significant excretion has been seen during the first few days after the injection.

The composition of the blood cell suspension varied considerably from study to study. Using an almost pure leucocyte suspension, Thakur et al. (1) found the liver uptake to be 34-39% and the spleen uptake 6-13% of the injected activity. The elimination from the blood was described by an effective halflife of 4.5-7.5 hrs. In one preparation with 5% erythrocytes and 95% leucocytes the distribution was 11-13% in the liver 12-16% in the spleen, with an effective halflife in the blood of 17 hrs. For granulocytes Weiblen (16) found a 12% uptake in the liver after one day and 19% in the spleen. The activity disappeared from the blood with an effective halflife of 5 hrs.

Goodwin et al. (17) also used an almost pure leucocyte preparation (80% neutrophils) and in 6 patients found 19 +/- 6% in the liver and 19 +/- 7% in the spleen. For "bad preparations" they recognized a considerable transient uptake (15%) in the lungs. These data are valid for the patients with normal scans.

Sokole-Buseman et al. (18) used a suspension composed of 49% leucocytes, 10% thrombocytes, 21% erythrocytes and 20% non cell bound 111-In. The liver uptake in 24 patients showed a mean value of 24% after 98 hrs. The spleen uptake was 15% and the estimated 111-In activity in the blood was 18%. The remaining activity was assumed to be present in the red bone-marrow.

Fueger (19) found +/- 20% of the activity in spleen, +/- 20% in liver, +/- 20% in bone-marrow and in blood 3-4 hrs after the

injection of a WBC suspension.   The urinary elimination   was   less
than 2% over 24 hrs.

Based on the data from the literature cited above, as well as
animal data (20,21,22), we have defined descriptive models for the
activity distribution after the injection of labelled blood cells
(Table 1).   For calculation of the total radiation absorbed dose
it is necessary to include a thrombocyte model which is based on
data from van Reenen et al.   (23,17,24,25).

Table 1.   Biokinetic Data Used in the Dosimetric Calculations

Blood cells	Organ	Fraction of adm.act.	Uptake T 1/2	Elimination T 1/2
Leucocytes				
	Lung	0.25	0	0.25 hrs
	Liver	0.20	0	30.0 d
	Spleen	0.15	0	30.0 d
	Bone marrow	0.25	0.25 hrs	30.0 d
	Remainder	0.40	0	30.0 d
Thrombocytes				
	Lung	–	–	–
	Liver	0.15	0	30.0 d
		0.165	4.5 d	
	Spleen	0.30	0	30.0 d
		0.055	4.5 d	
	Bone marrow	0.22	4.5 d	30.0 d
	Remainder	0.55	0	4.5 d (80%)
				30.0 d (20%)
"Free" 111-In				
	Liver	0.85	0	0
	Spleen	0.10	0	0
	Bone marrow	0.05	0	0
	Remainder	–	–	–

Several authors have found that some of the activity in the reinjected cell suspension is not cell bound. We have assumed that this activity is treated by the body in the same way as has been found for neutral indium (e.g. 113m-In) i.e. as a colloid. Furthermore, some erythrocytes have been labelled using existing techniques. For dosimetric purposes we have used the same effective dose equivalent for erythrocytes as for thrombocytes, since the latter model includes a biological halflife which is long compared with the physical halflife of the actual radionuclides.

In the calculation of the absorbed dose and dose equivalent for a typical WBC suspension we have assumed a composition of 50% leucocytes, 20% thrombocytes, 10% erythrocytes and 20% "free" 111-In (18).

15.3 CALCULATION OF THE ABSORBED AND EFFECTIVE DOSE EQUIVALENT

Using the biokinetic data given in Table 1, the cumulated activity of 111-In, 99m-Tc, 51-Cr and 97-Ru in various organs and in the remaining body have been calculated. The radiation absorbed dose in the organs was then determined using "S-values" given by MIRD (26). The effective dose equivalent, H(E) was calculated according to ICRP (27).

15.4 RESULTS AND DISCUSSION

The results of the absorbed dose calculations for pure leucocytes labelled with 111-In, 99m-Tc, 51-Cr or 97-Ru are given in Table 2. The effective dose equivalent is given for pure leucocytes as well as for a typical WBC suspension.

Table 2.	Absorbed Dose in Various Organs and Effective Dose Equivalent, H(E)			

"Pure" leucocytes

Radionuclide:	111-In	99m-Tc	51-Cr	97-Ru

Absorbed dose in organs
mGy/MBq

	111-In	99m-Tc	51-Cr	97-Ru
Spleen	3.4	0.12	2.1	1.8
Liver	0.68	0.023	0.61	0.39
Red bone marrow	0.55	0.021	0.34	0.28
Bone	0.16	0.0055	0.08	0.089
Lungs	0.14	0.0058	0.11	0.082
Pancreas	0.38	0.012	0.22	0.22
Kidneys	0.26	0.0082	0.16	0.15
Ovaries	0.13	0.0044	0.081	0.074
Testes	0.057	0.0020	0.047	0.033
Whole body	0.15	0.0049	0.099	0.085

Effective dose equivalent

mSv/MBq	0.43	0.015	0.28	0.23

Typical "WBC" suspension

Radionuclide:	111-In	99m-Tc	51-Cr	97-Ru

Effective dose equivalent

mSv/MBq	0.50	0.017	0.29	0.28

The highest mean absorbed dose is received in the spleen, followed by the liver, red bone-marrow and organs located close to the spleen e.g. the pancreas and the kidneys. The transient lung uptake gives only a minimal contribution to the absorbed dose in the lungs. The absorbed dose per unit injected activity is highest for 111-In followed by 51-Cr and 97-Ru. When using 111-In labelled cells the effective dose equivalent amounts to 0.4 and

0.5 mSv/MBq for pure leucocyte preparations and the mixed WBC suspensions respectively. When using biokinetic data given by Thakur et al (1) and Goodwin et al. (17) instead of our standard model we have found the effective dose equivalent to be 0.41 and 0.59 mSv/MBq respectively.

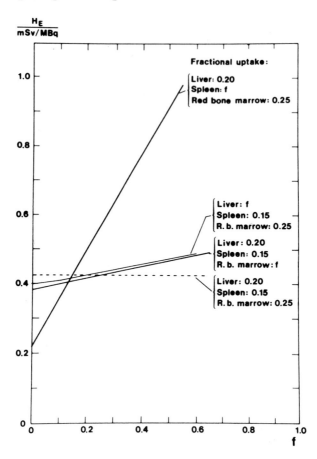

Fig. 1. Effective dose equivalent, H(E), for 111-In-labelled pure leucocytes for varying fractional uptake, f, in either spleen, liver, or red bone marrow.

If 51-Cr or 97-Ru is used the effective dose equivalent is reduced to 0.2-0.3 mSv/MBq. From the dosimetric point of view the most favourable radionuclide is 99m-Tc which gives an effective dose equivalent which is about 30 times lower than for 111-In.

The effective dose equivalent is highly dependent on the magnitude of the fraction of the injected activity which is accumulated in the spleen; this is illustrated in Figure 1. The figure shows the effective dose equivalent for 111-In labelled pure leucocytes for varying fractional uptakes in either spleen, liver or bone-marrow. The uptakes in the other two organs are assumed to be constant and numerically the same as in our standard model. When the organ uptake is increased, a corresponding decrease in the content of the remainder of the body occurs. As can be seen, an increase in spleen uptake from 15% to 30% will give an increase in H(E) from 0.43 to 0.63 mSv/MBq. A variation in liver and bone-marrow uptake gives comparatively smaller changes in H(E). A rise in the liver content from 20% to 40% gives, for example, an increase of H(E) from 0.43 to 0.46 mSv/MBq.

Variations in the composition of the actual WBC suspension has no drastic effect on H(E) as shown in Table 3.

Table 3. The Effective Dose Equivalent, H(E), for Different Compositions of the Blood Cell Suspension

Leucocytes	Thrombocytes	Erythrocytes	"Free" 111-In	Effective dose equi- valent H(E) (mSv/MBq)
100%	-	-	-	0.43
-	100%	-	-	0.65
-	-	-	100%	0.47
50%	10%	20%	20%	0.50

From this table it is clear that H(E) will only vary between 0.43 and 0.65 mSv/MBq assuming the most extreme variation in the blood composition.

When 111-In is used for labelling the WBC the mean absorbed dose in various organs as well as the effective dose equivalent is high compared with that of other present day nuclear medical procedures. The effective dose equivalent is further increased by between 6 and 36% due to 114m-In, which is a radionuclide impurity present in 111-In (28).

When lymphocytes are labelled with the various radionuclides the absorbed dose in the cells will be of special importance because these cells reproduce in the blood. Recent reports on labelling with 111-In have shown extremely high absorbed doses in the cells (29) and have given evidence for the possibility of some chromosome damage (30,31). Before the question of possible late malignancies has been further investigated it is recommended to keep the labelled lymphocyte fraction in WBC cell suspensions as small as possible.

From the dosimetric point of view it is obvious that it should be a great step forward to use 99m-Tc for WBC labelling instead of 111-In (32,33,9). The method used by Oberhausen, Schroth et al. (9) seems promising, especially since it may reduce cell damage during labelling.

This study has shown that there is a lack of biological data, and it is therefore difficult to construct a reliable functional model for labelled leucocytes in man. There is therefore an urgent need to collect more information among patients with various diseases as well as better information on the liver and bone-marrow uptake. The activity in the total body as well as the excretion via the urine and faeces should be determined during the weeks following the injection. In order to facilitate the comparison of results from various laboratories, it is also important that the composition of the actual cell suspension is given.

Acknowledgements:

This study has been supported by grants from the John and Augusta Persson's Foundation for Scientific Work, Lund.

SUMMARY

Published data on the biokinetics and radiation dosimetry of labelled leucocytes in man are reviewed and discussed together with some recent unpublished human and animal data from various laboratories.

Investigations with 111-In labelled blood cells give a comparatively high absorbed dose to the liver, spleen and bone marrow, and the effective dose equivalents for such investigations are among the highest for modern nuclear medical procedures or about 0.7 mSv/MBq.

REFERENCES

1. Thakur M.L., J.P. Lavender, R.N. Arnot, et al: Indium-111-labeled autologous leucocytes in man. J. Nucl. Med. 18:1012-1019, 1977.
2. Thakur M.L. and A. Gottschalk (Eds.): Indium-111 Labeled Neutrophils, Platelets, and Lymphocytes. Trivirum Publising Company, New York, 1980.
3. Chisholm P.M. and A.M. Peters: The effect of indium-111 labeling on the recirculation of rat lymphocytes. In: Indium-111 labeled Neutrofils, Platelets, and Lymphocytes, edited by M.L. Thakur and A. Gottschalk, pp.205-208. Trivirum Publishing Company, New York, 1980.
4. Uchida T. and S. Kariyone: Organ distribution of the Tc-99m labeled white cells. Acta Haematol. Jpn. 36:78-81, 1973.
5. Uchida T. and P.C. Vincent: In vitro studies of leukocyte labeling with technetium-99m. J. Nucl. Med. 17:730-736, 1976.
6. English D. and B.R. Andersen: Labeling of phagocytes from human blood with Tc-99m-sulfur colloid. J. Nucl. Med. 16:5-10, 1975.
7. English D. and B.R. Andersen: Organ distribution of canine leukocytes labeled with Tc-99m-sulfur colloid. J. Nucl. Med. 18:289-295, 1977.
8. Linhardt N., B. Bok, M. Gougerot, M.T. Gaillard and M. Meignan: Tc-99m labelled human leukocytes. An in vitro functional study. Acta Haemat. 63:71-80, 1980.
9. Schroth H.J., E. Oberhausen and R. Berberich: Cell labelling with colloidal substances in whole blood. Eur. Nucl. Med 6: 469-472, 1981.
10. Athens J.W., O.P. Haab, O.S. Raab, A.M. Mauer, H. Ashenbrucker, G.E. Cartwright and M.M. Wintrobe: Leukokinetic studies IV. The total blood, circulating and marginal granulocyte pools and the granulocyte turnover rate in normal subjects. J. Clin. Invest. 40:989-995, 1961.
11. Dresch C. and Y. Najean: Etude de la cinetique des poly-nucleaires apres marquage in vitro par le radiochrome. I. Etude critique de la methode et resultats obtenus chez les sujets normaux. Nouv. Rev. Franc. Hemat. 7:27-48, 1967.
12. Roevekamp M.H.: Indium-111 labelled leucocyte scintigraphy in the diagnosis of inflammatory disease. Thesis, Univ. Amsterdam, 1982.
13. Sinn H. and D.J. Silvester: Simplified cell labelling with indium-111 acetylacetone. Br. J. Radiol. 52:758-759, 1979.
14. Danpure H.J., S. Osman and F. Brady: The labelling of blood cells in plasma with In-111 tropolonate. Br. J. Radiol. 55:247-249, 1982.
15. Zakhireh B., M.L. Thakur, M.L. Malech, et al: Indium-111-labeled human polymorphonuclear leucocytes: viability, random migration, chemotaxis, bactericidal capacity, and ultrastructure. J. Nucl. Med. 20:741-747, 1979.
16. Weiblen B.J., L. Forstrom and J. McCullough: Studies of the kinetics of indium-111-labeled granulocytes. J. Lab. Clin. Med. 94:246-255, 1979.
17. Goodwin D.A., R.A. Finston and S.I. Smith: The distribution and dosimetry of In-111 labeled leucocytes and platelets in

humans. Proceedings Third International Dosimetry Radio-pharmaceutical Symposium, pp.88-101. Oak Ridge, 1980.
18. Sokole-Buseman E., D. Hengst and M.H. Roevekamp: Radiation dosimetry of In-111 oxinate labelled leucocytes. Symposium on blood cell labelling, pp.14-16. Nucleair Geneeskundig Bulletin I. 4 suppl., 1982.
    (Sokole-Buseman E.: Personal communication, 1982.)
19. Fueger G.F.: Personal communication, 1982.
20. Olsson P.I.: Personal communication.
21. Linhardt-Colas N., M. Meignan, B. Bok, et al: In vivo kinetics of 99m-technetium labelled leucocytes in dogs and the effects of an abscess. Biomedicine 32:133-139, 1980.
22. McAfee G.M., G.G. Subramanian, Z.D. Grossman, F.D. Thomas, M.L. Roskopf, P. Fernandes and B.J. Lyons: Distribution of leucocytes labeled with In-111 oxine in dogs with acute inflammatory lesions. J. Nucl. Med. 21:1059-1068, 1980.
23. Van Reenen O.R., M.G. Loetter, P.C. Minnaar, A.P. Heyns, P.N. Badenhorst and H. Pieters: Radiation dose from human platelet labelled with Indium-111. Br. J. Radiol. 53: 790-795, 1980.
24. Klonizakis I., A.M. Peters, M.L. Fitzpatrick, M.J. Kensett, S.M. Lewis and J.P. Lavender: Radionuclide distribution following injection of 111-indium labelled platelets. Br. J. Haematol. 46:595-602, 1980.
25. Peters A.M., I. Klonizakis, J.P. Lavender and S.M. Lewis: Use of 111-indium labelled platelets to measure spleen function. Br. J. Haematol. 46:587-593, 1980.
26. Snyder W.S., M.R. Ford, G.G. Warner and S.B. Watson: Absorbed dose per unit cumulated activity for selected radionuclides and organs, "S" (MIRD) Pamphlet No. 11, 1975.
27. ICRP publication 26. Recommendation of the International Commission on Radiological Protection. Pergamon Press, Oxford, 1977.
28. Bjurman B., L. Johansson and S. Mattsson: In-114m in In-111 radiopharmaceuticals and its contribution to the absorbed dose in the patient at investigations with In-111 labeled blood cells. Proc. Third World Congress of Nuclear Medicine and Biology, Paris, Aug.29-Sept.2, 1982, pp.2403-2406, 1982.
29. Silvester D.J.: Consequences of Indium-111 decay in vivo: Calculated absorbed radiation dose to cells labelled by Indium-111 oxine. J. Lab. Comp. Radiopharm. 16:193-194, 1979.
30. Danpure H.J. and S. Osman: Cell labelling and cell damage with indium-111 acetylacetone - an alternative to indium-111 oxine. Br. J. Radiol. 54:597-601, 1981.
31. Ten Berge R.F.M., A.T. Natarajan, S.L. Yong, et al: Labelling of human lymphocytes with In-111 oxinate. Symposium on blood cell labelling, pp.18-20. Nucleair Geneeskundig Bulletin 4, Suppl., 1982.
32. Subramanian G., J.G. McAfee, G.M. Gagne, R.W. Henderson and M. Rosenstreich: 99mTc-Oxine: A New Lipophilic Radiopharma-ceutical for Labeling Leukocytes and Platelets. Proc. 14th Internat. Meeting of the Soc. of Nucl. Med., Berlin, 1976.
33. Spitznagle L.A., C.A. Marino and S. Kasina: Lipophilic chelates of technetium-99m: Tropolone. J. Nucl. Med. 22: PB, 1981.

16 ANTIGENIC DETERMINANTS OF MIGRATORY CELLS

G.P. TILZ, H. BECKER AND G. LANZER

16.1 INTRODUCTION

This contribution describes the antigenic surface receptors of migratory cells of the body and gives an introductory overview of techniques of the analysis of such surface receptors.

Conceptually it appears desirable to radioactively label migratory cells by signal emitting antibodies directed specifically at certain surface antigens. Heterologous antibodies, however, some are potentially toxic to the recipient of the labelled cells and will have to be avoided. New techniques will be required to circumvent the problems of in-vivo immunologic reactions e.g. delayed hypersensitivity reactions.

Migratory cells are derived from stem cells (Fliedner, Chapter 3) They are comprised of the phagocytic complex and the lymphoid cells (Table 1). They share species-specific antigens and to some extent components of the human leucocyte antigen system (HLA). Furthermore, they acquire differentiation antigens and surface structures closely limited to their functions (Tables 1 and 2).

Table 1.   Migratory Cells

I.   Neutrophil granulocytes
          (polymorphonuclear phagocytic cells)

II.   Monocyte-macrophage complex
          (the mononuclear phagocytic system)

III.   Lymphocytes
          (mononuclear secretory system)

Fueger, G.F. (ed.), Blood Cells in Nuclear Medicine, Part II. ISBN 089838-654-3
©*1984 Martinus Nijhoff Publishers, Boston/The Hague/Dordrecht/Lancaster − Printed in the Netherlands*

Table 2.   The Mononuclear Phagocytic System

Cells   Localisation

Precursor cells   Bone marrow

Promonocytes   Bone marrow

Monocytes   Bone marrow, blood

Macrophages   Connective
                      tissue: histiocytes
                      Liver: "Kupffer cells"
                      Lung: alveolar macrophages
                      Spleen: free and fixed macro-
                                     phages
                      Lymph node: free and fixed macro-
                                     phages
                      Bone marrow: macrophages
                      Serous
                      cavities: pleural and peri-
                                     toneal macrophages
                      Bone tissue: osteoclasts?
                      Nervous
                      system: microglial cells?

16.2 MATERIAL AND METHODS

Animal models such as thymectomized mice, bursectomized chickens, repopulation and transfer experiments, and finally the human pathology of aplastic anaemia (A.A.) or severe combined immunodeficiency (SCID) have increased our understanding of the structure, function and markers of migratory cells (Tables 3, 4a and 4b).

Table 3.   Some Receptors or Antigens Used in General
            for the Detection of Migratory Cells

No.	Receptor Antigen	Detection	Method	T cells	B cells	L cells	M cells	other
1	Slg	anti IgG	IF	−	+	+*	+*	Polys
		IgM	Cytox		+			some
		IgD	Autoradio		+			T
2	C(3)	EAC-mouse	Rosettes					Polys
		AG-AB	Radiola-	−	+	−	+	some
			belling					T
		linked C(3)			(+)			+ RBC
3	Fc	EA (7S)	Rosettes	−	+/−	+TR	+	Polys
		Agg.IgG	IF	−	+/−	+	+	some
		AG-AB	Radiola-					T
			belled IgG	−	+/−	+	+	
4	T	E	Rosettes	+	−	−	−	
	HUTLA	anti-T	IF					
		anti-Thym.	Cytox	+	−	−	−	
		anti-brain						
		Mc-AB						
	Hu BLA	anti-B	IF	−	+	−	−	
	DR	anti-DR	Cytox					

*)   not incorporated in the cell membrane
**)   as part of the 0-cells

Table 4a.   Distribution of C-Receptors on
               Human Peripheral Blood Cells

Cell	C-Receptor						
	Clq	C3a	C3b-C4b	C3bi	C3d	C5a	C5b
T cell	−	−	−	−	−	−	−
B cell	+	−	+	−	+	−	+
Basophilic cell	−	+	?	−	−	+	−
Eosinophilic cell	−	+	+	−	+	+	−
Macrophage	−	?	+	+	+	?	−
Polys	−	+	+	+	+	+	?
Platelets	+	−	−	−	−	−	−
RBC	−	−	+	−	−	−	−

Table 4b.   Distribution of Fc-Receptors and Certain Biological
               Properties   of   Human   Peripheral   Blood   Cells

Cell	Fc-Receptor				Biology	
	IgG	IgM	IgA	IgE	Phagocyt.	Killing
T cell	+	+	+	+	−	+
B cell	+	+	+	+	−	
Basophilic cell	+	−	−	+	−	−
Eosinophilic cell	+	−	−	?	+	+
Macrophage	+	−	−	−	+	+
Polys	+	−	+	−	+	+
Platelets	+	−	−	−	−	−
RBC	−	−	−	−	−	−

326

Table 5.　　　　Evidence　of　A　Certain　Overlap　of
Antigenic Determinants of Migratory Cells

```
|---------------|----|----|----|----|----|----|----|----|----|----|
|   B-cells     |                                                    |
|               |                                                    |
|   FC(+)       |   2-18%                                            |
|               |--------|                                           |
|   CR          | 16-25%                                            |
|               |----------|                                         |
|   SIg(+)      |  8-20%                                             |
|               |--------|                                           |
|---------------|----------------------------------------------------|
|   T-cells     |                                                    |
|   E(+)        |                            50-75%                 |
|               |           |----------------------------------------|
|      T(+)     |                            60-80%                 |
|               |             |--------------------------------------|
|---------------|----------------------------------------------------|
|   L-cells     |                                                    |
|               |                                                    |
|   SIg(-)      |                                                    |
|   Fc  (+)     |                                                    |
|   E   (-)     |  5-33%                                            |
|               |----------------|                                  |
|---------------|----------------------------------------------------|
|   M-cells     |                                                    |
|               |                                                    |
|               |  - 5%                                             |
|               |---|                                               |
|---------------|----------------------------------------------------|
| "Null-cells"  |                                                    |
|               |                                                    |
|               |  - 3%                                             |
|               |--|                                                |
|---------------|----|----|----|----|----|----|----|----|----|----|
```

The introduction of heterologous antisera and the production of monoclonal antibodies have given access to knowledge of the behaviour of migratory cells under different physiological and pathological conditions.

With these antisera, immunofluorescence, cytotoxicity, radio- and enzyme-labelling are the methods of choice to characterize these cells in terms of surface antigens. However, cross-reactions, common receptors on different cell types and sharing of antigenic determinants are limiting factors to this approach. (Table 5).

Another way of characterizing some of the migratory cells consists of the incorporation of radioactive tracers followed by autoradiography of the cells or some of their molecules, when the cells have been lysed after the content has been subjected to polyacrylamid gel electrophoresis (PAGE). However, this procedure is limited to research purposes.

16.2.1 Animal experience

The following animals have been widely used in our laboratory: rabbits, guinea pigs, rats, mice, pigs, and horses. For the production of antilymphocytic globulins mice, rabbits, horses and pigs have been used. For so-called tumour-associated and membrane-associated antigens mice, rabbits and one horse have been used.

Injection: For many procedures rabbits can be handled very conveniently. Intraperitoneal, intramuscular injections or application of the antigen suspension through the ear veins have been used. For basic experiments or pilot studies, mice are the animals of choice. This is particularly true for the production of monoclonal antibodies.

Mice: The ALB-C-mice are the strain of choice used by us for these experiments. Mice are injected intraperitoneally and bled by orbital plexus puncture or heart puncture.

It is more complicated to use pigs. Piglets are used by us

between the fourth and sixth week of life and sacrificed after the third month. The reason for this is that the subcutaneous fat becomes very important and the activity of the grown animals makes the handling difficult. Injections into these piglets have been carried out behind the ear since the subcutaneous fat is negligible at that site. For horses, the intravenous route through the jugular vein has been used and is recommended by us as the method of choice. Bleeding is carried out again by puncturing the jugular vein. For guinea pigs, considerable practice is needed for puncturing the veins. It is worth trying to find the jugular route in an anaesthetized animal. Intracardial injection has a high mortality.

16.2.2   Selection of antigens and concentration

Proteous antigens, such as tumour associated factors or membrane isolated proteous antigens, are purified and selected after chromatographic or electrophoretic analysis or differential centrifugation. Crude precipitation can be carried out as a first step by ammoniumsulphate precipitation at 33% concentration. For IgG isolation, the DEAE-cellulose procedure is widely used, and for IgM preparation, gel filtration on Sephadex G 200 is the method used in our laboratory. Column or batchwise application of the gel is used depending on the quantity we needed.

For the preparation of high affinity antibodies, affinity chromatography is used. For this purpose we usually carry out a glutaraldehyde-fixation of the proteous antigen and split the absorbed antibody by acid buffers pH 2.8 to pH 3.2 with glycine buffer. Another method we use is the cyanide-bromide-sepharase (CNBr method) with the dissociation of the antigen antibody complexes with propionic acid.

For immunization several milligrams of proteous antigens or $5.0 \times 10E06$ to $10E07$ cells are used, depending on the type of antigen and primary or secondary response. Once we have found a good antiserum, the specificity is checked by cytotoxicity, agglutination, precipitation, and later, immunoelectrophoresis and immunofluorescence. The necessary absorptions are carried out with insolublized antigens. The necessary exchange dialysis and concentration is carried out in dialysis bags and Amicon ultrafiltration chambers. Optical analysis of the antibody solutions is carried out in our laboratory on a Zeiss spectrophotometer at 280 nm. Special attention is paid to stability, quality, and sufficient quantities before starting clinical diagnostic trials. As far as monoclonal antibodies are concerned, our laboratory procedure is given in detail below.

16.2.3 Cell hybridization

The principle of the technique is that particularly long-lived myeloma cells from the mouse are fused with sensitized lymphocytes (1). The resulting cell hybrids combine the qualities of both, namely longevity and sensitization, and produce a monoclonal antibody with a very narrow and high specificity. Immunized spleen cells are fused to NS-1-myeloma cells in the presence of PEG or Sendai-virus. In our laboratory, PEG is used alone. The myelomatous cell line NS-1 which is defective in the enzyme hypoxanthine-guanine-phosphoribosyl-transpherase (HGPRT) will not survive in tissue culture supplemented with hypoxanthine, aminopterin and thymidine (HAT). Aminopterin blocks the pathway for DNA synthesis. The outcome depends on the presence of the above mentioned enzyme. Non-fused cells will die in a tissue culture medium, only hybrids survive in a HAT-selective medium, since the myeloma contribute the growth potential, and the spleen cells the necessary enzyme HGPRT to overcome the aminopterin-block. Apart from NS-1 cells, the HGPRT-defective X-63-cells can be used.

16.2.3.1 Material -

Earle's balanced salt solution, Dulbecco's minimal essential
medium (MEM) supplemented with penicillin, streptomycin (100 units
per litre), L-glutamin (4 mM), sodiumpyruvate (1 mM) and 20%
heat-inactivated horse-serum, PEG (polyethylenglycol) MW 6 000,
Sendai-virus (1 000 haemagglutinating units), 10E07 myeloma cells
NS-1 oder X-63, 10E08 spleen cells, aminopterin (to 1.74 mg 25 ml
of distilled water with 1.2 ml of 2-n NaOH). Add distilled water
to 100 ml and neutralize slowly with 0.2 ml of 2-n HCl. This
yields a 100-fold concentrate. Hypoxanthine (100 x)
136.1 mg/100 ml: heat at 45 deg.C for 1 hour to dissolve.
Thymidine (100 x) 38.7 mg/100 ml; further equipment: microtitre
plates, wet incubator (CO-2, 37 deg.C)

The procedure of cell hybridization is respresented in the
following flow sheet (Table 6).

16.2.3.2 General results of cell hybridization -

Successful cell hybridization results in 30 to 60 hybrids of
which 40 to 60% produce new immunoglobulins of the IgM or IgG
classes, and 10% have a specificity for the antigen used for
immunization. Many antigens and cell lines have been used for the
immunization of mice and for the production of monoclonal
antibodies including T cells, tumour associated factors, leukemia
antigens, hormones, haptens and others. Successful fusions were
obtained in syngeneic, allogenic and xenogenic combination. The
advantage of using monoclonal antibodies lies in easier
standardization and reproducibility, by keeping the cells in
permanent lines, in tumours in mice and tissue cultures.

Table 6.   Flowsheet for the Production of Monoclonal Antibodies
----

Myeloma cells (NS I)   Sensitized spleen cells (Balbc)
                                                 in suspension
        count   count
Centrifuge (200g), 10 min   Centrifuge (200g), 10 min
     10E07 cells   10E08 cells

                        Ratio 1:1 - 1:10
                        (not very critical)

                Pool, centrifuge (200g), 5 min
        Add 1 ml drop by drop over 1 min PEG 50% in medium
                    (Water box, 37 deg.C)

        Resuspend after 1 min in medium without serum

        Centrifuge, resuspend in HAT + 10% FCS

                Plate in 100 ul/well

        Add feeder layers (1 mouse Balbc - 1 plate)
                Feed every 4-5 days
                Medium with HAT + FcS x 3
        but the third time (about day 10)
        no aminopterin byt thymidin + hypoxanthin
                than medium without HT
                day 14 - 20 -- assay
                    (RIA or IF or EIA)

                        Hybrids?
            Yes   No

        Continue feeding   Start again

Transfer cells in 24 well-plate, put
feeders, 1 mouse, 1 plate, wait 1 week,
change, wait another week, check clone:
good clones: 96 well plate + feeders,
wait, feed, assay again, choose best
well, go back to 24 well plate + feeders,
wait, assay and clone again.
Reclone if negative cells are on 96 well
plate, but no cloning if all 96 wells are
positive after one goes to flasks
Another possibility is to dilute 100 ul
from the 24 well plate in doubling
dilutions instead of putting back in 96
well plate.
Add feeders, assay first 2 rows
Go to 24 row well, assay and grow up in
mice Balbc (primed with 0.5 ml Pristane),
store, harvest, and freeze.

By this method, P. Beverley and Tilz (2) have studied extensively monoclonal antibodies e.g. Ly-1 and others. This Ly-1 reacts with early differentiation antigens of cells of the myeloid and lymphoid cell line. This marker helped us and still serves as a reference if an anaplastic tumour or undifferentiated carcinoma is to be differentiated from any type of malignant lymphoma. By this means, we could find a way of detecting and differentiating a metastasis from an anaplastic bronchial carcinoma which has been treated as a lymphoma previously in one case.

We possess a true battery of ten monoclonal antibodies to complete the diagnosis of antigenic determinants of migratory cells of the peripheral blood and bone marrow. Many tests, however, still use conventional techniques and reagents, e.g. from immunization of animals, bleeding, purification of gamma-globulins, preparation of F(ab')2 fragments and binding of different sorts of indicators, such as fluorescent dyes to the gamma-globulin.

16.2.4   Immunofluorescence (IF)

In the early 1940s, Coons described the coupling of fluorescent immunoglobulins. Reagents with high activity and specificity are critical for immunofluorescence. Many of the reagents are commercially available, nevertheless, the production of the investigator's own immunreactive preparations is a prerequisite for research and development in any laboratory. We have carried out at least a 10 000 immunofluorescence assays. We focus immediately on the purification of gamma-globulin without referring to immune adsorbent columns, as it has been done by CNBr-activated sepharose or the glutaraldehyde system of Avrameas (3).

The immunoglobulin fraction of an antiserum is prepared in our laboratory by precipitation with ammonium sulphate, followed by an anion-exchange chromotography. The antiserum is diluted in phosphate buffered saline (PBS) and cooled down. A volume of 3.2 M ammonium sulphate, equal to the volume of diluted serum is added drop by drop with consequent stirring. The final concentration will be 1.6 M corresponding to 33% saturation in the cool. The mixture is stirred for 30 minutes and centrifuged at 5 000 g for 20 minutes. We dissolve the pellet in PBS to the original volume and repeat the procedure twice, dialyse against 0.01 M phosphate buffer pH 7.5, and removed the denatured precipitate before applying the solution to the anion-exchange column. DEAE cellulose (0.6-0.7 milliequivalent per gram) is washed twice with the same buffer and the sediment packed into a column. The rough amount of cellulose used is approximately 1 g dry weight per 2 ml antiserum (starting volume). The gamma-globulin solution is loaded onto the column and the elution started after having connected the column with a through-flow photometer (UVICORD II from LKB). The outflow is connected with a fraction collector (Ultrorak) and 2-10 ml amounts are collected depending on the size of the column. The first peak represents the more basic IgG (gamma-globulin) which is followed by a second peak, if 0.01 M phosphate, and 0.05 M NaCl (pH 7.5) is used as an eluent. The two fractions are used isotonically, which can be done either by dialysis or the addition of concentrated (10 x) PBS. Again, we can concentrate by pressure dialysis (Amicon) or simple dialysis tubes. For the production of antilymphocytic globulin, very large amounts of fractionated gamma-globulins have to be concentrated. For this purpose we used a dialysis machine from our kidney unit. According to our experience, antibody activities almost equal the distribution of IgG fractions. Nevertheless, one should check before, since exceptions may occur.

When the Fc-portion of immunoglobulin might interfere with receptors of cells, we prepare our antibody fragments according to Nisonoff: The immunoglobulin preparation is dialysed against 0.1 M acetate buffer at pH 4.3. Crystalline pepsin at a gamma-globulin to pepsin ratio of 50 : 1 is added, and the pH checked. Then we leave the mixture at 37 deg.C for approximately 12 hours and cool it down. After having removed the denatured protein, we adjust the pH to 8 with 1-M NaOH in order to inactivate the pepsin, then we dialyse against PBS or concentrate with ammonium sulphate (see above), spin 30 minutes at 5 000 g, and dissolve in PBS. After having removed the sulphate ions, the preparation is checked for purity by anti-Fab or anti-Fc sera. If the digestion is incomplete, further digestion has to be carried out, or the native IgG molecule removed by gel-filtration (Sephadex 150).

According to our experience, rabbit immunoglobulin is completely digested to F(ab')2, which is not the case with sheep immunoglobulin. We have no experience with mouse immunoglobulins, but differences seem to exist from one subclass to another. Hence, we prefer rabbit, antimouse, F(ab')2 as a second layer in our immunofluorescence assays, especially as monoclonal antibodies are in the first layer of the sandwich.

Again, monovalent Fab prime fragments can be obtained from pepsin fragments by reduction and alkalisation. We have no personal experience, but in principle a reducing agent such as mercaptoethanolamine-HCl is added to a final concentration of about 0.01-0.015 M. The mixtures are incubated for 1-2 hours at 37 deg.C and stopped by iodoacetamide. In a final concentration of 0.022-0.036 M the mixtures are dialysed, concentrated and ready for use.

For conjugation we rely on our own experience with fluorescent-iso-thio-cyanate (FITC) and tritium-iso-thio-cyanate (TRITC), admitting that in the meantime new fluorescent dyes have become available, such as Texas red and others, not yet introduced in our laboratory. The protein concentration is about 5 mg/ml with the addition of 12.5 ug FITC or 15 ug TRITC per mg protein. The fragments are conjugated at lower fluorochrome concentrations, such as 10 ug fluorochrome per mg of protein or less. The required amount of fluorochrome is dissolved in 50 to 100 ul of 0.1 M bicarbonate buffer and the protein solution (ca. 2.5 ml) equilibrated with 0.1 M bicarbonate to reach a pH of 9. Then, the protein solution is added drop by drop to the fluorochrome; permanent stirring and low temperature (cool room) are necessary. We leave the mixture over night, centrifuge or dialyse and continue with purification and quality control. For purification, column chromatography on Sephadex G 500 (fine) with 0.01 M phosphate buffer pH 7.5 can be used. The alternative is dialysis and concentration. The gel filtration should be done by applying a flow-through photometer and a fraction collection device. Again, further purification on a DEAE column (0.01 M phosphate buffer pH 7.5, increasing concentration (0.2, 0.3, 0.4 M in NaCl) might be necessary.

Fractions with low salt concentration are generally hypo-conjugated. Fractions with a "normal conjugation" are eluted with NaCl solutions as concentrated as 0.4 M.

The protein concentration and the fluorochrome to protein ratio are critical and are calculated by the optical density at 280 nm and 495 nm for FITC. The calculation is carried out according to the following formula:

$$\text{protein concentration in mg/ml (FITC)} = \frac{A\,280 - (0.35 \times A\,495)}{1.4}$$

$$\text{Molar ratio FITC/ITG} = \frac{2.87 \times A\,495}{A\,280 - (0.35 \times A\,495)}$$

More detailed information regarding TRITC is available from the excellent textbook by Wick (4).

Conjugates are adjusted to a protein concentration of 0.5 mg/ml or may be used at even lower concentrations, particularly with purified high affinity antibodies. We sterilize by millipore filters, divide into aliquots, and store either at 4 deg.C or deep-freeze to lower temperatures.

For use, samples with a molar ratio of less than 1, are not good reagents, since the antibodies are not sufficiently labelled. Conjugates with a molar ratio of 2-3 are the reagents of choice in our hands if FITC is used; non-specific staining can result if rhodamine is used. The best way of quality control is a series of investigations on cells or frozen sections. Chess-board type titrations are highly recommended. If a very homogeneous distribution of the colour is obtained, it is a further indication of the non-specificity of the reagent prepared. Immuno-precipitation and haemagglutination are not sufficient to control the specificity of the antibodies used for immuno-fluorescence. Stainings for the detection of the capping-phenomenon on viable cells are particularly suited to indicate the specificity of the reagents obtained, if antigens of lymphoid cells are used to make the antibodies.

In our laboratory, membrane antigens of living cells are stained. 10-20 x 10E06 cells/ml are used, and immunofluorescence is done in the sandwich system in order to obtain satisfactory results. If, however, reagents and cells are of limited availability or expensive, we use a new micro-system with good results. Direct staining is carried out by using 50 ul of cell suspension and mixing with 10-50 ul of conjugated antiserum. After an incubation period of 20 minutes, the cells are washed 3-5 times in the cold, or eventually centrifuged against an albumin gradient to remove unbound fluorescence. Double staining is carried out under the same conditions, excepting the addition of a second layer after the last wash of the first labelling step. Further washing is needed after the incubation. For the capping-phenomenon cells are incubated for 20 minutes, and thereafter 1 ml of medium without sodium azide is added. The cells are incubated for 10 further minutes in the incubator, cooled down with 3-5 ml of medium containing sodium azide and washed. Thereafter a second staining is carried out with a marker characterized by a different fluorochrome. Every washing step has to be done at 4 deg.C and in the presence of sodium azide.

Difficulties with receptor bearing lymphocytes have been encountered when non-specific attachment or Fc-receptor dependent attachment of the labelled antibodies interfered. Under these conditions, the exposure of cells to F(ab')2 fragments or the application of a hapten-antihapten system can be helpful. After labelling, cells are resuspended in a phosphate buffered glycerol and placed on a slide, covered with a cover-slip or put into a micro-chamber as it is in current use in our laboratory. Fixation is also possible after drying the cell suspension. They are fixed in ethanol, re-hydrated in PBS, and mounted in glycerol. They can be kept ready for observation for several days. If an intracytoplasmatic antigen is relevant to detection, cells have to be fixed in order to allow antibodies to penetrate. Cytocentrifuged smears for ordinary bone marrow smears are also used. The cells are air-dried and fixed in ethanol-acidic acid (5%, 10 minutes), and washed 3-5 times in PBS. Thereafter, the antibody is added on the wet smear, and the preparation is incubated at room temperature, preventing desiccation. After labelling and further washing, (direct and indirect systems are suitable), the cells or cryostate sections are observed in a UV-microscope. Double staining is possible in a single step with a mixture of two reagents. Interferences between each other must be excluded beforehand.

A combination of both systems, namely the detection of intracytoplasmatic and membrane associated antigens can be done by labelling first the vital cells with a membrane-reactive antibody, and then fixing the cells and carrying out the second labelling procedure as mentioned above.

Rabbit immunoglobulins do not label so well with fluorochromes in comparison with sheep and goats. This is particularly the case if FITC-labelling is necessary, since FITC requires heavy labelling of the IgG-molecule.

For problems concerning theory, quantification, microscopy and other applications, the reader is referred to the textbook by Wick (4), for the preparation of antisera and purified antibodies to Weir's handbook (5), or Vorlaender (6).

16.2.5 Histocombatibility antigens

The labelling of specific membrane antigens on human migratory cells requires their differentiation from ubiquitous histocombatibility antigens. These can be detected by several techniques. In our laboratory the complement dependent cytotoxicity assay, as it has been described by Terasaki (7), and which has become the standard technique (NIH-2-step-technique), is the method of choice. Further details are given below: Human lymphocytes are separated from defibrinated blood after a density gradient centrifugation. The separated lymphocytes are incubated in standard trays with typing sera. These sera, obtained from patients after having rejected a kidney, or multiparous women, are distributed in 1 ml amounts. 2 000 cells are added to these trays and the mixture is incubated for 30 minutes. Thereafter, complement is added (5 ul), and another 60 minutes incubation period is added. Then, the mixture is decanted, and an indicator dye, such as eosin, at 5% concentration, is added. Dead cells indicate a positive cytotoxic reaction and appear in an inverted phase contrast microscope as dark or almost invisible ghosts, according to the intensity of the reaction. Negative reactions show the brilliant vital cells.

For the sake of convenience, repeating dispensors have been developed. This is also the case for automatic pipetting devices and oil-applicators, since all reactions have to be carried out under mineral oil in order to prevent evaporation. The results are given according to the A-, B-, or C-locus, and are of particular interest for all questions of transplantation, genetics, linkage, family studies and forensic problems. Monoclonal antibodies have been recently introduced into tissue typing. They are, however, limited, not only regarding the number of antigens, but they often seem to define a narrow part of the molecule. Hence, for the next few years, allo-antisera will remain the reagent of choice for the questions mentioned. The use of complement is critical; we normally use pooled and absorbed rabbit serum as a source of complement. However, the application of very large pools without absorptions is advisable, and has become standard in major transplantation centres.

For B cell antigens, the so-called D-related or DR-locus, another system is needed. DR-antigens are tested on B lymphocytes, hence the need for particular characterization of these cells in the test system used. B lymphocytes are a minor population in the normal peripheral blood and may be as low as 6-12%. This necessitates a modification of the cytotoxicity

assay, since 6-12% of dead cells could be indistinguishable from
the background of the assay. Another problem is, that human
antisera very often contain antibodies against A-,B-, and
C-antigens besides DR-antigens. This can be overcome by
absorptions with platelets which contain ABC-antigens, but not DR.
In our laboratory we use two systems: the double fluorescence
assay according to Van Root, and the various French systems which
rely on the isolation of B lymphocytes with consequent
cytotoxicity assay. B cells may adhere to nylon fibres and may be
washed out after the elimination of T cells through columns. The
purity of the assay has to be checked by a control system which
relies on fluorescent labelling of surface membrane
immunoglobulins. Another possibility is to attach B lymphocytes
on Petri-dishes covered with goat anti-immunoglobulin, and to
apply a separation buffer afterwards, to remove the attached
B lymphocytes. This system is particularly suitable, reliable and
rapid and can be easily standardized. Good immunological
reagents, however, are necessary.

Particular attention should be paid to complement in
B lymphocyte assays: B lymphocytes are very sensitive to rabbit
complement, and the source of complement has to be checked
beforehand, in order to prevent non-specific killing of
B lymphocytes, and hence missing DR-antigens.

16.2.6 Rosette forming cells (Figure 1)

By the use of the rosetting procedure T and B cells may be
differentiated and separated quantitatively and qualitatively for
further assays, such as DR-typing. Also, receptors, such as the
Fc-receptor, or complement-receptor, and others, can be determined
by the rosetting procedure. The sedimentation is a function of
the number of erythrocytes bound to the rosetting cell. Of
course, the cell itself may influence the rosetting procedure and
the sedimentation. For simple T cell assays, PBS will suffice to
carry out all the manipulations. However, if the method has to be

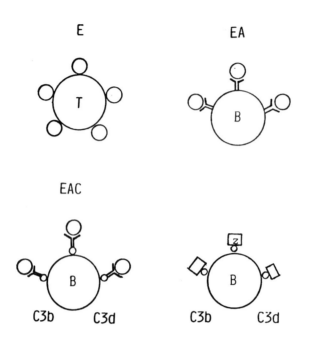

Fig. 1. Presentation of 3 Types of Rosettes and the Zymosan Reaction for the Characterization of Lymphocyte Population:

T cells react at 4 deg.C with sheep RBC and form E-rosettes. The Fc-receptor on B cells can be detected by IgG bound to indicator-RBC (EA). The complement-receptor can be characterized by the addition of complement to RBC + antibody (AB). In order to avoid interference with the Fc-receptor, IgM and complement with low agglutinating and lysing properties are used. This problem can be circumvented by using dextran pearls with additional zymosan + complement (15).

standardized and optimized, the use of buffer solutions and media is advisable. Eagle's minimal essential medium (MEM) buffered with TRIS-buffer is widely used, according to the following composition, yielding two liters:

Solution I: 120 g TRIS reagent, 17 g Na-2-H-PO-4 x 2 g H-2-O, 0.2 g phenol red.
Solution II: 4.92 g MgSO-4 x 7 g H-2-O, 5.8 g CaCl-2 x 2 g H-2-O.
Solution g III: 140 g NaCl, 9 g KCl.

The final solution is composed of equal volumes of solutions I, II, and III. Sodium azide (1%), furthermore, neuraminidase treatment is used in some experiments:
8.0-10.0 x 10E08 sheep erythrocytes (SRBC) are incubated in a solution of neuraminidase (50 units/ml in PBS, pH 7.4, 30 minutes, 37 deg.C). Cells are washed three times in 10 ml of MEM and rosette forming cells are added, consequently. SRBC are stored in our Alsever-solution. We normally use the cells on days 1-3 after the bleeding of the animal.

Many variables can alter the morphology of rosette forming cells (RFC). In our laboratory we use both a macro- and a micro-technique, details of which are given below. For the macro technique, rosettes are made in MEM with no serum present. 8.0 x 10E07 nucleated cells are mixed in 2 ml of MEM with 8.0 x 10E08 SRBC. The ratio of 10 : 21 for SRBC to nucleated cells has been found to be optimal. In some experiments, SRBC with neuraminidase treatment before rosette formation increased the sensitivity of the technique. The cell suspension is centrifuged at 4 deg.C in a 15 ml tube at 100 g for 6 minutes. The pellet at the bottom is incubated at 4 deg.C at least for 1 hour or over night, then gently resuspended by pipetting the suspension in a Burker-chamber.

For the micro-technique, 2 ul of lymphocytes at a concentration of 4 000 per ml are added to 2 ul of SRBC in a micro-tray as used for tissue typing. 2 ul of an albumin solution (2%) are added, and the system is incubated, as mentioned above. After the incubation period, 2 ul of a 1% glutaraldehyde solution is added, and the cells are incubated for another 30 minutes at 4 deg.C. Thereafter, the cells are transferred to another tray and diluted in buffered saline (1 ul of cell suspension and 2-3 ul of PBS). The cells are counted in an inverted microscope. As opposed to this T cell rosetting procedure, EA-rosettes and EAC-rosettes can be done, e.g. for B cell typing. EA means: erythrocytes + antibody, EAC stands for: erythrocytes + antibody + complement.

The former assays are particularly suitable if the Fc-receptor is required to be the site of reaction. EAC is used when the complement receptor has to be analyzed. The distribution of the various receptors on peripheral blood lymphocytes of humans is listed in Tables 3-5, in order to facilitate the selection of the appropriate assay for the characterization and quantification of migratory cells.

Another system of rosetting is obtained by the use of protein A: To detect cell surface antigens, one requires an antibody specific for the antigen. Having this antibody, one can label it with a fluorochrome, a radioisotope, carry out cytotoxic assays with complement, or carry out another rosetting system by binding this antibody to a carrier cell. This cell, again, can be a red blood cell, as it has been done, and brought to a unique sensitivity by Coombs (8). Another method is to attach protein A to the surface of red blood cells. This protein A has the unique property of binding specifically to the Fc-portion of immunoglobulin G. Hence, the antigen bearing cell can easily be seen in the microscope as a rosette. In detail, protein A is coupled to SRBC by the glutaraldehyde method or the chromium-chloride method. After an incubation period of approximately 4 minutes, the coupling procedure is stopped by adding 50 volumes of PBS. The coupled cells are washed and adjusted to a final concentration of 0.5% and stored until use. With this reagent, peripheral blood lymphocytes, and cultured cells are suitable for a rosetting procedure. Furthermore, the reagent can be applied for frozen sections with the disadvantage of interference with the detailed morphological structure. Antisera against cell surface antigens have to be applied at an optimal dilution. About 50 ul of cell suspension are mixed with the antiserum, washed, and added to the indicator SRBC, bound to protein A. The incubation mixture is centrifuged and left at 4 deg.C over night. Thereafter, the pellet is resuspended and put in a counting chamber. It has to be ascertained that the cells are still viable, since non-viable cells quite often do not rosette. The antiserum has to be an IgG, since IgM molecules do not react with protein A. With these reservations, the test is very suitable for some aspects of lymphoma typing the combination with autoradiography for the examination of surface antigens of dividing cells, or the isolation of cells bearing a given surface antigen. Again, the system is suitable for the development of a histocompatibility assay for DR-typing.

16.2.7   Separation of B lymphocytes on Petri-dishes

This technique is based on the binding of B cells on immunoglobulins fixed to a plastic surface. Passive absorption of antibodies or the fixation of these antibodies in gelatine are both possible. Batchelor (9) at the Hammersmith Hospital prefers the former technique, which is very simple, reliable, and suitable for the isolation of B lymphocytes for tissue typing. Another possibility is to use gelatine cells as the matrix. This allows the recovery of bound cells by melting the adsorbant. Melting of 10% gelatine occurs at physiological temperatures. Antibodies and haptenes can be coupled to gelatine without affecting the layer itself. Gelatine may be obtained from gelatine capsules. The concentration can be calculated from the light extinction at 215 nm, using an extinction coefficient of 17.5. Gelatine or haptene mixtures with gelatines are heated to 40 deg.C, and pipetted into sterile Petri-dishes. The dishes are incubated 5 minutes with 5 ml of glycine buffer (pH 2.2-2.5), and washed several times in the cool. Extensive washing procedures are essential to remove any gelatine from dishes which are not incorporated into the gel. If a cross-linking is necessary, the dishes are rinsed with a 2.5% solution of glutaraldehhyde (3). The glutaraldehyde is removed after 10 minutes, and the dishes are washed again with glycine buffer. Cells from the peripheral blood are added to these dishes and moved periodically or by means of a shaker. 10E08 lymphoid cells in a volume of 3-5 ml can be separated per dish (ca.3 cm diameter). 60 minutes of incubation period are sufficient. After 15 minutes already the greater part of the desired cells are fixed. The recovery of the non-fixed cells is good, provided that the immuno-adsorbant gelatine is not overloaded. After several washes a dissociation buffer at 37 deg.C is added. The gel melts, and the binding cell population is suspended in the medium. The cells are transferred into tubes, and used for further experiments. Adherent gelatine may be removed from the cell surface after the treatment with trypsine or collagenase. The use of highly purified collagenase is recommendable.

Specific B cells can be obtained by this technique. Furthermore, the technique is very useful for the isolation of B lymphocytes, if an anti-immunoglobulin is used in the immobilized phase.

16.2.8   Immuno-assay for monoclonal antibodies

Radioimmuno-assay and enzyme-immuno-assay are suitable for the indications given. Immunofluorescence can also be used, however, it is only suitable for laboratories with a smaller production of monoclonal antibodies. For the sake of completeness, some indications on the enzyme-linked immuno-assays are given: Antigen is immobilized on a plastic surface, and a supernatant from the medium from hybridoma cultures or from the ascites is added. The binding of the antibody is detected by a second layer with specificity for the monoclonal reagent linked to an enzyme or radioactivity. Both possibilities are used for the absorption of antigens: Protein can be absorbed non-specifically to plastics, or immobilized in gelatine gels, as mentioned above.

For antibodies against surface structures of cells, the screening is carried out on viable culture, peripheral blood, or fixed cells. Again, the cells can be fixed on a solid phase, and, in principle, an immuno-adsorbant test follows the initial step. Affinity-purified rabbit anti-mouse IgG can be made easily in every laboratory, according to the procedures given above. For immunization, up to 1 mg of mouse-IgG's are injected in weekly intervals with complete Freund's adjuvant into rabbits. The antiserum is purified by fractionation, and affinity purification, and bound to alkaline phosphatase, peroxydase or glucose-oxydase, according to the various laboratories' possibilities. In principle, we couple the purified enzyme with the affinity-purified antibody by glutaraldehyde (3). We dialyse and stabilize with bovine serum albumin. Target cells can be used in suspension, or attached to the microtitre PVC-plates by centrifugation in glutaraldehyde fixation. If, however, the cells are not tightly bound, a protein layer can be used to link this attachment. A photometer is useful for the quantification of the enzyme reaction and hence the monoclonal antibody activity. However, optical inspection will be also satisfactory for these screening purposes. Monoclonal antibodies are added to the different vials and will react with a strongly positive reaction when approximately 10E06 cells are fixed either directly or by the intermediate action of a protein matrix or a lectine layer. We also have carried experiments with microplates, as are used for tissue typing, and preliminary results show the usefulness of the method, at least in some experiments. After extensive washes, the second layer is added as in immunofluorescence and washed again. Visualization or counting of radioactivity gives an indication as to the specificity of the monoclonal product obtained. This given method is suitable for soluble antigens, such as hepatitis products, or membrane-antigens on cells.

Many other techniques should be discussed, such as the Jerne-technique for plaque-forming cells, helper and suppressor cell assays, in-vitro immunization of cells (according to the Michel-Dutton-technique), micro-culture techniques for the assessment of the average clone size of the progeny of precursors, which are rare cells indeed, culture techniques for the establishment of lymphoid and tumour cell lines in-vitro semi-solid media, viral immunology for the detection of receptors, transformations and immortalization of some B cell lines, long-term culture of specific helper cells, assays for cytotoxic cells, all types of immune complex assays, the characterization of antibodies specific for various tissue antigens, and cell antigens, gel electrophoresis, ELISA-technique, and EIA-techniques. Their discussion would go beyond the scope of this chapter. For details, the reader is referred to Weir's Handbook of Experimental Immunology (5).

16.3 RESULTS OF ANTIGEN DETERMINATIONS ON MIGRATORY CELLS

The results of the distribution of antigenic determinants and receptors of migratory cells and some of the reagents used are summarized in Tables 3, 4a and 4b; additional details and exceptions to the scheme are given in Table 5.

16.3.1 Stem cells

They are discussed in the review by Fliedner (Chapter 3). No further comments are needed.

16.3.2 Monocytes (Macrophages)

We were unable to find quantitative antigenic determinants between macrophages and lymphocytes by standard techniques with heterologous antisera in the mouse. Techniques have since changed and, with monoclonal antibodies, Nancy Hogg (10) from the Imperial Cancer Research Foundation has shown that at least two types of macrophages exist in humans (Table 7).

Table 7.   Reaction of New Monoclonal Antibodies from
            the Mouse with PB Monocytes and Polymorphs

	MONOCYTES	POLYMORPHS
AG		
1	+	+
2	+	
3		+
4	Some 80 %	

These consist of a large subset of about 80-85% and a smaller
subset of cells. According to Hogg's (10) investigations, another
new classification of macrophages seems to be a realistic
assumption.   It is similar to the former classification of T and
B lymphocytes. Further differences between macrophages and
lymphocytes are summarized in Tables 3, 4a and 4b: Briefly,
macrophages have complement- and Fc-receptors and possess
surface-membrane-immunoglobulins which are not incorporated into
the cell membrane. The cells adhere to plastic and glass surfaces
(A-cells) and can easily be separated from lymphocytes by this
method. Due to the intracytoplasmic enzymes macrophages are
potent inducers of inflammatory lesions.

16.3.3 Neutrophilic granulocytes

There is no need to search for surface antigens to distinguish
these cells from their other migratory companions. Their
microscopic appearance is characteristic: They have a short life
span, are vulnerable and easier to manipulate than monocytes.
Neutrophilic granulocytes dominate quantitatively in the
peripheral blood, which enables us to label them for various

clinical questions such as imaging purposes.

Work is under way to analyse their antigens. Knapp from the Vienna Institute of Immunology, has shown the existence of antigens specific to myeloid cells. Consequently, such markers have come into use for typing leukemias and studying the development of the myeloid cell lines. Apart from these and HLA-antigens, polymorphs possess receptors for complement, IgG and IgA which enable the cells to fulfill their function, namely migration, adherence, phagocytosis and killing (Tables 3, 4a,b).

16.3.4 Eosinophilic granulocytes

They have receptors for some complement fractions and IgG. Specific antigens have not been classified on an international basis.

16.3.5 Basophilic granulocytes

The same seems to be the case with basophilic cells. They possess however a receptor of unique affinity for IgE giving the cell a central role in anaphylactic reactions. The antigenic determinants of these receptors have not been elaborated very clearly. Presumably they exist.

16.3.6 Lymphocytes

Data on lymphocytes and their antigenic determinants are extensive (Tables 8-12, Figure 2), and exceed the range of this presentation. Within the scope of the labelling of migratory (blood) cells some limitations on the data of lymphocytes have to be made.

Table 8.   Selectivity of Lymphocyte Mitogens
                for T and B cells

                                          Human
                                        T   B

Lectins:

PHA   +   ?
Con A   +   -
PWM   +   +
LPS   -   -

Other:

Anti-immunoglobulin sera   -   +
PVP   n.s.

Table 9.   Distribution of Cells in the Lymphnodes
             if Obtained with the Relevant Markers

Marker   % in the P.B.   % in the nodes

E-Receptor   65 +/- 11   45 +/- 20

C-Receptor   12 +/- 10   20 +/- 13

S.I.G.   20 +/- 8   25 +/- 13

IgG   8 +/- 6   8 +/- 6

IgA   2 +/- 2   3 +/- 2

IgM   7 +/- 4   12 +/- 9

IgD   4 +/- 3   10 +/- 9

Ig kappa   10 +/- 3   18 +/- 12

Ig lambda   8 +/- 6   12 +/- 9

Table 10.   Subpopulation of T-Lymphocytes and Their Markers

Suppressors T(s)	Helpers T(h)
Fc-Receptor for IgG	Fc-Receptor for IgM
essentially large lymphocytes	essentially small lymphocytes
abundant cytoplasma with mito- chondria, endoplasmatic reti- culum and Golgi-Apparatus	scarce cytoplasma with few organelles
non-specific esterases 0 - + (granular)	non-specific esterases ++ - +++ with dots
Microvilli	more smooth membranes
Phagocytoses of IgG covered RBC	no phagoocytic activity
Monoclonal antibodies e.g. 2a, OKT8, UCHT4, RFT8	Monoclonal antibodies e.g. 3a, OKT4

Beverley, Janoszy, Prentice

Table 11.   Cytochemical Differences between T, B, and M Cells

----

Enzyme	T cells	B cells	M cells
Alpha-naphtyl-butyrase (non-specific esterases)	(+)	-	+
Acid-phosphatase	(+)	-	+
Tartrate-resistant acid phosphatase	-	++	+
Muraminidase (lysozyme)	-	-	+

Table 12. Functional Characteristics of
Peripheral Human Lymphocytes

Response	Test	T cells	B cells	L cells
1. Proliferation				
PHA	blasts in the smear or incorporation of tritiated thymidine	++	(+)	–
Con A	– " –	++	(+)	–
PWM	– " –	+	++	–
Endotoxin	– " –	–	–	–
Soluble antigens (PPD, SK, SD)	– " –	+	+/–	–
Allogeneic cells	MLC: responder cells	++	+/–	–
	stimulator cells	+	++	+
	CML:	++	–	n.d.
2. Ig-production	take up of labelled amino acids	–	+	–
3. Lymphokine production	MIF	++	+	n.d.
4. Cytotoxicity on targets (killing) a) Ab-undependent = direct cyto- toxicity	cytotoxicity	++	–	–
b) Ab-dependent = ABCIL or ADCC	cytotoxicity	–	+/–	++
5. Suppression and regulation	suppression of Ig-synthesis	++	–	n.d.
	suppression of mitogens	++	–	n.d.
6. Helper function	Ig-synthesis	+	–	n.d.
7. Anamnestic response	proliferation after relevant antigen	+	+	n.d.

Fig. 2. The 5 Types of cell mediated immune reactions (15):

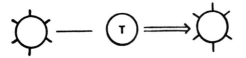

1. Histo-incompatible cells are destroyed by activated T cells.

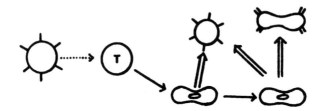

2. The activation of T cells leads to the production of further activating factors (interleukins), macrophages are activated and destroy T cells and tumour-associated cells.

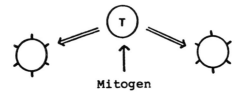

3. Non-specific activation of T cells by mitogens, and, consequently, destruction of targets related to the cells.

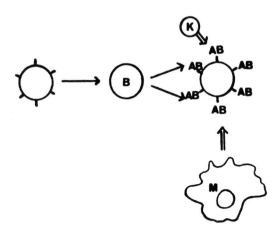

4. AB-dependent cell mediated cytolysis: antibodies adherent to the targets interfere with the Fc-receptor of killer cells. The destruction of the targets follows.

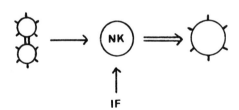

5. Natural killer (NK) cells are activated by rapidly and randomly proliferating cells and are able to respond to this stimulus. Another possibility of activating NK-cells follows Interferon.

Lymphocytes may be separated conveniently by gradient centrifugation and can be further analyzed by the E-Rosette-technique.

T gamma and T my cells may be used to separate suppressor and helper cells from each other. Another even more comfortable way of characterizing these subpopulations of cells is the use of monoclonal markers for the relevant surface antigens (Tables 13-17).

Table 13. Some Commercially Available Markers I: Their Range of Detection

---

OKT 3:	Pan:	Mature peripheral T cells
OKT 4:	Ind:	Helper inducer T
OKT 6:	Thy:	"Common thymocytes"
OKT 8:	Sup:	Suppressor cytotoxic T lymphocytes
OKM 1:		Blood monocytes + 0 cells
OKT Ia:		Human DR framework B cells, 0 cells, activated T cells

---

Table 14. Some Commercially Available Markers III: Activity on Peripheral Blood Lymphocytes

		TH (1)	TH (2)	B
OKT 8 =	Leu-2 a	20-40%		
OKT 4 =	Leu-3 a		40-60%	
OKT Ir =	DR			10-20%

Suppressor   Helper

Table 15a. Monoclonal Antibodies for Identifying
Cells of the Human Immune System

Antibody	Cellular distribution	C-fix	Clinical applications
OKT 3	greater than 95% of T lymphocytes 20% of thymocytes 30% of splenocytes	+	Identification of human peripheral T lymphocytes Pan T
OKT 4	65% of peripheral T lymphocytes 75% of thymocytes 15% of splenocytes	+	Identification of of human inducer/ helper T lymphocyte subclass
OKT 6	70% of thymocytes	-	Identification of human "common" thymocytes
OKT 8	35% of peripheral T lymphocytes 80% of thymocytes 15% of splenocytes	+	Identification of human suppresor/ cytotoxic T lymphocyte subclass
OKT 9	Reactive with pro- liferating cells in- cluding early haemato- poietic stem cells, activated lymphocytes, and many neoplastic cells	-	Identification of transferrin receptor
OKT 10	Reactive primarily with early haematopoietic stem cells, including prothymocytes, thymo- cytes and some normal monocytes, TdT cells and B cells in bone marrow, myeloblasts, promyelo- cytes, activated T and B lymphocytes and circulating null cells	-	Identification of precursor haemato- poietic cells and activated lymphocytes
OKM 1	78% of adherent mononuclear cells 18% of non-adherent mononuclear cells (null cells)	+	Identification of human monocytes, null cells, and granulocytes
OKIa 1	90% of B lymphocytes and monocytes, 20% of null cells, activated T lymphocytes	+	Identification of B lymphocytes, activated T lymphocytes, and some monocytes

Table 15b. Some Commercially Available Monoclonal
            Antibodies for Lymphocyte Typing from NEN   (11, 12)

Mc-Antibody	Specificity
Anti-human Lyt-antibody	Recognizes 87-93% of peripheral blood T lymphocytes, greater than 95% of thymocytes, T leukemias, T leukemia cell lines, and chronic lymphocytic leukemia cells. Recognizes a multimeric polypeptide complex of 65 and 67 kilodaltons. Does not react with normal B cells, B cell lines, monocytes, or bone marrow cells.
Anti-human Lyt 1 antibody	Reacts with 50-80% of peripheral blood T lymphocytes 20-50% of thymocytes, a proportion of T leukemias and T leukemia cell lines. Recognizes a single-chain polypeptide of 45 kilodaltons on helper T cells and certain killer T cells Does not react with B cells.
Cytotoxic/ suppressor T lymphocyte	Reacts with appr. one third of mature human peripheral blood T cells which includes the cytotoxic/ suppressor T cell subset. Does not bind to B cells, null cells, monocytes, or non-T cell malignancies. Blocks the activity of antigen positive cytotoxic T cells. The antigen complex recognized is composed of subunits of appr. 32 and 45 kilodaltons expressed on the surface of human cytotoxic and suppressor T cells.
Anti-human T lymphocyte antibody	Reacts with mature human T cells, but not with null cells, monocytes, B cells, nor non-T cell leukemias. Recognizes an antigen complex with subunits of approximate molecular weight of 19-29 kilodaltons expressed on all mature human T cells. Directly mitogenic to human T cells and blocks both the activity of cytotoxic T cells and and T cell proliferative responses.
Anti-human helper/ inducer T lymphocyte	Reacts with appr. 50-60% of human peripheral blood T cells, including the helper/inducer T cell subset. Recognizes an antigen with a molecular weight of 55 kilodaltons expressed upon the helper/inducer subset of human T cells.

Table 15c. Some Commercially Available Monoclonal Antibodies for Lymphocyte Typing from Becton Dickinson

Mc-Antibody	Specificity
Anti-Leu-1	pan T
Anti-Leu-2a	cytotoxic suppressor
Anti-Leu-2b Anti-Leu-3a	cytotoxic/suppressor helper/inducer
Multi-Clone (TM)	Anti-Leu-3a + Anti-Leu-3b
Anti-Leu-4	pan T, mitogenic
Anti-Leu-5	E-Rosette-Receptor
Anti-Leu-6	Thymocytes, Langerhans' cells of the epidermis
Anti-Leu-7	K/NK cells
Anti-Leu-8	80% of Leu-3 (+) cells 60% of Leu-2 (+) cells
Anti-Leu-9	pan T, T-ALL associated
Anti-Leu-10	B cells
Anti-Leu-M1	greater than 80% of circulating monocytes, greater than 95% of mature granulocytes
Anti-Leu-M2	60-95% of circulating monocytes
Anti-Leu-M3	80-95% of monocytes
Anti-Leu-M4	neutrophils
Anti-Leucocyte	HLe, pan leucocyte
Anti-HLA-DR	Ia, non-polymorphic

Table 16.   Markers   for   Leukemia   Typing

Anti TdT: Coulter, NEN, Becton, Dickinson, Ortho

"   kappa/lambda: Seward

"   Calla: Greaves, Knapp, Janoszy-Prentice,
                         Coulter

"   Pan T, E-Receptor: Beverley, OKT 11, Leu 5, Coulter 9.6,
                         Prof. Prentice, Janoszy (RF)

"   Pan T: p.20   OKT 3, BD Leu 4, UCHT 1

"   Helper: OKT 4 = Leu 3a

"   Suppressor: OKT 8 = Leu 2a = UCHT 4 RFT 8
                         Prof. Prentice + Janoszy

"   Pan B: B 1 - Coulter

"   Myeloid: Knapp, P. Beverley

"   Monocytes: UCHM 1, BD. Mac 120, Hogg

"   Erythroid,
      Glycophorin: Paul Edwards

Table 17.   Monoclonal Markers for Leukemia Typing
(non-commercial, M-seria)

This seria is completed by some commercial products.

M1 = monocytic
M2 = granulocytic
M3 = suppressor
M4 = Pan-T
M5 = Ly-1, which reacts with lymphocytes and myeloid cells,
         and is used to differentiate between undifferen-
         tiated metastases from carcinomas and lymphomas.
M6 = IA, DR
M7 = RF P2 = anti-acute lymphoplastic leukemia
M8 = antisuppressor
M9 = Calla
M10= antimacrophage marker.

These markers have been developed in P. Beverley's Laboratory
(University College Hospital, London), and in the laboratory of
Prof. Prentice and Janoszy at the Royal Free Hospital in
Hampstead, London (13).

Further commercial reagents are employed such as helper-cell
markers, light-chain reagents, and others, see Tables 13-15.

360

Some of the functional characteristics of lymphocytes are summarized in Table 8. Complement receptors are in general not present at the cell surfaces of T-lymphocytes.

B-cells carry surface membrane immunoglobulins and complement receptors (Table 9). They are active in the antibody dependent cell-mediated cytolysis (ADCC) and in fact Coombs (8) is convinced that 0-cells are part of the B-cell or M-cell pool. The data are deduced from experiments with his very sensitive technique of the mixed cell agglutination with B , 0 and M cells. A synopsis of the relevant receptors is shown in Tables 3, 4a and 4b. The name of some monoclonal markers used by us, their significance and their distribution among some of the cells in the peripheral blood are presented in Tables 13-17.

16.4 CONCLUSION

Migratory cells are a heterogeneous group of cells with some overlap of antigenic surface markers. The method of cell separation is dependent on what the Nuclear Physician wants to do with these cells, whether he needs large amounts of cells or highly purified suspensions. For analytical questions fluorochrome labelling and related techniques using monoclonal markers are most widely applied giving very satisfactory results in our hands.

For large scale preparations of small subsets more sophisticated methods such as step by step purification on gradients or the more expensive and time consuming FACS-system will be necessary.

For reprints, please write to G.P. Tilz, Med. Univ. Klinik, A-8036 Graz, LKH.

This work has been partially supported by the Austrian National Fund for Scientific Research (Fonds zur Foerderung der wissenschaftlichen Forschung, Wien).

SUMMARY

This work describes relevant antigenic determinants of migratory cells and the techniques used for their detection in our laboratory. The experiences from animal work are communicated, and the ways of antigen preparation, purification and application presented. The same applies to the purification of antibodies by simple precipitation, chromatography or immunoadsorband columns. Furthermore, the production of monoclonal antibodies is discussed and labelling techniques by fluorochromes and related stains are shown. The rosetting tests, cytotoxic assays for histocompatibility antigens complete the methods.

With these tools, antigenic determinants of migratory cells are analysed and discussed with respect to their importance and relevance to clinical standard diagnosis. A synopsis of the receptors of migratory cells completes the article.

REFERENCES

1. Koehler G. and C. Milstein: Continuous cultures of fused cells secreting antibodies of predefined specificity. Nature 256:495, 1975.
2. Tilz G.P., P. Beverley, H. Becker and G. Lanzer: Zellhybridisierung: Die Entwicklung eines monoklonalen Antikoerpers zur haematologisch-ontologischen Diagnostizierung. Acta Med. Austr. 8C:85-87, 1981.
3. Avrameas S.: Immuno-enzyme techniques: enzymes as markers for the localization of antigens and antibodies. Int. Rev. Cyt.27:349-359, 1970.
4. Wick G., S. Baudner and F. Herzog: Immunfluoreszenz, pp.89-113. Medizinische Verlagsgesellschaft, Marburg/Lahn, 1976.
5. Weir D.M.: Experimental Immunology. Vol.I, Ch.15, pp.15-1 - 15-30. Blackwell Scientific Publications, Oxford, London, Edinburgh, Melbourne, 1976.
6. Vorlaender K.O.: Immunologie. Thieme, Stuttgart, 1983.
7. Terasaki P.J., D. Bernoco, M.S. Park, G. Ozturk and Z. Iwaki: Testing for HLA-A-BC and D-Antigens. Am. J. Clin. Path. 69: 103-119, 1978.
8. Coombs R.R.A., A.B. Wilson, E. Eremi, B.W. Gurner, D.G. Haegert, Y.A. Lawson, S. Bright and A. Munro: Comparison of the direct antiglobulin reaction with the mixed antiglobulin rosetting reaction for the detection of immunoglobulins on lymphocytes. J. Immunol. Methods 18: 45-49, 1977.
9. Batchelor R.: Personal communication, 1983.
10. Hogg N. and M. Susarenko: Monoclonal antibody with specificity for monocytes and neurons. Cell 24:875-884, 1981.
11. Knapp W. (Ed.): Leukemia Marker. Academic Press, London, New York, 1981.
12. Knapp W.: Monoclonal antibodies against differentiation antigens of myelopoiesis. Blut 45:301, 1982.
13. Beverley P.: The application of monoclonal antibodies to the typing of lymphoreticular cells. Proc. Royal Soc. Edinb. 81B, p.221, 1982.
14. Tilz G.P.: Haematologische Diagnostik. In: Haematologische Diagnostik, edited by H. Begemann. Urban Schwarzenberg, Muenchen (in press).
15. Tilz G.P.: Immunohaematology. In: Klinische Haematologie, edited by H. Begeman. Thieme, Stuttgart, 1984.

FURTHER READING

1. Aisenberg A.C.: Malignant Lymphoma, N. Engl. J. Med. 288:833-941, 1976.
2. Albegger K.W. and G.P. Tilz: Der menschliche Lymphocyt und seine Oberflaeche. Arch. Oto-Rhino-Laryng. 206:319-335, 1974.
3. Albert D.E. and S. Scholtz: Das Haupthisto-kompatibilitaetssystem (HLA) des Menschen: Serologie, Genetik und Klinische Bedeutung: Immunforschung in Klinik und Labor, pp. 77-105, Wiss. Information Fresenius Stiftung, Bad Homburg, Sonderband August 1979.
4. Albrechtsen D., A. Bratlie, E. Kiss, B.G. Solheim, A.B. Thoresen, N. Winter, E. Thorsby: Significance of HLA matching in Renal Transplantation. Transplantation 28:280-284, 1979.
5. Allison A.C.: Interactions of antibodies, complement components and various cell types in immunity against viruses and pyogenic bacteria. Transplant. Rev. 19:3-55, 1974.
6. Avrameas S.: Immuno-enzyme techniques: enzymes as markers for the localization of antigens and antibodies. Int. Rev. Cyt.27:349-359, 1970.
7. Bach F.H., M.L. Bach and P.M. Sondel: Differential function of major histocompatibility complex antigens in T-lymphocyte activation. Nature 259:273-281, 1976.
8. Becker H.: Maligne Non-Hodgkin-Lymphome: Patho-morphologische Grundlagen. Hautarzt Supplement III (Retikulosen und Lymphome der Haut aus heutiger Sicht):21-29, 1978.
9. Begemann H.: Lehrbuch der klinischen Haematologie, Thieme, Stuttgart, (in press).
10. Berendt M.J. and R.J. North: T-cell mediated suppression of Anti-Tumor immunity. J. Exp. Med. 151:69-79, 1980.
11. Bjoerklund B. and J. Paulsson: Studies of hemagglutination as means for assay of malignant and normal human tissue antigens. J. Immunol. 89:759-766. 1962.
12. Bjoerklund V. and B. Bjoerklund: Localization of Synthesis of TPA in Normal Malignant Human Tissues by Immunohistological Techniques. In: Protides of the Biological Fluids, edited by H. Peeters, pp. 229-232 Pergamon Press, Oxford, 1979.
13. Blaylock W.K., W.E. Clendenning, P.P. Carbone et al.: Normal immunologic reactivity in patients with the lymphoma mycosis fungoides. Cancer 19: 233-236, 1966.
14. Block K.J. and C. Angevine: Mast cells and mast cell sensitizing antibodies. In: The Immunochemistry and Biochemistry of Connective Tissue and its Disease States, edited by J. Rotstein, Karger, Basel, 1970.
15. Braun-Falco O., G. Burg and H.H. Wolff: Kutane Lymphome und Pseudolymphome. Therapeut. Umschau 33:543-550, 1976.
16. Broder S., D. Poplack and J.-Whang-Peng: Characterization of a suppressor cell leukaemia. N. Engl. J. Med. 298:66-72, 1978.

364

17. Buffe D.,   C. Rimbaut,   D. Erard   and   G.P. Tilz: Immunosuppressive activity of alpha 2 H "Isoferritin" as compared to normal crystallized Ferritin.   Scand.   J. Immunol. 8 (Suppl. 8):633-640, 1978.
18. Burg G.:   Fortschritte der Diagnostik kutaner   Lymphome. Fortschritte der Medizin 94:1089-1098, 1976.
19. Cochrane C.G.   and D. Koffler: Immune complex disease in experimental animals and man. Advanc. Immunol. 16:185-256, 1972.
20. Coombs R.R.A.,   A.B. Wilson,   E. Eremi,   B.W. Gurner, D.G. Haegert,   Y.A. Lawson,   S. Bright   and   A. Munro: Comparison of the direct antiglobulin reaction with the mixed antiglobulin rosetting reaction for the detection of immunoglobulins on lymphocytes. J.   Immunol.   Methods 18:45-49, 1977.
21. Cooper D.A., V. Petts, E. Luckhurst, J.C. Biggs and R. Peny: T and   B cell   populations   in blood   and lymphnodes in lymphoproliferative disease.   Br.   J.   Cancer 31:550-558, 1975.
22. Cooper M.D., L. Moretta, S. Webb et al.:   Diversity of defects of B-cell differentiation. In: VII Int. Symp. Immunopathology,   edited by P.A. Miescher, PP.   343-354, Benno-Schwabe, Basel, 1977.
23. Dausset J.:   Le   complexe   HL-A.   Implication   en transplantation et en transfusion. La Nouvelle Presse Med. 22:1341-1348, 1976.
24. Dausset J.   and   J. Colombani: Histocombatibility Testing. Munksgaard, Copenhagen, 1976.
25. Dixon F.J.:   Pathogenesis of   immunologic   disease.   J. Immunol. 109:187-191, 1972.
26. Dunsford J.   and J. Grant: The anti-Globulin   (Coombs)-Test. Oliver and Boyd, Edinburgh, 1959.
27. Eijsvogel V.P.:   Lymphocyte   function testing.   In: Blood leucocytes,   functon and   use   in   therapy,   edited by C.F. Hoegmann,   K. Lindahl-Kiessling   and   H. Wigzell,   pp. 7-10, Almquist + Wiksell International, Stockholm, 1977.
28. Evans R.   and P. Alexander: Cooperation of   immune lymphoid cells   with   macrophages   in   tumor   immunity.   Nature 228:620-621, 1970.
29. Furt R., Z.A. Cohn, J.G. Hirsch, J.H. Humphrey, W.G. Spector and H.L. Langevoort: The   mononuclear phagocyte system: a new   classification of   macrophages,   monocytes   and   their precursors. Bull. Wld. Hlth. Org. 46:845-852 1972.
30. Gerard-Marchant R.,   I. Hamlin,   K. Lennert,   F. Rilke, A.G. Stansfeld   and   J.A.M. van Unnik: Classification of non-Hodgkin's Lymphomas. Lancet II: 406-408, 1974.
31. Good R.A.:   Manipulation of the immune response system.   In: Blood Leukocytes function and use in therapy, edited by C.F. Hoegman,   K. Lindahl-Kiessling   and   H. Wigzell,   pp. 87-93, Almquist + Wiksell International, Stockholm, 1977.
32. Goetze D.:   Somatische Zell-Hybridisierung: Methoden und Anwendung.   Immunforschung   in Klinik   und   Labor, pp. 5-36 Wiss. Information Fresenius Stift., Bad Homburg, Special

Edition, August 1979.

33. Greaves M.F., J.J.T. Owen and M.C. Raff: T- and B-Lymphocytes: origins, properties and roles in immune responses. American Elsevier Publishing Co. Inc., New York, 1974.
34. Greaves M.F.: Recent Progress in the Immunological Characterization of Leukaemia Cells. Blut 43:349-356, 1977.
35. Hansen J.A. and R.A. Good: Malignant disease of the lymphoid system in immunological perspective. Human Pathology 5:567-599, 1974.
36. Horwitz D.A. and M.A. Garrett: Distinctive functional properties of human blood lymphocytes: A Comparison with T-lymphocytes, B-lymphocytes and monocytes. J. Immunol. 118:1712-1719, 1977.
37. Huber C., A. Asamer and H. Huber: Zur funktionellen Differenzierung lymphatischer Zellen. Lymphocyten mit Immunglobulindeterminanten und Bindungsfaehigkeit fuer Immunkomplexe bei der Maus. Z. ges. exp. Med. 156: 34-37, 1971.
38. Huber Ch. and G. Michlmayr: Surface markers on lymphoid cells. In: Blood leukocytes, function and use in therapy, edited by C.F. Hoenigman, K. Lindahl-Kiessling and H. Wigzell, pp. 1-6, Almquist + Wiksell International, Stockholm, 1977.
39. Huhn D., P. Meister, E. Thiel, R. Bartl and H. Theml: Maligne Histiozytose. Dtsch. Med. Wschr. 103:55-61, 1978.
40. Humphrey J. and R.G. White: Kurzes Lehrbuch der Immunologie. Thieme, Stuttgart, 1971 (2.Ed. 1972).
41. Humphrey G.B. and J. Lankford: Acute leucemia: The use of surface markers in classification. Seminars in Oncology 3:243-250, 1976.
42. Jaeger L., J.H. Kersey and K.J. Gail: T- and B-lymphocytes in humans. A review. Am. J. Pathol. 81:446-457, 1975.
43. Jaeger L.: Klinische Immunologie und Allergologie (Parts I and II), VEB Fischer, Jena, 1976.
44. Knapp W.: Charakterisierung der Lymphozyten- Subpopulationen des Menschen. Dtsch. Med. Wschr. 102:802-806, 1977.
45. Kersey J.H., W. Tucker and P.D. Le Bien: Childhood leukemia-lymphoma heterogeneity of phenotypes and prognosis. Am J. Clin. Pathol. 4 (Suppl. 2) 72:746-752, Oct. 1979.
46. Lachmann P.J. and D.K. Peters: Clinical Aspects of Immunology, Vol.I., Blackwell, Oxford, 1982.
47. Lachmann P.J. and D.K. Peters: Clinical Aspects of Immunology. Vol.II. Blackwell, Oxford, 1982.
48. Lambert P.H. and R. Zuebler: La formation de complexes immuns: Roles physiologique et manifestation pathologiques. In: Transplantation and Clinical Immunology, edited by J. Jaeger, pp.10-15, Sinep, Ville Urbanne, 1977.
49. Lambert P.W. and M.B.A. Oldstone: Host immuno-globulin G and complement deposits in the choroid plexus during spontaneous immune complex diseases. Science 180:48-410, 1973.

50. Lennert K.: Klassifikation und Morphologie der Non-Hodgkin-Lymphome. In: Maligne Lymphome und monoklonale Gammopathien, edited by H. Loeffler. J.F. Lehmanns Verlag, Muenchen, 1975.
51. Lennert K., N. Mohri, H. Stein and E. Kaiserling: The histopathology of malignant lymphoma. Br. J. Haematol. (Suppl.) 31:193-203, 1975.
52. Lennert K. and H.K. Mueller-Hermelink: Lymphocyten und ihre Funktionsformen: Morphologie, Organisationsform ud funktionelle Bedeutung. Verh. Anat. Ges. 69:19-62, 1975.
53. Lerner R.A. and F.J. Dixon: The human lymphocyte as an experimental model. Scientific American 228:82-91, 1973.
54. Lukes R.J. and R.D. Collins: Immunologic characterization of human malignant lymphomas. Cancer 34 (Suppl. 4):1488-1503, 1974.
55. Masson P.L.: Dosage de complexes immuns circulants par inhibition de l'activite agglutinante du facteur rheumatoide ou du Clq sur les particules couvertes d'IgG. In: Transplantation and Clinical Immunology, edited by J. Traeger. Sinep, Ville Urbanne, 1977.
56. Mathe G., H. Rappaport, G.T. O'Conor and H. Torloni: Histological and cytological typing of neoplastic diseases of haematopoietic and lymphoid tissues. Internat. Histol. Classification of Tumors No.14, WHO, Geneva, 1976.
57. Melwicz F.M., S.L. Shore, E.W. Ades and D.J. Phillips: The mononuclear cell in human blood which mediates antibody-dependent cellular cytotoxicity to virusinfected target cells. J. Immunol. 118:567-573, 1977.
58. Miescher P.A.: Autoantibodies against thrombocytes and leucocytes. In: Textbook of Immunopathology, edited by P.A. Miescher and E. Mueller, Grune + Stratton, New York, 1978.
59. Mowbray J.F. and E.J. Burton: Clinical relevance of the determination of circulating immun complexes. In: Transplantation and Clinical Immunology, edited by J. Traeger, pp. 35-43, Sinep, Ville Urbanne, 1977.
60. Munro A. and S. Bright: Products of the major histocompatibility complex and their relationship to the immune-response. Nature 264:145-152, 1976.
61. Perlmann P.: Antibody induced K-cell mediated cytotoxicity. In: Blood leukocytes, function and use in therapy, edited by C.F. Hoegman, K. Lindahl-Kiessling and H. Wigzell, pp.22-23, Almquist + Wiksell International, Stockholm, 1977.
62. Peters D.K. and P.J. Lachmann: Immuno deficiency in pathogenesis of glomerulonephritis. Lancet I:58-60, 1974.
63. Resch K.: Das Immunsystem. Internist 18:233-247, 1977.
64. Ross G.D.: Surface markers of B and T cells. Arch. Pathol. Lab. Med. 101:337-341, 1977.
65. Ryder L.P., E. Anderson and A. Svejgaard: HLA and disease registry. (Special Edition: Tissue-Antigens, 3rd report), 60 pages, Munksgaard, Copenhagen, 1979.
66. Salfner B.: Primaere Defektimmunopathien. Internist 18:248-254, 1977.

67. Schoorl .R., A. Brutel de la Riviere, A.E.G. von dem Borne and T.M. Feltkamp-Vroom: Identification of T- and B-lymphocytes in human breast cancer with immunohistochemical techniques. Am. J. Pathol. 84:529-538, 1976.
68. Schuhmacher K.: Sekundaere Defektimmunopathien. Internist 18:255-263, 1977.
69. Seligmann M.: Lymphocyte membrane markers in human leukaemias and lymphomas, pp.4-27, Leukaemia Research Fund, London, 1976.
70. Slavin S., Z. Fuks, S. Strober, H. Kaplan, K.J. Howard and D.E.R. Sutherland: Transplantation tolerance across major histocompatibility barriers after total lymphoid irradiation. Transplantation 28:359-361, 1979.
71. Steffen C., H. Ludwig and W. Knapp: Collagen, anti-collagen immune complexes, rheumatoid arthritis, synovial fluid cells. Z. Immun.-Forsch. 147:229-235, 1974.
72. Stein H.: Immunologische und immunochemische Techniken und ihre Bedeutung fuer die Klassifikation lymphatischer Neoplasien. Verh. Dtsch. Ges. Path. 59:510-522, 1975.
73. Tack J.L., F. Beucher, J. Maillard and G.A. Voisin: Triple pathway of induction of chemotaxis in neutrophil leucotytes by guinea pig immune complexes of different Ig-classes. Int. Arch. Allergy 74:609-622, 1974.
74. Tappeiner G., G. Heine, J.C. Kahl and R.E. Jordan: Clq binding substances in pemphigus and bullous pemphigoid. Clin. Exp. Immunol. 28:40-48, 1977.
75. Tilz G.P., D. Buffe and C. Rimbaut: Immunochemische Diagnostik gastrointestinaler Erkrankungen mit besonderer Beruecksichtigung der Tumorimmunologie. Med. Klinik 68:994-999, 1973.
76. Tilz G.P.: Immunologie heute: einige Moeglichkeiten und neue Trends. Prakt. Arzt 354:1401-1415, 1976.
77. Tilz G.P., D. Buffe, C. Rimbaut and H. Pickel: Immunological investigations of the carcinome of the cervix. In: Cervical Pathology and Colposcopy, edited by E. Burghardt, pp.88-97, Thieme, Stuttgart, 1978.
78. Tilz G.P.: Immunotherapie I, Entwicklung und Testung von Antilymphocytenglobulin. In: Med. Klinik 69:200-205, 1974.
79. Tilz G.P., H. Vollmann, G. Lanzer and I. Teubl: Indikationen und Anwendungen der therapeutischen Komponentenseparation. Med. Klinik 73:1351-1355, 1978.
80. Tilz G.P.: Neue Erkenntnisse ueber das lymphocytaere System am Menschen: Das ALG und Lymphoid-Zell-Panel. Dtsch. Med. Wschr. 98:2179-2183, 1973.
81. Tilz G.P.: Neue Erkenntnisse ueber das lymphocytaere System am Menschen II. Die Charakterisierung von T- und B-Lymphocyten und deren Bedeutung fuer die praktische Medizin. Dtsch. Med. Wschr. 99:518-523, 1974.
82. Tilz G.P., St.Cyr. De Vaux and P. Grabar: New Antigens in cells transformed by the Sv 40 Virus. Evidence of their cytoplasmic localization in a cell line of hamster fibroblasts transformed by SV 40. Int. J. Cancer 4:641-647, 1969.

83. Tilz G.P. and H.L. Seewann: T-Zell-Leukaemien der Erwachsenen. Dtsch. Med. Wschr. 102:1848-1850, 1977.
84. Tilz G.P.: A microtest for rosette formation. Clin. Exp. Immunol. 32:366-369, 1978.
85. Tilz G.P., H. Becker, H. Vollmann and G. Lanzer: Diagnostischer T-Lymphozyten-Nachweis mittels eines neuen Mikrosystems. In: Internationale Arbeitstagung ueber Lymphknotentumore, edited by A. Stacher, Urban Schwarzenberg, Muenchen, 1979.
86. Tilz G.P., S. Saler and R. Heschl: Histokompatibilitaets-testung vor Transplantationen. Wiener Ztschr. Inn. Med. 50:134-137, 1969.
87. Tittor W.: T-Zell-Subpopulationen in der Lymphozyten-Mischkultur. Fortschritte der Medizin 95:2779-2784, 1977.
88. Uchiyama T., K. Sagava and K. Takatsuki: Effect of adult T-cell leukaemia cells on pokeweed mitogen induced normal B-cell differentiation. Clin. Immunol. Immunopathol. 10:24-34, 1978.
89. Vorlaender K.O.: Praxis der Immunologie. Thieme, Stuttgart, 1976.
90. Vorlaender K.O.: Immunologie, Thieme, Stuttgart, 1983.
91. Vyas G.N., D.P. Stites and G. Brecher: Laboratory diagnosis of immunologic disorders. Grune + Stratton, New York, 1973.
92. Waksmann B.H.: Atlas of Experimental Immunobiology and Immunopathology. Yale University Press, London, 1970.
93. Whiteside T.L. and D.T. Rowlands: T-cell and B-cell identification in the diagnosis of lymphoproliferative diseases. A review. Am. J. Pathol. 88:854-790, 1977.
94. Wick G., J.H. Kite jr., R.K. Cole and E. Witebsky: Spontaneous thyreoiditis in the obese strain of chickens: the effect of bursectomy on the development of the disease. J. Immunol. 104:45-52, 1970.
95. Wick G., R.S. Sundick and B. Albini: The obese strain of chickens: an animal model with spontaneous autoimmune thyreoiditis. Clin. Immunol. Immunopathol. 3:272-300, 1974.
96. Wigzell H.: Aspects on future therepeutical possibilities. In: Blood leukocytes, function and use in therapy, edited by C.F. Hoegman, K. Lindahl-Kiessling and H. Wigzell, pp. 16-21, Almquist + Wiksell International, Stockholm, 1977.
97. Yefenof E., G. Klein, M. Jondal and M.B.A. Oldstone: Surface markers on human B- and T-lymphocytes. IX. Two-colour immunofluorescence studies on the association between EBV receptors and complement receptors on the surface of lymphoid cell lines. Int. J. Cancer 17:693-700, 1976.
98. Yu D.T.Y., R.J. Winchester, S.M. Fu, a. Giofsky, H.S. Ko and H.G. Kunkel: Peripheral blood Ia-positive T-cells. J.Exp. Med. 151:91-100, 1980.

17 COMPARATIVE EVALUATION OF SEPARATION AND LABELLING METHODS OF MIGRATORY BLOOD CELLS

Round Table Discussion

M.R. HARDEMAN AND G.F. FUEGER, EDS.

17.1   INTRODUCTION

This chapter represents a summary of a round table discussion chaired by M.R. Hardeman (Amsterdam) and held among the following participants:

Colas-Linhart (Paris), Danpure (London), Egger (Graz), Fliedner (Ulm/Donau), Fueger (Graz), Goodwin (Palo Alto), Hofer (Tallahassee), Moisan (Rennes), Oberhausen (Homburg/Saar), Schell-Frederick (Brussels), Thakur (Philadelphia).

17.2   METHODS OF CELL SEPARATION AND LABELLING

The following variations in the methods of separating and labelling neutrophil preparations were presented to the participants of the round table discussion:

Table 1.   Methods of Neutrophil Preparation

	1	2	3
Blood Collection	4 ml HES + 2 ml saline + 800 iu heparin + 50 ml blood	2 x (49 ml blood + 1 ml heparin + 5 ml HES)	30 ml blood + 150-200 iu heparin
Sedimentation	60 min/ 20 deg.C	45-60 min/ 20 deg.C	30-60 min/ 20 deg.C
Remove Supernatant			
Centrifugation	5 min at "speed 4.5"	5 min/450 g	5 min/450 g
Supernatant			
PPP WBC - Pellet	30 min at "speed 9-10"	15 min/1000 g	-
Washing	-	-	5 ml saline
Centrifugation	-	-	-
Resuspended in:	3 ml saline	2x3 ml saline	5 ml saline

Labelling

1) Stanford University Medical Center
2) Palo Alto V.A. Medical Center
3) Yale School of Medicine

4	5	6	7
2x (5 ml ACD+ 20 ml blood)+ 1 ml methyl cellulose	4 ml ACD + 36 ml blood + 7 ml HES	2x (5ml ACD + 25 ml blood) + 1 ml methyl cellulose	3x (5 ml Macrodex + 0.1 ml heparin + 20.0 ml blood)
45-60 min/ 20 deg.C	60 min/ 20 deg.C	45-60 min/ 20 deg.C	45-60 min/ 37 deg.C
10 min/130 g	5 min/450 g	10 min/500g	5 min/150 g
10 min/500 g	-	-	10 min/1000 g
-	10 ml saline	-	-
-	4 min/180 g	-	-
2 ml PBS	5 ml saline	2 ml PBS	0.5 ml PBS

4) Byk-Mallinckrodt, Petten
5) Syracuse
6) University of Amsterdam
7) Graz

Table 2.   Neutrophil Preparation (Wissler)

Blood + Heparin (10 iu/ml)

Methylcellulose (50ul/ml)

20-35 min/10-20 deg.C

Remove Supernatant = PRP

10 min/10 deg.C/400 g (ca. 1200 rpm)

Leuco-pellet

resuspended in hypotonic, phosphate buffered
glucose - citrate - saline pH = 7.1
30 sec/0 deg.C

hypertonic, phosphate-buffered
glucose - citrate - saline pH = 7.1   (0 deg.C)

10 min/400 g (ca.1200 rpm)/0-10 deg.C

A)   Leuco-pellet

Labelling

B) Cellular ghost element - and protein -
containing supernatant salt solution

Table 3. Neutrophil Preparation (McAfee)

30-100 ml blood, 8 ml ACD or
250-1000 heparin/50 ml
5-15 ml 6% HES or 1.5 ml 2%
methylcellulose

60 min/20 deg.C

remove supernatant

5 min/450 g (ca. 1400 rpm)
5-8 min/150 g (ca. 800 rpm)

Metrizamide cushion, density 1.19

remove plasma

wash and spin cells one or two times

resuspend cells in 5.0 ml saline

Labelling

Table 4. Neutrophil Preparation (Danpure)

7.5 ml ACD (NIH A) + 42.5 ml blood

30-60 min at 37 deg.C

Remove supernatant

5 min 100 g -- supernatant
(platelet-rich-plasma, PRP)
1000 g 10 min
cell-free-plasma

Mixed leucocyte pellet

A) If neutrophilic patient:
Resuspend in 0.5-1.0 ml cell-free plasma
for labelling with 111-In-tropolonate

B)   Otherwise:
Resuspend pellet in appr. 5 ml PRP
Layer on discontinuous density gradient of
Percoll/plasma or Metrizanide/plasma

150 g, 5 min

Remove granulocyte band
Add 5 volumes cell-free plasma

100 g, 5 min

Remove supernatant
Resuspend pellet in 0.5-0.1 ml cell-free plasma
for labelling with 111-In-tropolonate

Table 5.

Routine Procedure of Phagocytotic Labelling

(Oberhausen)

1 vial tin-II-chloride (RCC Amersham)

add 100 mCi 99m-Tc-O-IV in 3-5 ml

Rotation, 30-60 min, 20 deg.C

add 10 mCi of 99m-Tc-Sn-colloid
to 10 ml heparinized WHOLE blood

Rotation, 30-60 min, 20 deg.C

add 1 ml 3.1% sodium citrate colution

Rotation, 30-60 min, 20 deg.C

Centrifugation, 3000 g/10 min

Remove supernatant
Resuspend cells with normal saline

Reinjection

Table 6.   Neutrophil Preparation (Moisan)

50 ml blood + 500 iu heparin (or 8 ml ACD)

A: 10 ml for PPP (400g/10 min)
B: 40 ml + 10 ml DEXTRAN (or 10% Plasmagel)

37 deg.C Sedimentation

Remove PRP, dilute with RPMI-MEDIUM

10 ml Ficoll-Metrizoate (LYMPHOPREP or MSL)

200 g/10 min/30 deg.C

Remove lymphocytes and plasma

Add 10 mm medium
5 min incubation

150 g/2min/30 deg.C

Resuspend in 3-5 ml medium

Labelling

Table 7. Neutrophil Preparation (Ficoll)

A) PREPARATION OF THE GRADIENT

gradient I (density = 1077)
layered on
gradient II (density = 1097)
Volume = 1:1

B)   CELL SEPARATION:

20 ml blood + 5 ml ACD
layered on top of methyl
cellulose solution (2:1)

60 min/20 deg.C

LRP layered on top of the two gradients (2:1:1)

20 min/1200 g

collect granulocytes
(at the interface between the two gradients)

Washing procedure
1) 1% HSA-solution
2) Saline

5-10 min/150 g

Resuspended in saline

Labelling

Ref.: Pfeiffer G., J. Eiten and K. Deubelbeiss: Iodation of granulocytes and labelling with In-111-oxine sulphate. Eur. J. Nucl. Med. 7:195-196, 1982.

Table 8. Neutrophil Preparation (Percoll)

10 ml 70% (v/v) Percoll in 0.15 M NaCl (1.086 g/ml

15 min/20 000 g

remove 2 ml gradient material from the bottom of the tube

2 ml 50% heparinized blood in 0.15 M NaCl
were layered on top of the gradient

5 min/400 g

remove plasma layer and replace with saline

15 min/800 g

density determination with density MARKER BEADS

Collection of leucocytes

Washing with 5 ml saline

2-10 min/200 g

Labelling

17.3   COMPOSITION OF CELL PREPARATIONS

(Hardeman) The first part of the discussion dealt with the comparison of the various methods for the preparation of neutrophil suspensions on the basis of a survey made by C. Barowitsch (Graz). For a fair comparison a distinction has to be made between methods aiming at a pure neutrophil preparation and those resulting in a "mixed cell" preparation; the first, predominantly in use for cell- kinetic studies applies an extra density-gradient centrifugation step and 1 or 2 wash steps before the final suspension in saline was made.   In the survey, the McAfee-procedure, using metrizamide (Sp.g. 1.19) was shown as an example of such a method.   The majority of the participants, however, agreed that the so called "mixed cell" preparations after labelling and re-injection sufficiently matched the demands for abscess detection, although these suspensions contained besides granulocytes also lymphocytes, erythrocytes and platelets in varying amounts.   Danpure commented on the tremendous variation in cell-separation methods used for labelling cells with 111-In, and considered the composition of the cell preparations for clinical and biological studies: Except for the Hammersmith group all use "crude" leucocytes for their studies.   Hammersmith use "pure" granulocytes containing 5-20% erythrocytes.   Hardeman uses "crude" leucocytes containing 50% platelets, lymphocytes and erythrocytes. Cellular composition will vary depending on the choice of sedimenting agent and g-force used to spin the cells.

17.4   CELL SEPARATION   BY DIFFERENTIAL CENTRIFUGATION

All examples of the method of cell separation by differential centrifugation included in the survey, did not differ principally: 1 g sedimentation (with or without an erythrocyte aggregating substance) followed by the separation of the "leucocyte- and platelet-rich plasma" (LPRP), centrifugation and resuspension of the cell pellet in normal or phosphate-buffered saline.

17.4.1 Anticoagulants

Regarding the anticoagulant used, the discussion focussed on the choice between heparin and ACD. It was agreed that EDTA should not be used for these studies due to its proven deleterious effect on cell viability and swelling of the cells. Thakur pointed out that many investigators have shown that EDTA was not an acceptable anticoagulant particularly for blood from which platelets have to be separated, since EDTA completely depletes calcium from plasma. Furthermore, when 111-In-oxinate is to be used, even a small trace of EDTA would dissociate 111-In from oxinate and no cell labelling would take place.

Although it was argued that heparin is not well defined (significant differences between various commercial preparations) and might have some platelet aggregating effect, the majority of the methods still use this anticoagulant for the preparation of granulocyte suspensions, while others use ACD (NIH.formula A).

Regarding the choice of an anticoagulant Danpure concurred that ACD was best because of its uniformity, provided all used the same formula (NIH formula A is used at Hammersmith). With respect to pH changes: 1.5 ml ACD to 8.5 ml whole blood does not lower the blood pH.

17.4.2 Erythrocyte separation

With respect to the separation of the bulk of erythrocytes, most methods use an erythrocyte-aggregating substance like hydroxyethyl starch (HES), Macrodex or methylcellulose. Of these polysaccharides only HES has been approved by the American FDA. In many cases it is, however, not necessary to use any of these substances because of an elevated erythrocyte sedimentation rate (E.S.R.) of the patients to be studied. The geometry and type of material of the blood-container as well as the angle under which the sedimentation takes place may influence the sedimentation rate (Thakur). Thakur did not use a sedimenting agent to facilitate the leucocyte separation from patients' blood, since the spontaneous rate of red cell sedimentation in patients' blood is frequently high.

Ambient temperature (i.e. 20 deg.C) was considered most suitable for these procedures by all participants.

As to erythrocyte sedimenting agents, dextran, methylcellulose, hydroxyethyl starch or nothing at all have been used. It was of interest that Fueger found Macrodex phagocytosed by neutrophils - but still this did not seem to impair in-vivo function. Danpure disagreed with Thakur that it does not need a sedimenting agent: With normal volunteers you do. If the donor has a high E.S.R. you do not.

17.4.3 Centrifugation conditions

Regarding centrifugation conditions, Danpure suggested that in some laboratories cells are centrifuged too hard. She found 100 g for 5 min sediments leucocytes very satisfactory. For cells to be labelled with 111-In-oxinate some groups wash their cells before labelling, others do not. Danpure pointed out that many people could separate leucocytes much more carefully and by gentler methods. Linhart-Colas stated that there is no completely perfect method to obtain pure and viable neutrophil populations after separation. She considers some manipulations as quite toxic, for example 450 g centrifugation and changes of temperature during preparation (10 deg. and 37 deg.C). Low g results in low platelet contamination.

17.5 DENSITY GRADIENT CENTRIFUGATION

Hofer (Tallahassee) pointed out that density gradient centrifugation has for many years been an established method for the separation and purification of cells, viruses and subcellular particles. Differences in density and/or size can be exploited to separate particles under relatively mild conditions, e.g. Ficoll, a synthetic high molecular weight polymer of sucrose and epichlorohydrin, or Percoll, a silicasol with non-dialysable PVP coating, may be used for cell separation. Details of such a method are given by Danpure (Table 10 and Chapter 8), Moisan (Chapter 9), Pfeiffer (Table 11 and reference, 1982). Linhart-Colas also prefers a separation with plasmagel and Ficoll-Paque. Haemolysis is realized with NaCl 0.2% and NaCl 1.2% at her laboratory.

Appreciable cell lethality was observed only when the cells were allowed to aggregate or when the density gradient was deliberately overloaded. It is difficult to offer a satisfactory explanation for the severe mortality induced by cellular aggregation or overloading of the gradient. Physical trauma due to the "wall effect" or due to packing of too many cells at the buoyant density peak may be one of the factors responsible for the decline in viability thus observed.

No loss of cellular viability was observed unless
a) the cells were allowed to aggregate in a medium free of anti-agglutinin;
b) the Ficoll gradient was deliberately overloaded;
c) the volume of the gradient tube was reduced without a concomitant reduction in the number of cells; or
d) the duration of the centrifugation was increased from 45 min to 3.5 hrs. In all other experiments the viability of cells subjected to Ficoll gradient separation was identical to that of untreated control cells. (Warters and Hofer, 1974).

17.6 CELL SEPARATION BY ELUTRIATION

The value of the elutriating technique for cell isolation was briefly discussed. The counter streaming centrifugation method developed by Lindahl in Uppsala in the late 1940's requires a specially built centrifuge and separation chamber. The cells (or other particles) are subjected to two opposing forces within the separation chamber: the centrifugal field generated by the spinning rotor, and the counterflow of fluid in the opposite (centripetal) direction. Each cell tends to migrate to a zone where its sedimentation rate is exactly balanced by the flow rate of the fluid through the separation chamber. It is a relatively gentle means of separating cells, e.g. 400 g at 2000 rpm. There is no exposure to the deleterious effects of pelleting, or osmotic effects of special media such as those used for density gradient centrifugation. This technique has been proven to be very successful for stem cell separation (Fliedner). It was thought it would not damage the cells. Although cells can be separated efficiently with this technique (on the basis of their size rather than their density) and in a way which avoids the peletting and resuspension of the cells, the obtained suspensions are too dilute for effective labelling (Hardeman). However, another design of the separation chamber combined with the use of density gradients in the continuous counter flow may result in a very elegant method for the isolation of viable granulocytes (Hardeman). Danpure emphasized the need to concentrate the cells after separation and before labelling.

17.7 OTHER METHODS OF CELL SEPARATION

Thakur briefly mentioned fluorescein separated cells but said the method was rather slow. Obviously new methods of separating cells must be investigated (Danpure).

17.8   SEPARATING VIABLE FROM DEAD CELLS

17.8.1   Neutral density centrifugation

Hofer (Tallahassee) discussed the reduced cell viability due to centrifugation and suggested the use of Ficoll for the actual separation of living and dead cells by neutral density centrifugation. Basically, neutral density centrifugation takes advantage of the fact that dead cells (which have lost membrane function) admit Ficoll into their interior, live cells exclude Ficoll. Thus, a mixture of dead and live cells can be suspended in Ficoll of appropriate density (usually between 20-30% w/w) and subjected to centrifugation. If the correct w/w percentage is chosen, the dead cells will sink to the bottom of Ficoll, the live cells will rise to the top. For details see Warters and Hofer, 1974.

In many cases it is even possible to separate different cell types by this procedure. It might be possible to place 2-3 ml of 30% w/w Ficoll at the bottom of centrifuge tubes and layer the labelled cell suspension on top of the Ficoll. All living cells would collect at the top of the Ficoll layer and could be harvested from there with a syringe. This may prevent cell damage due to compression of cells at the bottom of the tube. Hundreds of tubes with Ficoll solution could be prepared at a time and frozen for later use (Hofer).

17.8.2   Biological filtration

The problem of non-specific uptake or retention of radioactivity in the liver or spleen may be due to dead cells in the labelled cell population. This used to be a problem in Hofer's mouse work with 125-IUdR pre-labelled cancer cells which were used to investigate tumour cell metastases in living hosts.

In mice, this problem was solved by Hofer by injecting 125-I-labelled cells into temporary host mice and recovering the viable cells from those mice after 12-15 hours. During this time, host phagocytes destroyed the dead cells and removed the radioactive debris, so after 12-15 hours only fully viable cells were recovered. Obviously, this procedure is not applicable to humans, but with additional research an equivalent procedure might be established in-vitro.

Oberhausen presented biodistribution data obtained after such biological filtration in rats (Chapter 11).

17.8.3 Cell sorting by surface charge

An alternate method might be separation of live and dead cells by surface charge. Laminar flow cell sorters are available which separate cells by electrical charge. Since a continuous laminar flow is used, very large cell samples can be processed in relatively short time periods, making this approach potentially much more useful than the single cell separation techniques commonly used for cell separation.

17.9 METHODS OF CELL LABELLING

The round table discussion continued by considering the various labelling methods currently in use for migratory cells. As a matrix against which the various methods can be evaluated the following criteria were accepted for the ideal labelling method (Hardeman).
1. high labelling efficiency
2. no elution of the label, either in-vitro or in-vivo
3. no re-utilization of the label after cell destruction
4. no exchange of the label with unlabelled compounds in the body stores

5. availability of a suitable radionuclide
6. maintencance of cell viability i.e. the capacity to stay in the circulation with a normal survival
7. maintenance of cell function(s) i.e. those function(s) thought to be relevant for the type of study
8. short, technically simple routine procedure
9. no toxic substances

Regarding the radio-nuclide for (migratory) cell labelling, the following criteria were used as a matrix for discussion:
1. radiation dose to the patient as small as possible
2. gamma emitter (positron emitter for emission tomography)
3. radiation yield sufficiently high for in-vivo detection
4. radio-active T 1/2 in the same order as biological T 1/2
5. suitable complex forming properties
6. low toxicity (in-vivo cell viability and function)
7. binding to intracellular components
8. radio-nuclide purity

17.9.1 111-In-chelates

The labelling techniques using 111-In-oxinate and 111-In-tropolonate met with very little controversy and accordingly were not discussed in extenso. Danpure's method of labelling in plasma was accepted as a distinct advantage since it was thought to ease the procedure and protect cellular viability. Thakur's new compound for labelling white cells, 111-In-2-mercapto-pyridine-n-oxide (MERC) was not discussed with respect to its biological effect on WBC's (viability, survival time, chemotaxis, chemo-kinesis etc.), but Danpure questioned the superiority claimed for it by Thakur over tropolonate. With respect to cell labelling, the details of labelling were not discussed excepting the need for relatively high cell concentrations - but whether cells are washed or not after labelling was discussed. Some wash in saline, some in plasma. Danpure agreed that plasma must be added after

387

labelling to complex unbound 111-In and loosely bound activity must be removed from the cells.

Thakur said that he washed leucocytes only once before suspending them in isotonic saline for labelling and that he added autologous plasma to the saline at the end of the incubation period, but before centrifugation and injected labelled cells in plasma.

(Hardeman)

In order to limit the overall dose to the patient, the use of shorter living radio-nuclides like 113m-In could be used in combination with tropolone since this method enables the visualization of abscesses already 4 hours following injection (Danpure).

17.9.2 Sn-pyrophosphate/99m-Tc-pertechnetate (PYPE)

The use of PYPE for WBC labelling for abscess localisation and similar applications has also been investigated (Colas): After PYPE labelling, the stability in-vitro and in-vivo is satisfactory. All viability tests and morphological studies are quite normal but there are other problems. Particularly the kinetics of labelled white cells in-vivo, in dogs, were not completely normal and the important liver uptake was considered abnormal (Linhart-Colas).

Some questions remained unanswered, however, regarding labelling efficiency and the intracellular stability of the label. Furthermore, 99m-Tc might be too short-lived an isotope for abscess detection (see below, Oberhausen's method). Maximal uptake of labelled granulocytes is at 24 hours following injection, and is very important for adequate scintigraphic detection (Goodwin). This, however, may vary from patient to patient; patients with high degrees of leucocytosis visualize their suppurative lesions earlier than those with no leucocytosis (Fueger). On the other hand, 99m-Tc can be used at much higher doses, compared to 111-In (Oberhausen).

17.9.3 99m-Tc-Sn-colloid

99m-Tc-Sn-colloid is in use for the labelling of phagocytes. Since the principle of this method is phagocytosis, the procedure can be performed in whole blood instead of in a suspension of isolated or mixed cells (Oberhausen). The specificity of this method appeared to be superior since it will not affect lymphocytes in contrast to the 111-In-ligand methods.

Oberhausen presented his method of phagocytic labelling of monocytes and neutrophils.   The procedure is given in detail in Chapter 11 of this book.

The phagocytotic technique using 99m-Tc-tin-colloid favours rather selectively the labelling of monocytes. Despite their predominating infiltration with neutrophil (and other) granulocytes, the visualization of abscesses is possible with labelled monocytes for the following reason (Oberhausen):

Whole blood contains a concentration of about $1.0 \times 10E06$ per 10 ml;   the   addition   of 10 mCi 99m-Tc-Sn-colloid yields a reasonably high concentration of label in the monocytes. Therefore, even a small number of cells suffices to visualize such lesions. The shorter halflife of 99m-Tc (in comparison to 111-In) raises the question whether or not septic lesions may be visualized with this radionuclide if 24 hours are required for sufficient infiltration with leucocytes. Neglecting biological elimination and distribution which is the same for 111-In and 99m-Tc-labelled WBC's an activity of 600 uCi 99m-Tc can be expected to be present in the body at 24 hours, respectively 4 halftimes after injection. Of 1 mCi 111-In, about 780 uCi will remain after the same time interval. Since the physical properties of 99m-Tc are more favourable for scintigraphic imaging than those of 111-In, statistically better images may be obtained from 600 uCi 99m-Tc than from 780 uCi 111-In.

Oberhausen's 99m-Tc-tin-colloid for specific cell labelling in whole blood met with great interest from all the research workers present. His clinical results were considered very good.

17.9.4 Biodistribution of cells labelled by phagocytosis

Egger questioned whether phagocytosed cells are stimulated as a result of the labelling. Although it was concluded that with a low number of monocytes in the blood the activity on each cell would result in a very high radiation dose to each cell - even so the monocytes localize in inflammatory sites very well. Danpure agreed with Oberhausen that he had not labelled neutrophils because the particle size was not optimal for neutrophils.

After injection of phagocytes i.e. monocytes labelled with 99m-Tc-Sn-colloid, however, 50-70% of the activity is accumulated in the spleen and liver. It is not clear whether this means appreciable cell damage (cell stimulation?) or a normal distribution of the labelled monocytes between a marginal and circulating pool. It was emphasized, though, that 99m-Tc-Sn-colloid, as such, is normally used for liver and spleen scintigraphy. Since monocytes may divide further, cellular damage due to a high dose of 99m-Tc may reveal another problem, parallel to that described for lymphocytes (Fliedner). Pathologists normally do not find many monocytes in abscesses in contrast to neutrophils (Kirkpatrick). This, however, does not necessarily mean that there are no monocytes involved in abscesses, they might have been overlooked due to less specific staining methods (Hardeman).

Thakur observed that there was no conclusive evidence to Oberhausen's claim that only monocytes were labelled with 99m-Tc, since monocytes were difficult to separate from whole blood. Thakur questioned the seemingly poor survival of the cells in circulation and the intense radioactivity into the spleen and liver. Someone had raised (perhaps Hofer) doubts as to how one could be sure if it was the infiltration with labelled cells that carried the radioactivity into the abscesses (Thakur).

17.9.5 99m-Tc-sulphur-colloid

Schell-Frederik observed that 99m-Tc-sulphur-colloid (TcSC) has been recommended as a suitable label for in-vivo detection of inflammatory foci. She reported having investigated the mechanism of cell labelling by TcSC and advanced the hypothesis that clearance of free 99m-TcSC by the reticuloendothelial system occurs largely by endocytosis. In non-elicited mouse peritoneal macrophages, TcSC labelling was markedly though not completely inhibited by cytochalasin B (CB) and by low temperature factors which both inhibit phagocytosis and micropinocytosis. In contrast, neutrophils were labelled at their surface and not by endocytosis. Labelling persisted in the presence of CB and was increased at 0 deg.C. The mechanism of neutrophil labelling did not appear to depend on particle size, at least in the 40-400 nm range tested.

The failure of granulocytes to ingest colloid particles which appear to be actively taken up by macrophages was explained as follows: The inhibitory effect of CB and low temperature on macrophage labelling suggested energy-requiring endocytosis, i.e. macropinocytosis. The 30% labelling remaining under these conditions may represent non-energy requiring micropinocytosis and/or surface binding. Circulating leucocytes apparently did not recognize TcSC as a phagocytic particle, even when the diameter was greater than 100 nm and when opsonizing factors were present. This may have been caused by the presence of gelatine which is weakly charged at a neutral pH and not readily engulfed.

17.9.6 Cell specific labels

The need for and desirability of cell-specific labelling
techniques was agreed upon by all participants. Danpure mentioned
111-In-BLEDTA (Goodwin) as a method for specific labelling of
neutrophil granulocytes. Peptides stimulating leucocyte
chemotaxis or binding to neutrophil receptor sites, as well as
monoclonal antibodies to surface antigens were considered obvious
areas of research. No specific possibilities or results were
advanced by any of the participants.

17.9.7 Radiobiolocigal damage to labelled cells

Danpure agreed that viability and function of labelled cells
must be maintained if cell labelling is to be worthwhile.
Therefore she stressed the importance of careful cell separation.
She agreed that 111-In causes radiation damage to cells from Auger
electrons, therefore it should not be suitable for
radiation-sensitive cells like lymphocytes. If lymphocytes are
killed there is no problem; but a potential problem might develop
if there is oncogenic transformation of the lymphocytes. Danpure
suggested workers should use "pure" granulocytes for cell
labelling although it involves a little more in-vitro manipulation
because no lymphocytes are labelled by this method. She also said
that using indium-tropolonate to label granulocytes, 113m-In could
be used instead of 111-In because the labelled cells very rapidly
localize in inflammatory sites. Goodwin disagreed because he said
24 hours was optimal. He said the physical halflife of the
radionuclide should be approximately 0.7 relative to the
biological halflife. Danpure still thought that 113m-In would be
useful because their 40 minute and 3 hour images were good.

It was stated, referring to a dutch study (ten Berge et al.)
that 111-In, the nuclide which is mostly in use now to label blood
cells for diagnostic applications, was found to induce chromosome
breakage in lymphocytes, straight after labelling with 10 uCi.

This is presumably due to Auger electrons having very short ranges and high energy transfer (see Hofer's article, Chapter 12). Although more study is needed here, the general feeling by the participants of this round table conference was that there is no immediate reason for big alarm for several reasons:
- in the normal individual 3-5% of the chromosomes are abnormal, an additional 0.01% due to the injection of 111-In-labelled lymphocytes does not matter (Thakur)
- chromosome aberrations do not necessarily mean oncogenic transformations (Goodwin)
- re-evaluation of the follow-up studies performed on atomic bomb survivors has revealed no increase in leukemia etc. (Hofer)
- lymphocytes with damage from energy deposition due to radiation do not replicate beyond a few cycles (Fliedner).

Thakur had asked for suggestions from the floor as to what experimental model one could use to study the possible consequences in patients receiving labelled lymphocytes (radiation effects). There were no concrete suggestions. Thakur pointed out two references (both in: Annals of Rheumatic Diseases. Vol. 22, 1973) by Stephenson and Dawson who had reported no adverse effects in patients who have had chromosome aberration as a result of intense radiation they had received.

17.10 CONCLUSION

It was not possible to end the discussion with a general con-clusion regarding the best labelling method for migratory cells. Since satisfying clinical results have been reported for 111-In-oxinate, 111-In-tropolonate as well as for 99m-Tc-Sn-colloid, the ultimate choice might depend on local circumstances i.e. having a technician available for the more laborious, but relatively cheap tropolonate-method rather than the money to buy the commercially available 111-In-oxinate. If there is no money and no technician available and one could overcome the disadvantages mentioned above, the 99m-Tc-Sn-colloid method is suggested (Oberhausen).

LARGE SCALE TECHNIQUES AND BIOTECHNIQUES FOR THE PRODUCTION AND ISOLATION OF LEUCOCYTIC EFFECTOR SUBSTANCES OF REGENERATIVE TISSUE MORPHOGENESIS BY CULTURING CELLS IN SERUM-FREE, SYNTHETIC FLUIDS: DESIGN, PREPARATION AND USE OF A NOVEL MEDIUM

J.H. WISSLER

Dedicated to Professor Dr. Eckhard Buddecke
University of Muenster,
On His 60th Birthday

1.0   INTRODUCTION: BASIC PROBLEMS AND DEFINITIONS

1.1   Basic problems in culturing cells in media

For the culture of different cells, tissues and organs, various media are known and are in use. In principle, for in vitro or in situ cell-biological work, an ideal medium would be equivalent to extracellular biological fluid synthetically composed and chemically defined. It should
   a. represent the physiological environment of a cell in interactive tissues;
   b. allow the cell to adapt to its changes terms of viabiliby and functional expressions; and it should
   c. react in its parameters (at least in part) to chemostatic reactions (1, 2) of the cells (such as are maintained in structure, function and life expressions in vivo).
For mammalian cells, in most cases, the variable compositions of the different biological fluids, like plasma (or, less ideally, serum), amniotic fluid, aqueous humour of the eye, etc. (3-6), would be close to such an ideal, physiological cell culture medium: They are the normal biological fluids of interstitial spaces as selected by evolution.
However, our knowledge of the diversity, structure and functions of physiological constituents of biological fluids is far from being sufficient to fulfil practical aspects of ideal viewpoints. Therefore, at least two different approaches have been taken towards these ideal criteria in cell-biological work: Biological fluid- (serum-) containing media AND (serum-) free, fully synthetic, chemically defined media have been composed. Basically, both groups of media normally are aqueous solutions. They may contain a more or less large variety of chemical compounds of different structural classes. The main constituents of these cell culture media may be salts, sugars and their metabolites, amino acids, nucleosides and nucleotides, vitamins, vitaminoids, co-enzymes, steroids and further additives, such as tensides (pre-

Fueger, G.F. (ed.), Blood Cells in Nuclear Medicine, Part II. ISBN 089838-654-3
©1984 Martinus Nijhoff Publishers, Boston/The Hague/Dordrecht/Lancaster — Printed in the Netherlands

sumably used in some culture media to dissolve hydrophobic compounds), heavy metal salts, indicator dyes and cellular activators etc. The compositions of customary (component-richer or poorer) cell culture media and salt solutions, like "Eagle's", "Hanks'", "Earle's", "Ham's", "McCoy's", "Leibovitz'", "Trowell's", "Waymouth's", "Iscove's", "Sato's", "Dulbecco's", "Medium 199", "NTCT", "RPMI", "Alsever's", etc., are presented in detail, re-evaluated or reviewed in several references (5-30, 78, 79, 143).

Since their constituents are described, in principle, they fulfil the definition of (component-richer or poorer) fully synthetic media. More problematic to state for any fluid is its chemical definition. In principle, to define a fluid chemically, not only the main constituents should be known, but also, the contaminants and dissolved gases, etc., that is every intrinsic and extrinsic component in equilibrium with each other. Evidently, none of the media ever to be composed shall be investigated in full for rigorous treatment according to this ideal viewpoint. Some recent approaches for the analytical determination of the trace components in media represented by contaminants like metal ions and others (4-6,31), clearly illustrate the difficulties inherent to a full chemical definition of any fluid. In this work, too, only an approach to a "chemical definition" of a component-rich, fully synthetic, serum-free medium can be made. Whether or not fully synthetic or chemically defined, however, a composition given for a medium has to be understood only as a momentary, valid starting description of any cell-biological work since addition to cells and their interaction with the fluid components brings about an alteration of the original chemical definition of the medium by turnover of its distinct individual constituents and addition of new components by cellular exudation or secretion. The cells chemostatically adapt the biological fluid in its own microenvironment to a large extent, and vice versa (Figure 1).

 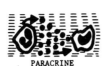

AUTOCRINE   PARACRINE   ENDOCRINE

MEDIATORS   HORMONES

ACTIVATORS, TRANSMITTERS
INHIBITORS, CHALONES, STATINES
AUTACOIDS, PARAMONES, CYBERNINES

●Cell-derived and ☰☰fluid molecules.

Fig. 1. Schematic presentation of relations and terms intrinsic to interaction of cells with their microenvironment; in-vivo in terms of interstitial fluid and biological structures; in-vitro on culture in terms of neighbour cells and fluid with special reference to biological (autocrine, paracrine and endocrine) information transmission mechanisms (1). Neural mechanisms are omitted, but are discussed extensively elsewhere (2, 34, 148).

1.2   Regenerative morphogenesis: terms, mechanisms, effectors

As a result of this interaction, not only ions and "simply" structured organic molecules (in the form of metabolites of some of the components of the extracellular fluid) are produced, transported, and turned over in the culture. One expression for this is the hydrogen production of cultured viable cells. A large variety of polypeptides of different molecular properties and with specific biological activities are also formed and exuded by cells. Each cell represents a highly sophisticated chemical factory. One example of the formation and turnover of biologically active polypeptides in cell cultures are the changes in patterns of enzyme activity provided by extracellular and intracellular conditions (32, 33). Another example represents the production and exudation of effector (cytokine) substances (mediators and hormones) (1, 2, 34) by cells in vivo and in vitro on their culture. In consideration are especially those of white blood cells and vessel cells in their functional expressions basic on the immune, haematopoietic and cardiovascular systems in inflammation and wound healing. Together with effectors of humoral origin (1, 2, 34, 93-103) they operate chemical mechanisms for cellular reactions and communication for the organized renewal of tissue or cellular distribution patterns in regenerative morphogenesis as represented by inflammatory and wound healing processes (1, 2, 34). Amongst them are polypeptide effectors as a so far little known and investigated structural group of natural chemical signals regulating organized cellular behaviour, displacement, topochemical guidance in the formation of the different tissue pattern types (1, 2). Chemopoiesis, chemorecruitment, chemokinesis, chemotaxis, chemotropism and chemostasis of cells are the major categories of chemical mechanisms, each consisting of several subgroups, intrinsic to the cellular organization processes in morphogenetic reactions. The definitions of such mechanistic terms have been presented elsewhere (1, 2), in relation to the formally distinguishable morphogenetic patterns of cellular and molecular structures which might be formed upon. Schematic illustrations of cellular patterns and functions basic to the immune, haematopoietic and cardiovascular systems concerning chemical mechanisms involved in regenerative morphogenesis by inflammation and wound healing processes, have been presented (1, 2, 34, 145). The polypeptide effectors triggering these mechanisms are transiently existing, mostly labile trace components of tissues, blood or culture supernatant solutions, comparable to known hormones of classical endocrine glands. They occur and express their biological activity at minute concentrations below the nanomolar range or femtomol amounts. Thus, they may transmit their information by autocrine and paracrine as well as endocrine and neural mechanisms as inflammatory or wound mediators and hormones, respectively (1, 2, 34). Figure 1 refers to such relations and terms which have been defined and further detailed elsewhere (1, 2, 34, 45).

These properties of polypeptide effectors regulating the organization of cellular and molecular structures in reactions of regenerative tissue morphogenesis allow an estimate as to how much viable cell material to be prepared and/or cultured is necessary as starting material for the production and isolation of physical (milligram) quantities of a natural trace polypeptide effector, as a prerequisite for its further physical, chemical, biological and clinical investigations. Such an estimate is summarized in Table 1 for natural polypeptide mediators and hormones exuded by leucocytes. As mobile "secretory leucocytic tissue" (1, 2, 34, 45), they are a main source for such cytokines formed ("leucokines", "monokines", "lymphokines").

FACTS AND BASIS OF CALCULATION:

A. MAXIMUM CONCENTRATION OF ACTIVE CYTOKINE IN CULTURE $\ll 10^{-8}$ MOL/L

B. A. IS EQUIVALENT TO $\ll 6 \cdot 10^{15}$ CYTOKINE MOLECULES/LITER $\ll 10^{15}$ MOLECULES/L

C. ONE ACTIVE CELL MAY MAINTAIN (STEADY STATE) MAXIMUM OF $\sim 10^{4}$ MOLECULES/L

D. MAXIMUM YIELD OF PURIFICATION PROCEDURE (8 - 9 STEPS) $\gtrless 10$ %

E. RANGE OF MOLECULAR WEIGHT OF CYTOKINES ($<$30'000 DALTON) $\sim 10^{4}$ DALTON

F. MINIMUM REQUIRED QUANTITY OF CYTOKINE FOR RELIABLE WORK $\sim 1 - 10$ MILLIGRAM

G. ONE KILOGRAM (LITER) BLOOD CONTAINS MAXIMUM ~ 5 GRAM OR $\gtrless 10^{10}$ LEUKOCYTES

CALCULATION AND RESULTS:

1. $\ll 10^{-8}$ MOL/L $\hat{=} \ll 10^{-1}$ MILLIGRAM/L $\hat{=} \ll 10^{15}$ MOLECULES/L $\hat{=} \gg 10^{11}$ CELLS/L

2. FOR 1 - 10 MILLIGRAM OF PROTEIN CYTOKINE, $>$100 - 1'000 LITER CULTURE SOLUTION WITH $>10^{13} - 10^{14}$ CELLS ARE NECESSARY

3. THEREFORE, FOR $\sim 10^{14}$ ($\sim$50 KILOGRAM) LEUKOCYTES, A MINIMUM OF $>$10 TONS OF BLOOD TO BE PROCESSED ARE NECESSARY

Table 1.

How much viable cell material is necessary for the isolation of a highly purified polypeptide cytokine of white blood cells in physical (milligram) quantities?

1.3 Cytokine effectors: Basic problems of their preparation

The calculation shows that for the preparation of 1-10 mg of a highly purified polypeptide effector substance, obtained with an (optimum) average yield of 10% of total activity, present in a crude tissue extract or cell culture supernatant solution by a purification in multiple steps, as starting material, at least 100 trillions (10E14) or 50 kg of cells, or suitable tissue with physiological effector production capacity are required. Still, it is conceivable that 1-10 mg of a polypeptide cytokine with a molecular weight larger than 2000 represents a modest amount; in considering the demands for a future, intensive investigation not only of their structure-function-turnover relations, but also for the possible pharmaceutical and clinical usefulness of novel cytokines elaborated, when considering the probable clinical relevance as summarized in Table 2. It is apparent from some introductory studies achieved (35, 36, 190-194).

Table 2. Probable clinical relevance in future as evident from introductory studies achieved (35, 36, 190-194) of novel, highly purified humoral and cellular polypeptide effectors operating chemical mechanisms for cellular reactions and communication in regenerative tissue morphogenesis intrinsic to inflammation and wound healing. For definition of terms, see references (1, 2, 34), where further quotations are presented.

Highly purified

MEDIATORS OF INFLAMMATION
and
WOUND HORMONES

are models of potential natural pharmaceuticals whose specificity of action has been selected in evolution.

This requirement in terms of amounts needed of a novel substance is also best reflected by the intensive efforts presently made in research on new biotechnical procedures to approach larger preparation or production capacities for many natural, already known biologically active substances, including polypeptide hormones; or as exemplified by interferons as representing one of the numerous polypeptide cytokine families (34, 37-45). The efforts disclose some similarities of problems intrinsic to present research on polypeptide effectors triggering chemical mechanisms for cellular reactions and communication in inflammation and wound healing, on one hand, and to classical hormone chemistry (46), on the other hand. There is a variety of novel substances with intriguing biological and chemical properties to be detected, if considered for the development of appropriate biotechnical and analytical methods. This became apparent from the disclosure of the existence of leucocytic wound hormones (1, 2, 45, 47-50). To verify production and purification of leucocytic polypeptide effectors, suitable amounts (Table 1) of conditioned (inflamed) tissues (e.g. ischaemically damaged, infarcted heart muscle sites), or of isolated, cultured leucocytes themselves, have to be at hand. Several aspects are worth considering: as basic problems, on one hand, they concern the technical procedures applied. On the other hand, they concern the criteria intrinsic to a cell culture medium useful for combined large scale and analytical work necessary during the production and preparation of (polypeptide) effector substances.

2.0 AVAILABLE TECHNICAL PROCEDURES FOR EFFECTOR PREPARATION

Different technical and biotechnical procedures are presently available for the production and preparation of highly purified, biologically active effector molecules operating chemical mechanisms for cellular reactions and communication in regenerative tissue morphogenesis intrinsic to inflammation and wound healing. They are summarized in Table 3.

---

1. THE CLASSICAL PROCEDURE:
   ISOLATION FROM NATURAL CELLS, TISSUES AND FLUIDS (WITH OR WITHOUT IN VITRO MANIPULATION, E.G. CULTURE)

2. CHEMICAL SYNTHESIS AND ISOLATION

3. ISOLATION FROM SELECTED AND CULTURED (HYPERACTIVE) CELL LINES (MOSTLY TUMOR CELL LINES)

4. SYNTHESIS BY HYBRIDOMA SELECTION TECHNIQUES AND ISOLATION

5. SYNTHESIS BY GENETIC ENGINEERING AND RECOMBINANT SELECTION AND ISOLATION TECHNIQUES

Table 3. Compilation of presently available technical procedures for the production and the preparation of (polypeptide) effector molecules operating chemical mechanisms for cellular reactions and communication in regenerative tissue morphogenesis with functional expressions intrinsic to the immune, haematopoietic and cardiovascular systems in inflammation and wound healing.

As alternatives to the classical preparation mode (procedure 1, Table 3) of mediators and hormones (in particular those of polypeptide nature) by isolation from (conditioned) animal and human tissues and cells, procedures 4 and 5 (Table 3) are relatively novel ones. They became available only recently; i.e. they are still in a phase of development (39-41). Both these alternative methods may have the possible advantages of high production capacity, variability in operational properties, technical practicability, optional automatization versatility and economy, especially when performed on the elaborated technical scales. In addition to these favourable characteristics, the two methods may also be superior to others due to their unique feature for the production and processing of biologically active substances of human origin and of complex structure; especially also of polypeptides of even higher molecular weight. Therefore, they probably are the techniques of choice and of the future for the production and preparation of already identified and known effector substances of human origin and structure, provided their structural features are not complicated by posttranslational modifications along their biosynthesis.

Similar characteristics are met by the procedures 2 and 3 (Table 3). Chemical synthesis is a method of choice for the preparation of peptides and small polypeptides whose structure is believed to be known. Then, this method may be developed and optimized for the production of such molecules even on kilogram scales. The chemical synthesis of somatostatin stands as an example for such a possible performance (51). However, it has to be considered that performance of chemical synthesis of polypeptide structures with molecular weights larger than 4000, or with several histidin residues consecutive in sequence (52), is still rather a matter of scientific art than a commonly established, realizable technical process. This is obvious from the known intensive efforts made for chemical synthesis of known biologically active polypeptide hormones, like insulin and glucagon (52, 53). This is also suggested by the preference presently given to the development of alternative methods (procedure 5, Table 3); or to combinations of different methods, like chemical modification of a similar sequence, or partial chemical synthesis of certain domains of a sequence, combined with their coupling to fragments or subunits of a natural substance already available. Procedure 3 (Table 3) has many aspects in common with the classical method; except that the availability of a hyperactive cell line is a prerequisite for the production and isolation of biologically active polypeptides. Such availability might sometimes be a matter of chance rather than a result of planned research.

Besides the advantages of the procedures 2-5 (Table 3), they also have several disadvantages in common: Firstly in principle, as such they are neither thought suitable in general for the preparation, nor for the discovery of yet unknown, novel natural effector substances of physiological origin. Secondly, for any biologically active product obtained by them, its identity concerning structure and function with the natural substance of physiological origin has to be demonstrated. In particular, concerning the clinical use in diagnosis and therapy, its possible constraints have to be elaborated, especially in terms of its comparable turnover, pharmacological and toxicological properties with the natural substance. Thus, for example, it is still an open question, whether or not a biologically active polypeptide mediator or hormone produced by tumour cell lines might be identical in properties to the corresponding one, exuded by normal, physiological cells. Thirdly, all these methods normally have in common that for every single biologically active substance under consideration, a separate, often laborious and, therefore, expensive production and preparation process has to be developed. This represents one major reason for the tremendous investment and production costs such procedures presently require, in particular in their early phase. This fact may be best exemplified by the production processes of interferon under investigation by genetic engineering (procedure 5, Table 3) (39, 43, 44). Fourthly, a mutual disadvantage of all the procedures 1-5 (Table 3) is the necessity for purification of every single, biologically active substance under investigation from a crude extract (homogenate or culture supernatant solution) in which it is produced and contained. This crude extract may also contain a variety of structurally and biologically diverse substances, but normally not a pure material. However, the difficul-

400

ties inherent to purification of the active substance investigated
and its separation from this variety of accompanying substances,
on one hand, may largely also depend on the nature and the mutual
similarities in the structure and function of the components present. On the other hand, it may depend on the stability of the
biological activity of the substance under investigation. It may
constitute a major contribution to the difficulties existing in
the purification methods to be applied. These reasons taken together explain the fact that, at present, still the classical
method 1 (Table 3) is predominantly used. In many cases, it still
has its economic basis under optimum performance, and may even be
favoured for promising developments in the production and preparation of mediators and hormones in the future (37-39, 42-45).

Nevertheless, in addition to the one previously mentioned
disadvantage of the classical procedure 1 (Table 3), namely the
requirement for purification of the biologically active substance
under investigation from a crude mixture of constituents, which it
has in common with all other methods (Table 3), two further drawbacks intrinsic to this method have to be recalled. Firstly, human
tissues or cells, as starting material for the production and isolation of a biologically active substance, are mostly not accessi-
ble, or only at high costs, and not in the amounts needed
(Table 1) for obtaining the required quantities of the investigated substance. Hence, mainly, the classical procedure has to rely
on the use of animal tissue, or cells, as starting material for
the isolation procedure of the required substance, at least in the
research and developmental, high risk phase of the investigation.
Therefore, the structural equivalent of human origin of a natural
substance may often be evaluated only with some delay, i.e. when
the processes for the production and isolation have already been
worked out on animal models. Secondly, the preparation of natural
trace substances is subject to the handling and processing of
large quantities of starting material and intermediary fractions
thereof (Table 1).

Although these three drawbacks in the use of the classical
method exist for the production and preparation of mediators and
hormones, in particular when of polypeptide nature, it has to be
the method of choice and to be applied for this purpose for the
following unsurpassable advantages:

a. The classical procedure as such allows detection, isolation and evaluation of the function and structure of a
variety of possibly existing, unknown, novel natural substances, either concomitantly or sequentially, from the
same crude starting material.

b. The classical procedure, and its use according to a), as
such, is a prerequisite for the later evaluation of
alternative processes for the preparation of a natural
substance, when possible at all.

The three mentioned possible disadvantages of the classical procedure 1 (Table 3) are balanced by the advantages, especially in the research and developmental, high cost and risk phase of new natural substances. An example is the first description of leucocytic wound hormones and other new mediators of inflammation and healing processes (1, 2, 34, 36, 45, 47-50, 54-59, 70-74). Intensive work is needed in the preparation and isolation processes on large scales (Table 1) for obtaining highly purified, biologically active, natural trace substances in physical amounts, by the classical procedure 1 (Table 3). But it is balanced by the possibility of evaluation of an evidently existing variety (1, 2, 34, 45) of costly, novel natural substances, from the same starting material which otherwise as yet are inaccessible (Figures 3-13).

Therefore, the classical procedure not only was the method of choice - or of necessity - in the period of classical hormone chemistry (46). In this period, steroid hormones had been isolated, for example from more than 20 tons of urine by Butenandt and his associates, and from about 1.5 tons of porcine ovaries by Doisy and co-workers (46). In addition, in this period, enzyme chemistry was developed similarly (46). For reasons of the subjects discussed before and by others (37), the classical procedure is still one of the methods of choice. On one hand, it allows an evaluation of the nature and variety of so far unknown, novel natural substances produced by normal cells. It also permits their distinction from similarly active substances produced by malignant, transformed or artificial cells. On the other hand, under optimum biotechnical performance, this method may be achieved economically and efficiently for this purpose. In the performance of all the techniques considered using cell cultures, however, a useful culture medium is a prerequisite and has to be at hand.

3.0 CULTURE OF CELLS IN MEDIA OF BIOLOGICAL FLUIDS (SERUM)

Implications of the use of cell culture media containing biological fluids, e.g. serum for the production and preparation of polypeptide cytokine effectors (of regenerative tissue morphogenesis):

Cell culture media are often complemented with a biological fluid, in particular serum, referred to as "serum-containing" media. Thus, when culturing cells for longer than one hour, or for certain purposes, in practice, usually (mostly heterologous, e.g. foetal calf or horse) serum in varying amounts is added to the culture medium. It accounts for and mimics an approach to physiological conditions of the previously mentioned ideal criteria. Due to some of the serum constituents so far evaluated, under investigation or still unknown (3-6, 11, 38, 75-80), its addition may be favourable in some instances for the maintenance and expression of cellular life and functions.

However, several difficulties may arise in the use of serum-containing media in cell-biological work, biochemical and clinical investigations on cell cultures, and in terms of their cell-interfacial, intracellular or extracellular properties. With respect to the latter, the medium must not only comply to the needs of cell survival and functions, as most known media do (5-30, 78, 79), but it also has to meet the concerns of cell-exuded substances like endogenous effector molecules of regenerative tissue morphogenesis. In particular, also the problems of their efficient and economic biotechnical and analytical processing in the production, preparation and biological testing must be met. To mention a few examples, in serum-containing media, due to the interaction of many of the serum proteins or lipids with cellular membranes (2, 34, 81-85), investigations of cellular membrane dynamics with fluorescent markers of distinct regions of the interfacial architecture may be tedious to achieve and to interprete, if not completely impossible. The same concerns other relations, for example, the dependence of cellular metabolism and transport on the extracellular fluid in which the cell under investigation will be maintained (5, 6, 86-92). Especially, numerous problems arise in investigations of cellular secretory or metabolic products exuded or already present in the extracellular fluid when they are in a form of a serum-containing medium. Such problems may be best exemplified in the biotechnical and analytical processing of polypeptide effectors (mediators and hormones) with labile biological activities exuded by leucocytes which operate chemical mechanisms for cellular reactions and communication in regenerative morphogenesis reactions (1, 2, 34, 47-50, 54-59, 70-75). The involvement of serum in the culture of leucocytes further complicates the anyway difficult preparation of such trace polypeptides for several reasons:

Firstly, the numerous "foreign" compounds making up the complex mixture of serum contained in a culture medium have to be separated from the labile, biologically active, newly formed or turned over extracellular trace substances. Secondly, the numerous components and enzymes of serum are not biologically inert with regard to the extracellular trace products. Thus, it might be difficult, if not impossible, to distinguish whether or not the cultured cell or the serum constituents prime the effect under investigation. Thirdly, under such conditions, upon addition of serum to a cell culture medium, it is laborious, if possible at all, to recognize the origin of such extracellular effectors. Hence, it may remain an open question whether or not a specific effector is of humoral (serum-derived), or cellular (e.g. leucocyte- or endothelial cell-derived) origin (1, 2, 34, 45, 93-103). Fourthly, in (mostly heterologous) serum-containing culture media, the demonstration of the species origin from which such a required effector substance stems, provides further problems. An effector polypeptide may be derived from the species whose cells have been cultured; or, alternatively, it may be derived from the species from which the added serum stems. Fifthly, standardized serum suitable for cell culture work has become very expensive recently. Hence, in summary, all the criteria mentioned below for the suitability of a serum-free, fully synthetic and chemically defined medium composition also apply to serum-containing media.

4.0 CRITERIA FOR THE DESIGN OF SYNTHETIC CELL CULTURE MEDIA

Implications of the use of fully synthetic, chemically defined media containing no biological fluid- (serum-) additive:

Known media used without serum likewise have drawbacks, for both the culture of cells and for the preparation of extracellular products, like the polypeptide effectors (operating chemical mechanisms for cellular reactions and communication in regenerative tissue morphogenesis by inflammation and healing). Thus, some of the media may be too poor in components for the full expression of cellular functions. Or they may contain some tensides, heavy metal salts or dyes which may be detrimental to the cells. These components may damage or irreversibly contaminate the trace polypeptide effectors to be isolated from the extracellular fluid in which they have been formed or are turned over by cells.

Criteria of cellular reactivity and functional integrity: In principle, beside the more specific aspects regarding the handling and limiting the applicability of a medium, several general criteria (for a fluid to be useful as a culture medium) have become obvious in recent investigations. Thus, some of the serum-free, component-poor media lack essential constituents which are necessary for maintaining the structural and functional viability of the cells as well as their life expressions on stimulation. As far as is known for some cell types of the haematopoietic, immune and cardiovascular systems (e.g. leucocytes, endothelial and heart muscle cells, etc.), for one example, Iscove and Melchers (14) found that the effects expressed by cells on addition of insulin, transferrin and serum albumin in a distinct (component-richer) medium, are not apparent in another (component-poorer) medium. This example shows that cellular behaviour is dependent not only on single components of a medium, but also on its whole composition.

Analytical criteria: Furthermore, despite the large number of existing and defined chemicals relatively few substances of cell-biological relevance are known which are clearly analytically defined; and whose different production lots provide a comparable or identical cellular reactivity, and functional integrity criteria for a culture medium. Thus, for example, although sensitive analytical methods are at hand, certain preparations of otherwise well defined chemicals which normally may be beneficial components in a medium, might also express some inhibitory activity on cellular reactions; whereas other preparation lots of the same chemical do not. Such behaviour has been found exemplified for some enzyme (e.g. trypsin) and indicator dye lots (e.g. phenol red) (5, 6) added to some media.

Criteria of component interaction: On the other hand, analytically defined and reactively constant lots of components added to a solution during the composition of a synthetic medium may interact and neutralize their intrinsic chemical functions before coming into interaction with cells in the culture. This is the case when their association parameters lead to a stable (soluble or insoluble) complex with other chemicals or cell-biological units. However, such interplay may also be a useful effect in the composition of a cell culture medium. The example applies to some vitamins as well as to fatty acids, etc. Free fatty acids, for example, normally are soaps which may not be favourable to cell-biological structures and functions investigated in a culture (84, 104). However, when associated and physically (multivalently) bound to serum albumin below its saturation point of 8 binding sites per molecules (105), fatty acids, in particular unsaturated ones, may exert physiological functions as essential components of cell biological fluids. This criterium also applies to the sequence by which chemically defined constituents of a medium during its composition are mixed together, with respect to their solubility as well as to their reactivity.

Preparative criteria: In addition, some of the chemically defined components used in the composition of media, like tensides, heavy metal salts, and/or dyes, may not only be detrimental to cells or tissues in culture. They may also damage, irreversibly alter or contaminate extracellular trace components exuded or secreted by cultured cells in or below the nanomolar concentration range (Table 1) (1, 2, 34, 45). Thus, heavy metal-sensitive polypeptides, not only in the form of enzymes, are commonly known and physiologically abundant. Additionally, in the biotechnical processing of extracellular, biologically active trace polypeptides, isolation could yield, for example, an artificially stained polypeptide preparation by irreversible adsorption of an indicator dye which initially has been a component of a synthetic cell culture medium. Such an experimentally possible result would mimic misleading properties of the polypeptide substance produced and isolated under intensive work and at high costs.

Economic criteria: For serial analytical and biotechnical work, larger volumes of cell culture media are required. Thus, costs of any (serum-containing or -free) medium come into play. It is evident from Table 1 that for the culture of technical (up to kilogram) quantities of cells, and the extensive biological analytics intrinsic to such processing, a suitable medium must also fulfil the economic criterium. The total volume of medium needed for the culture of, for example, about 50 kg (about 10E14) of cells at a maximum density of 10E08 cell/ml, is at least 1 cubic metre; whatever the method is, and the possible techniques are for the preparation and culture of these amounts of cells.

5.0 PREPARATION AND PROPERTIES OF A NEW SYNTHETIC MEDIUM

Fully synthetic and chemically defined, serum-free cell
culture media compositions for applied large scale and
serial analytical biotechniques:

From the discussion so far, it is evident that a universally
useful medium for the culture of all cell types existing and for
the variety of culture purposes possible cannot be designed as
such. However, for serial analytical and large scale work involving the production and isolation of trace polypeptide mediators
and hormones of white blood cells the problems concerning the evaluated criteria have been resolved by the composition of a suitable cell culture medium. It is useful for leucocytic polypeptide
mediators and hormones with biological activities basic to functional expressions of the immune, haematopoietic and cardiovascular systems in inflammation and wound healing which trigger chemical mechanisms for cellular reactions and communication in regenerative tissue morphogenesis. Tables 4 and 5 present its constituents and their properties. It is a component-rich basic medium
containing a combination of 91 constituents. Furthermore, normally, it may contain variable additional and alternative components
from which three are detailed also in Table 4. In Table 5, the
single components are described in their known properties and
sources to allow the preparation of constant properties of the
medium. In the following, a detailed description of the preparation mode and of the features of the culture medium is presented.

5.1 Material and methods for the preparation of the medium

The medium (Table 4) is prepared from concentrated stock solutions of groups of components which are termed ST-A to ST-T.
Their concentrations in terms of multiples of the final concentrations of components in the medium are summarized in Table 5 together with the characteristics of chemicals used to compose the
medium. Complementing the footnotes of Tables 4 and 5, these stock
solutions are prepared in the following manner:
Each of the different stock solutions ST-A to ST-N is made
from the weighted multiples of amounts of the single components
no.1 to no.72 by dissolving one after the other in the numbered
sequence given within one stock solution, in about 2/3 of a final
volume of sterile, pyrogen-free, ultrapure water of ASTM-1 quality
(106-108) (component no.47, Tables 4 and 5, preparation described
below) at about 37 deg.C; except for stock solutions ST-I, ST-J,
ST-K and ST-L which are first prepared in water of such quality
having about 90 deg.C. After cooling to 20 deg.C, the formed clear
solutions of the highly pure substances are adjusted to their desired volume (e.g. 1 or 100 1) by the water component no.47 of
20 deg.C. The stock solution ST-O is prepared in the same manner;

but at variance, the single components no.73-79 are first dissolved in warm (about 37 deg.C) 0.01 to 0.05 mol/1 NaOH, made up
(wearing goggles!) of the same water quality to about a pH of
12 +/- 0.5. After having been neutralized to pH 7.40 by the addition of a few drops of 0.5 mol/l HCl prepared from ASTM-1 water
quality, the clear solution is processed to its final volume unit
as given for the other stock solutions at 20 deg.C. All these
stock solutions ST-A to ST-O may be stored at about -30 deg.C, unless not used immediately. Some precipitates formed upon freezing
will readily dissolve again after thawing and transiently warming
up to 37 deg.C in maximum while gently shaking (for ST-G, see
below).

Stock solutions ST-P, ST-Q and ST-R are prepared together as
follows. Firstly, the weighted multiples of amounts of components
no.81-85 are dissolved as single substances one after the other in
the numbered sequence added (Table 4) while gently stirring to
about two-third of a chosen final stock solution volume of
water-free, non-denatured, (about 80 deg.C to boiling) hot ethanol (analytical grade quality, 99.8 w/v%, no.972/983, Merck,
Darmstadt, Germany). Prior to use, it was further purified to the
quality described below and made pyrogen-free by the process mentioned below. After cooling of the formed clear stock solution
ST-P of the components no.80-85 to about 37 deg.C, the weighted
multiples of amounts of the single components no.86-88 (Tables 4
and 5) are then sequentially further added in the same manner, resulting the combined stock solution ST-P-Q. Then, this clear solution is freed from dissolved air by gently stirring under low
pressure at 20 deg.C for about 30 minutes, after which it is
further handled in an atmosphere of heat-decontaminated,
pyrogen-free, filtersterilized, analytical grade nitrogen prepared
as described below for the processing of sterile, pyrogen-free air
(oxygen). Subsequently, under further handling in an atmosphere of
this nitrogen quality, to the ST-P-Q stock solution, the weighted
multiples of amounts of the labile unsaturated fatty acid components no.89-91 are added at 37 deg.C while gently stirring. Conveniently, components no.89 and 90 may be added as already available in a 80:20 mixture, as specified in Table 5. After a clear
solution has been formed, ethanol of the described quality is
added to correct for the desired final volume unit. The combined
stock solution ST-P-Q-R results. Unless used immediately, it can
be stored at or below -25 deg.C for at least 2 years in the dark
in an atmosphere of the described nitrogen quality.

Polypeptide and polysaccharide stock solutions ST-S and ST-T
are prepared as given for ST-A, except that pyrogen-free, sterile
physiological (1.5 mmol/1) Na, K-phosphate-buffered, (0.15 mol/1 =
= 0.9 w/v%) NaCl solution, pH 7.40, is used at about 37 deg.C to
dissolve the weighted multiples of the amounts of components
no. 92-93 and no.94, respectively. Conveniently, the ST-S stock
solution components are available mixed commercially and may be
used as such (Table 5); if not self-made from similar sources,
such as analytical grade benzylpenicillin G (potassium salt, puri-

ty higher than 99%, activity about 1320 IU/mg, no.13750) and streptomycin sulphate (purum, activity: about 780 IU/mg, no.85880) from Fluka, Neu-Ulm, Germany, respectively, which gave identical results. When other additional or alternative, variable components are added to the basic medium, their stock solutions are prepared in a similar manner. Salt solutions in use are made sterile and pyrogen-free as described for the preparation of water. Prior to storage or use, polypeptide and polysaccharide stock solutions like St-S, St-T and St-G (serum albumin), are sterilized by filtration (0.2 um pore size), whether prepared in salt solutions (like ST-S and ST-T) or in water (like ST-G).

Ultrapure, sterile and pyrogen-free water of ASTM-1 quality (106-108) which is used throughout in all processes of preparation of the medium and all solutions, was provided and handled in heavy metal-free installations and materials made up of polypropylene, polyethylene, polyvinyl chloride, polycarbonate, polymethylpentene, teflon, silicone and lead-free soda-lime or borosilicate glass like Duran quality (Schott, Mainz, Germany; Wheaton, Millville, New Jersey; Bellco Glass, Vineland, New Jersey; Schuett, Goettingen, Germany; Science Services - Nalge Company, Munich, Germany; Bel Art, Pequannock, New Jersey; Fischer, Schaffhausen, Switzerland). This water quality was produced from tap water at a maximum flow of 10 l/min in a system consisting of a charcoal column, a reverse osmosis reactor and a regenerable ion exchange column in sequence with a Millipore (Bedford, Massachusetts) Super-Q-4-recycling ultrapurification system (109, 110). It is composed of a one-way-used, non-regenerable charcoal, two ion exchange and one filter sterilization (0.2 um pore size) cartridge columns in sequence. In these first sequential steps, highly purified, presterilized water with an average specific electric conductivity of 0.055 uS/cm (about 18 Mega Ohm.cm) is obtained. Prior to use, this highly purified water was processed further to ultrapure, pyrogen-free, sterile water by a Millipore-Super-Q-3-ultrapurification cartridge system (109, 110). It consists of one charcoal, one ion exchange and one sodium hypochlorite- (0.1% NaOCl-) sterilized, tenside-free filter sterilization (0.2 um pore size) columns in sequence, followed by an ethylene oxide-sterilized pyrogen elimination system in the form of ultrafiltration in a Millipore Pellicon Membrane Casette system (111). It was equipped with tenside-free Millipore PTGC 00005 ultrafiltration membranes having a nominal exclusion limit range for hydrodynamic equivalents of molecular weights of 1 000 to 10 000. For the latter purpose, ultrafiltration systems of Amicon (Witten, Germany) equipped with tenside-free, sterilized UM10-membranes (115) (or similar exclusion limits), were in use, too, when smaller volumes of water or all types of salt solutions had to be freed from exogenous pyrogen contaminants. Sterilization of such smaller volumes of solutions was achieved, if possible, either by steam autoclaving, but mostly by filtration on tenside-free or -freed membranes (0.2 um pore size) (Millipore, Neu-Isenburg; Sartorius, Goettingen, Germany).

Pyrogen-free, absolute, non-denaturated ethanol was made from the mentioned quality (no.972/983, higher than 99.8%, Merck, Darmstadt, Germany) by fresh distillation according to common procedures (112) over magnesium metal chips (analytical grade Grignard, no.805817, Merck, Darmstadt, Germany) in a silver-coated, vacuum-jacketed separation column (1200 x 30 mm) filled with stainless steel (V4A) Raschig rings (3 x 3 mm with stick, 1500 meshes/sq.cm, no.58830, Brand, Wertheim, Germany). The final quality of the pyrogen-free ethanol has been further established in terms of its density (rho 20 deg.C/4 deg.C = 789.33 g/l), as measured in a DMA60/601 Kratky-Paar digital density measurement apparatus (Anton Paar, Graz, Austria) (113); and its refractive index n(D) 20 deg.C = 1.36155, as measured in an Abbé refractometer (Zeiss, Oberkochen, Germany); or, as relative value with reference to a standard solution, in a laser differential refractometer KMX-16 (Chromatrix, Sunnyvale, California) (114). The ethanol prepared in this way could be kept on stock over pyrogen-free, heat decontaminated, filter-sterilized phosphorous pentoxide-dried nitrogen which, prior to use, was prepared from analytical grade nitrogen as described below for air (oxygen).

Preparation of other chemicals: Heat-decontaminated, pyrogen-free, sterile air-oxygen was used throughout and prepared by flushing 0.2 um pore size filter-sterilized air at low flow (about 5 l/hr) through a silica tube of about 200 ml (160 x 40 mm) which was kept at a minimum temperature of about 500 deg.C. After cooling, this heat-decontaminated air was washed twice by bubbling (diameter of bubbles < 1 mm) through sterile, pyrogen-free water of ASTM-1 quality. In the same manner, other gases of analytical grade quality (like nitrogen, carbondioxide, etc.) have been heat-decontaminated and made sterile and pyrogen-free. If necessary, they were dried over analytical grade phosphorous pentoxide. Unless otherwise specified, all other usual chemicals mentioned were also of analytical grade quality (e.g. HCl, NaOH, etc.). They were not further controlled on specifications given by the purchasing companies, when methods were reproduceable.

Mixing of the stock solutions and preparation of the final medium: To about 2/3 of the desired final medium volume unit of sterile, pyrogen-free, ultrapure water of ASTM-1 quality (ST-M, component no.47, Tables 4 and 5), the stock solutions ST-A, B, C, D, H, I, J, K, L, N, and O are sequentially added at 20 deg.C, diluted and mixed by gently stirring in their appropriate volume units. These volume units of stock solutions are dictated by their concentration factors (Table 5) with reference to the final composition (Tables 4 and 5) and the desired final volume of the ready made medium. Thus, they are, e.g., 2 ml (1) ST-A, 50 ml (1) ST-B, 20 ml (1) ST-C, 10 ml (1) ST-D, ST-I, St-J, St-K, St-N and ST-O, 5 ml (1) ST-H, 1 ml (1) ST-L which are added to about 660 ml (1) water, if the desired final medium volume is to be 1000 ml (1). Then, sequentially, in the same manner, stock solutions ST-E and ST-F are added one after the other which means 10 ml (1) ST-E and 50 ml (1) ST-F in the volume example of 1000 ml (1) given for the final medium. During this procedure, the pH should be kept below 7.80 by continuous registration and possible correction by a few drops of 1.0 mol/l HCl which was made up of pyrogen-free, sterile water. Possible contamination with exogenous pyrogens brought in this partial medium solution by the commercial components dissolved in the stock solutions on addition to the pyrogen-free water, are eliminated by ultrafiltration by ethylene oxide-sterilized, tenside-free membranes with a nominal exclusion limit range for hydrodynamic equivalents of molecular weights of 1 000 to 10 000, as described in detail for the preparation of ultrapure, pyrogen-free water (e.g. Millipore PTGC 00005 or Amicon UM10, PM10 or equivalents) (111, 115).

Prior to further processing of this pyrogen-free solution for the final medium, stock solutions ST-G (serum albumin, no.24, Tables 4 and 5) and ST-P-Q-R (components no.80-91) are made ready for use by dropwise stirring in at about 20 deg.C of 60 ul (ml) of the ethanol stock solution ST-P-Q-R into 25 ml (l) stock solution ST-G, if the desired final medium volume is to be 1 000 ml (l). Homogeneous distribution of the hydrophobic substances contained in ST-P-Q-R and their adsorption to the albumin in ST-G is complemented by a sequence of 5 ultrasonic pulses of 10 s and 100 W of a temperature-(PT-100)-controlled sonifier (Labsonic 1510, Braun, Melsungen, Germany). During this procedure, the temperature is allowed to be a maximum of 20 deg.C. No foaming of the serum albumin solution ST-G should occur during and after the adsorption process of the hydrophobic, water-insoluble substances no.81-91) in St-P-Q-R to the serum albumin. Then, the combined clear stock solution ST-G-P-Q-R containing the water-dissolved serum albumin charged with the hydrophobic molecules (45,74,75), is added while stirring to the pyrogen-free, already combined, diluted solution of the other stock solutions. Finally, the volume of this diluted mixture of components no.1-91 (Table 4) is corrected to the desired final medium volume by addition of ultrapure, pyrogen-free, sterile water. The desired pH (e.g.7.10, component no.45) ist adjusted by the addition of a few drops of either sterile, pyrogen-free 1 mol/l HCl or NaOH. At variance, during culture, the pH of the medium is kept constant either by dropwise addition of sterile, pyrogen-free 0.1 mol/l acetic acid (analytical grade, non-denaturated quality, 100 w/v/%, no.63E Merck, Darmstadt, Germany) as an alternative component to no.15 (Table 4), or by sterile, pyrogen-free 0.2 mol/l sodiumbicarbonate (component no.23, Table 4). This may be achieved automatically by autotitration of the culture fluid through the control of addition of acid or base by magnetic valves. Prior to the use of this basic medium of 91 components, it is equilibrated with heat-decontaminated, sterile, pyrogen-free air-oxygen (component no.46, Table 4) and kept constant at its saturation concentration by electrode-controlled flushing at 20 deg.C (37 deg.C during culture) with fine bubbles (< 1 mm) of air at low flow (about 5 l/hr), as described above, while further stirring (60 rpm) for 3 hrs (or continuously during culture) and concomitant registration and possible correction of the desired pH to a constant. Immediately prior to use or storage, the basic medium is sterilized by filtration (0.2 um pore size). Unless used immediately, the ready made medium may be stored at 4 deg.C for shorter periods (up to 2 months) in the dark over the heat-decontaminated, sterile, pyrogen-free air atmosphere; or in the same manner, but in small batches, it may be kept frozen below -25 deg.C in the dark. Thawing and warming up to 37 deg.C with slow circular shaking results again in a clear medium solution. The variable, alternative or additional components, like no.92-94 (Tables 4 and 5), are added to this basic medium immediately prior to use directly from their sterile, pyrogen-free stock solutions, e.g. ST-S (no.92-93) and ST-T (no.94), to give first the reference culture medium (REF) (components no.1-93) and, then, the production culture medium (e.g. CON) (component no.1-94). The volume concentration error introduced by this manipulation through the final addition of the concentrated stock solutions to the other dissolved components, remains in the small range of about +/- 1.5%. These prepared medium forms are free of exogenous pyrogens, when submitted in doses up to 10 ml/kg rabbit to the standardized pyrogen assay (158), described in detail elsewhere (measurement of rectal temperature of rabbits prior, during and after intravenous probe application) (2). The media have an average osmotic pressure of 290 mOsm/kg, as expressed by freezing point depression measurement (Knauer, Berlin, Germany). If variable alternative components are to completely replace one of the components of the basic medium, the final medium is prepared by omitting the addition of the appropriate stock solution and replacing it by another (e.g. normal thymidine by tritium-labelled thymidine as component no.44, Table 4).

Table 4. Composition of serum-free, fully synthetic, chemically defined medium for culture of cells on analytical and biotechnical scales (45, 75)

NO.	COMPONENT	MOL/L	NO.	COMPONENT	MOL/L
1*	DISODIUM HYDROGENPHOSPHATE	0.8 m	48	L-ALANINE	0.2 m
2*	POTASSIUM DIHYDROGENPHOSPHATE	0.2 m	49	L-ARGININE	0.1 m
3	POTASSIUM CHLORIDE	5.0 m	50	D,L-CARNITINE CHLORIDE (BT)	50.0 μ
4	SODIUM CHLORIDE	120.0 m	51	L-CARNOSINE	5.0 μ
5	SODIUM SULFATE	0.2 m	52	CYANOCOBALAMINE (B12)	0.5 μ
6*	D-GLUCOSE	5.0 m	53	L-CYSTEINE	0.2 m
7	L-ASCORBIC ACID (C)	0.2 m	54	L-GLUTATHIONE REDUCED	3.0 m
8	CHOLINE CHLORIDE	50.0 μ	55	GLYCINE	0.2 m
9	2-DEOXY-D-RIBOSE	5.0 μ	56	L-HISTIDINE	0.1 m
10	D-GALACTOSE	0.5 m	57	L-HYDROXYPROLINE	10.0 μ
11	D-GLUCURONO-γ-LACTONE	0.1 m	58	L-LYSINE MONO HCl	0.2 m
12	GLYCEROL	50.0 μ	59	L-METHIONINE	0.1 m
13	MYO-INOSITOL	0.5 m	60	D,L-MET METHYLSULFONIUM Br (U)	1.0 μ
14	D-RIBOSE	20.0 μ	61	D,L-MEVALOLACTONE	5.0 μ
15	SODIUM ACETATE	0.2 m	62	NICOTINIC ACID AMIDE (PP)	20.0 μ
16	SODIUM CITRATE TRI Na	50.0 μ	63	L-ORNITHINE MONO HCl	50.0 μ
17	SODIUM PYRUVATE	0.1 m	64	D-PANTOTHENIC ACID Ca (B5)	5.0 μ
18	SUCCINIC ACID	0.1 m	65	L-PROLINE	0.1 m
19	XYLITOL	10.0 μ	66	PYRIDOXAL HCl	5.0 μ
20	D-XYLOSE	20.0 μ	67	PYRIDOXIN HCl (B6)	2.0 μ
21	CALCIUM CHLORIDE	2.0 m	68	SARCOSINE (N-METHYLGLYCINE)	50.0 μ
22	MAGNESIUM CHLORIDE	1.0 m	69	L-SERINE	0.1 m
23	SODIUM HYDROGENCARBONATE	10.0 m	70	TAURINE	0.1 m
24	SERUM ALBUMIN (HUMAN) 0.5MG/ML	7.3 μ	71	THIAMINE HCl (B1)	5.0 μ
25	L-ASPARAGINE	0.1 m	72	L-THREONINE	0.2 m
26	L-GLUTAMINE	1.0 m	73	ADENINE (B4)	50.0 μ
27	ADENOSINE	50.0 μ	74	FOLIC ACID (Bc)	5.0 μ
28	4-AMINOBENZOIC ACID	2.0 μ	75	GUANINE	5.0 μ
29	L-ASPARTIC ACID	0.1 m	76	GUANOSINE	20.0 μ
30	D-BIOTINE (H)	1.0 μ	77	HYPOXANTHINE (6-HYDROXYPURINE)	5.0 μ
31	CYTIDINE	50.0 μ	78	RUTIN (P)	5.0 μ
32	L-GLUTAMIC ACID	0.1 m	79	XANTHINE (2,6-DIHYDROXYPURINE)	5.0 μ
33	L-ISOLEUCINE	0.2 m	80	ETHANOL (60 μl/l)	1.0 m
34	5-METHYLCYTOSINE	5.0 μ	81	CHOLESTEROL	1.0 μ
35	L-PHENYLALANINE	0.1 m	82	ERGOCALCIFEROL (D2)	0.5 μ
36	RIBOFLAVINE (B2)	1.0 μ	83	D,L-α-LIPOIC ACID	2.0 μ
37	THYMINE (5-METHYLURACIL)	5.0 μ	84	MENADIONE (K3)	0.2 μ
38	L-TRYPTOPHANE	50.0 μ	85	D,L-α-TOCOPHERYL ACETATE (E)	1.0 μ
39	L-TYROSINE	0.1 m	86	COENZYME Q10 – UBIQUINONE 50	0.1 μ
40	URACIL	5.0 μ	87	3-PHYTYLMENADIONE (K1)	0.2 μ
41	URIDINE	20.0 μ	88	RETINYL ACETATE (A)	1.0 μ
42*	L-LEUCINE	0.2 m	89	LINOLEIC ACID (F)	1.0 μ
43*	L-VALINE	0.2 m	90	LINOLENIC ACID (F)	5.0 μ
44*	THYMIDINE	20.0 μ	91	OLEIC ACID (F)	5.0 μ
45*	HYDROGEN IONS (pH 7.1)	79.4 n	92*	BENZYLPENICILLIN K 50 IU/ml	0.1 m
46*	OXYGEN (AIR SATURATION, 37 °C)	0.2 m	93*	STREPTOMYCIN SULFATE 50 IU/ml	0.1 m
47	WATER (ASTM 1, PYROGEN-FREE)	55.4	94*	ACTIVATOR(S): CONCANAVALIN A	50.0 n

*) Footnote see page 414

Table 5a. Mode of preparation of the serum-free, fully synthetic, chemically defined cell culture medium: Specification of components and stock solutions. Number in first column refers to number of components of Table 4 (omitting names). Other details are given in the context and the footnote * (continued next page).

NO.	MOLECULAR WEIGHT	FINAL MEDIUM CONCENTRATION MG/L	STOCK SOLUTION NO. ST-	X - FOLD OF MEDIUM CONCENTRATION	SPECIFICATION/QUALITY /GRADE	SOURCE *	ORDER NO.
1	177.99	142.40	A	500 - x	x2H$_2$O, analytical	Merck	6580
2	136.09	27.22	A	500 - x	anhydrous, analytical	Merck	4873
3	74.56	372.75	B	20 - x	anhydrous, analytical	Merck	4936
4	58.44	7 012.80	B	20 - x	anhydrous, analytical	Merck	6404
5	142.04	28.40	B	20 - x	anhydrous, analytical	Merck	6649
6	180.16	900.80	C	50 - x	anhydrous biochemical	Merck	8337E
7	176.13	35.23	D	100 - x	crystalized, USP XIX	Merck	500074
8	139.63	6.98	D	100 - x	>99 %, crystaline	Sigma	C-1879
9	134.13	0.67	D	100 - x	purum, melting:~85 °C	Fluka	31170
10	180.16	90.08	D	100 - x	anhydrous, pfs, 99%	Sigma	G-0625
11	176.13	17.61	D	100 - x	purum, melting ~175°C	Fluka	49340
12	92.10	5.29	D	100 - x	87 %, analytical *	Merck *	4094
13	180.16	90.08	D	100 - x	puriss., ~99 %	Fluka	57570
14	150.13	3.00	D	100 - x	pfs, crystaline, 99%	Sigma	R-7500
15	82.04	16.41	D	100 - x	anhydrous,puriss. 99%	Fluka	71180
16	294.10	14.71	D	100 - x	x2H$_2$O,analytical,99%	Merck	6448
17	110.05	11.01	D	100 - x	biochemical, 99 %	Merck	6619
18	118.09	11.81	D	100 - x	puriss., >99.5 %	Fluka	14079
19	152.15	1.52	D	100 - x	puriss., pyrogen-free	Fluka	95649
20	150.13	3.00	D	100 - x	puriss., > 99 %	Fluka	95730
21	147.02	294.04	E	100 - x	x2H$_2$O, analytical>99%	Merck	2382
22	203.31	203.30	E	100 - x	x6H$_2$O, analytical, 99%	Merck	5833
23	84.01	840.10	F	20 - x	anhydrous, analytical	Merck	6329E
24	69'000	500.00	G	40 - x	homogeneous, natural*	Behring *	ORHA-20
25	150.14	15.01	H	200 - x	x1H$_2$O, biochemical,99%	Merck	1566
26	146.15	146.15	H	200 - x	biochemical, 99 %	Merck	289
27	267.20	13.36	I	100 - x	crystalized, 99 %	Böhringer	102083
28	137.14	0.27	I	100 - x	puriss., >99.5 %	Fluka	06930
29	133.10	13.31	I	100 - x	biochemical, 99%	Merck	126
30	244.32	0.24	I	100 - x	pfs, ~98 %	Sigma	B-4501
31	243.22	12.16	I	100 - x	puriss., >99 %	Fluka	30270
32	147.13	14.71	I	100 - x	biochemical, 99 %	Merck	291
33	131.18	26.24	I	100 - x	biochemical, 99 %	Merck	5362
34	125.13	0.63	I	100 - x	purum, ~96 %	Fluka	66581
35	165.19	16.52	I	100 - x	biochemical, 99 %	Merck	7256
36	376.38	0.38	I	100 - x	pfs, ~98 %	Sigma	R-4500
37	126.12	0.63	I	100 - x	purum, >97 %	Fluka	89310
38	204.23	10.21	I	100 - x	biochemical, 99 %	Merck	8374
39	181.19	18.12	I	100 - x	biochemical, 99 %	Merck	8371
40	112.09	0.56	I	100 - x	pfs, crystaline,>99%	Sigma	U-0750
41	244.20	4.88	I	100 - x	crystalized, 98 %	Böhringer	109975
42	131.18	26.24	J	100 - x	biochemical, 99 %	Merck	5360
43	117.15	23.43	K	100 - x	biochemical, 99 %	Merck	8495
44	242.23	4.84	L	1'000 - x	pfs, crystaline, > 99%	Sigma	T-9250
45	1.00	79.40·10^{-6}	M	1 - x	analytical *	*	
46	32.00	6.40	M	1 - x	pyrogen-free air *	*	
47	18.00	997.00·10^{+3}	M	1 - x	ASTM-1, pyrogen-free	*	

*) Footnote see page 414

Table 5b.

NO.	MOLECULAR WEIGHT	FINAL MEDIUM CONCENTRATION MG/L	STOCK SOLUTION NO. ST-	X - FOLD OF MEDIUM CONCENTRATION	SPECIFICATION/QUALITY /GRADE	SOURCE *	ORDER NO.
48	89.09	17.82	N	100 - x	biochemical, 99 %	Merck	1007
49	174.20	17.42	N	100 - x	biochemical, 99 %	Merck	1542
50	197.66	9.88	N	100 - x	chloride, purum, ~ 99%	Fluka	22020
51	226.24	1.13	N	100 - x	N-ß-Ala-His, purum>99%	Fluka	22030
52	1'355.39	0.68	N	100 - x	puriss., crystaline	Fluka	95190
53	121.16	24.33	N	100 - x	free base biochemical	Merck	2838
54	307.30	0.92	N	100 - x	GSH crystalized >98 %	Böhringer	127744
55	75.07	15.01	N	100 - x	biochemical, 99 %	Merck	4201
56	155.16	15.52	N	100 - x	biochemical, 99 %	Merck	4351
57	131.13	1.31	N	100 - x	puriss., > 99 %	Fluka	56250
58	182.65	36.53	N	100 - x	x1HCl, biochemical 99%	Merck	5700
59	149.21	14.92	N	100 - x	biochemical, 99 %	Merck	5707
60	244.16	0.25	N	100 - x	bromide, purum, >98 %	Fluka	64380
61	130.14	0.65	N	100 - x	purum, salt-free,~98 %	Fluka	69761
62	122.13	2.44	N	100 - x	puriss., > 99 %	Fluka	72340
63	168.62	8.43	N	100 - x	x1HCl, puriss., >99 %	Fluka	75470
64	476.54	2.38	N	100 - x	calcium salt, purum	Fluka	21210
65	115.13	11.51	N	100 - x	biochemical, 99 %	Merck	7434
66	203.63	1.02	N	100 - x	x1HCl, puriss., >99 %	Fluka	82860
67	205.69	0.41	N	100 - x	x1HCl, purum, >98 %	Fluka	95180
68	89.10	4.46	N	100 - x	puriss., ~99 %	Fluka	84530
69	105.09	10.51	N	100 - x	biochemical, 99 %	Merck	7769
70	125.15	12.52	N	100 - x	>99 %, pfs crystaline	Sigma	T-0625
71	337.27	1.75	N	100 - x	x1HCl, purum,~4% water	Fluka *	95160
72	119.12	23.82	N	100 - x	biochemical, 99 %	Merck	8411
73	135.10	6.76	O	100 - x	crystalized, >98 %	Böhringer	102067
74	441.41	2.21	O	100 - x	99-100 %, pfs	Sigma	F-7876
75	151.13	0.76	O	100 - x	grade II, crystaline	Sigma >99%	G-0506
76	283.25	5.67	O	100 - x	crystaline, pfs, > 98%	Sigma	G-6752
77	136.11	0.68	O	100 - x	anhydrous, crystaline	Sigma	H-9377
78	610.53	3.32	O	100 - x	purum, ~8 % water *	Fluka *	84028
79	152.11	0.76	O	100 - x	crystaline, 99-100 %	Sigma	X-0626
80	46.07	46.07	P	20 000 - x	absolute, analytical*	Merck *	972
81	386.67	0.39	P	20 000 - x	puriss., >99 % USP	Fluka	26740
82	396.66	0.20	P	20 000 - x	puriss. crystaline 99%	Fluka	95220
83	206.33	0.41	P	20 000 - x	purum, > 98 %	Fluka	62320
84	172.19	0.04	P	20 000 - x	purum, ~97 %	Fluka	67900
85	472.76	0.47	P	20 000 - x	purum, ~ 97 %	Fluka	95250
86	863.37	0.09	Q	20 000 - x	pure, >99 % (HPLC)	Serva	17404
87	450.68	0.09	Q	20 000 - x	purum, 98 %	Fluka	95271
88	328.50	0.33	Q	20 000 - x	acetate, purum, 95 %	Fluka	95140
89	280.46	1.68	R	20 000 - x	pract, natural 80:20 (no. 90:89), ∑6µmol/l	Fluka *	62170
90	278.44		R	20 000 - x			
91	282.47	2.01	R	20 000 - x	Erg. B6, ~70 % *	Fluka *	75093
92	372.48	37.20	S	100 - x	5'000 IU/ml solution*	Flow *	7010-D
93	728.70	72.90	S	100 - x	5'000 IU/ml solution*	Flow *	7010-D
94	104'000 *	5.20	T	200 - x	crystalline, research	Serva	27648

*) Footnote see page 414

414

Footnotes of pages 411-414:

*) (Table 4) The components 6, 45, and 46 are continuously meas-
ured and corrected to constant during culture. The components
92-94 are variable, alternative components added to the basic medium of the first 91 constituents. Correspondingly, they may be replaced or intensified in their action by other substances, or omitted, such as in the reference medium for no.94. The buffer components 1 and 2 may be replaced or intensified in their capacity
by other suitable buffer systems. For tracer methods, the components 42-44 may be replaced correspondingly. Letters in brackets
refer to vitamin nomenclature (60) added to the systemic name.
Group division of components refer to combinations of substances
in stock solutions having 20 - 20 000-fold concentrations: soluble
in water are at 37 deg.C no.1-26, 45-72, and 92-94; at 90 dec.C
no.27-44; in $\leq$ 0.05 Mol/l NaOH (pH 12.0) at 37 deg.C no.73-79;
in warm ethanol at 37 deg.C no.86-91, and at 78 deg.C no.80-85.
For further details see Tables 5a,b.

*) (Tables 5a, b) Sources of chemicals: Merck, Darmstadt, Germany;
Sigma, St.Louis, Missouri; Fluka, Neu-Ulm, Germany; Boehringer,
Mannheim, Germany; Serva, Heidelberg, Germany; Flow, Bonn,
Germany; Behring, Marburg, Germany. Purity grade abbreviations and
further specifications, see company catalogue identifications. Molecular weight quoted for human serum albumin (no.24), benzylpenicillin K (no.92), streptomycin sulphate (no.93), and concanavalin
A (no.94) are from references (3, 61-63). Natural, non-defatted
serum albumin used for this medium was homogeneous in electrophoresis and chromatography; as judged by electrophoresis (Figure 2)
in 10% acrylamide under denaturing and dissociating conditions
(0.1 w/v % sodium dodecylsulphate and 0.1 mol/l 2-mercaptoethanol)
performed according to Porzio and Pearson (64), and by gel filtration on Ultrogel AcA34 and AcA44 (LKB-Instruments, Bromma, Sweden)
(65). It contains about 1-2 mol fatty acid (hydrophobic) residues
already bound per mol serum albumin, as determined after extraction on an Extrelut column (no.11737, Merck) (66) by gas chromatography (67-69). Sterile, pyrogen-free water (no. 47), air-oxygen
(no.46), ethanol (no.80) are prepared and pH (no.45) adjusted as
described in section 5.1. Compound concentrations corrected for
water content, when containing (greater than or equal) 4% water.

5.2 Properties of the serum-free, synthetic, chemical medium

Certain features of the newly designed serum-free, fully synthetic, chemically defined medium became evident from investigations of the culturing of some cell types of the immune, haematopoietic and cardiovascular systems, e.g. the different leucocyte types, blood vessel (endothelial) cells, bone marrow cells, fibroblasts and heart muscle cells (2, 34, 45, 74, 75):

a. The basic medium of 91 components (Tables 4 and 5) has been found biologically "quiescent" in a variety of biological assay systems in-vivo and in-vitro. It is neither toxic, nor injurous to cells and tissues. Nor does it provoke an inflammatory response or shock reaction, when applied in-vitro or in-vivo to assay systems in-situ or systemically, respectively. We use the basic medium as a reference fluid in the assays for angiogenesis (1, 2, 194), enhancement of capillary permeability in the skin (94), chemotaxis and chemokinesis (2, 34, 73, 74, 96, 97), febrile reactions (2) and others (50, 57, 58): sensitive physiological morphogenic patterns and functions of tissues and cells apparently remain normal and intact (Figures 10-13). Except for chemokinesis in-vitro and short term, transient, low grade vasodilatory effects in-vivo (discussed below), cellular activation needs to be induced by additional, specially added components. It is not a function of the basic medium composition which serves for the maintenance of cells.

b. Nevertheless, the basic medium of 91 components contains certain well defined, natural substances important for cell function (3, 31, 38, 60, 120-122, 128-135, 142). So far, they have not been generally considered in cell culturing, in particular with media poorer in components (5-29, 78, 79, 143). These constituents include among others (Table 4 and 5), L-carnosine, carnitine, one flavanoid (134) (preferably rutin, vitamin P, with the rhamnoside rutinose as constituent), mevalolactone, ubiquinone 50 (co-enzyme Q10), vitamin U (D,L-methione-methylsulfonium bromide), etc. In addition, it contains otherwise unusual combinations with other basic substances, such as with different types of unsaturated fatty acids, sugars and sugar derivatives, polyols, uronic acid, amino acids, amino acid derivatives, nucleosides and nucleoside bases, vitamins, vitaminoids, specific co-enzyme derivatives, steroids, phytyl derivatives, salts and defined peptides and polypeptides, e.g. glutathione, carnosine, serum albumin, etc.

c. The basic medium of 91 components may be easily "upgraded" for other specific purposes by the addition, replacement or omission of components without loss of its fully synthetic, chemically defined nature. Such variation is indicated in

Table 4 by the division into groups of components in different stock solutions from which several modifications of fluid
compositions may be easily prepared. Thus, for example, if
the pH is not constantly controlled by the usual means or
medium renewal, the inorganic buffer capacity (mainly phosphate and bicarbonate) can be increased or replaced by the
addition of an organic buffer system, if necessary.
HEPES-buffer systems, (N-2-hydroxy-ethyl)-piperazine-N'-2-
ethane sulfonic acid, (127) in a usual concentration of
0.01 mol/l have been found useful for analytical purposes;
although, they are too expensive for use on biotechnical
scales. Furthermore, labelled substances may be exchanged for
non-labelled, normal constituents of the basic medium, if required; for example, the components no.42-44, Table 4, for
studies of the metabolic turnover or of cells in their mitotic cycle by double marker techniques. Another example is the
omission of calcium and magnesium ions (no.21 and 22) for investigations of normal, non-aggregated thrombocytes (126,
139). In contrast, the nucleoside adenosine (component no.27)
is added at a (threshold) concentration at which it may display its short lasting, transient vasodilatory effects
(196-197), when the complete medium is used (e.g. for perfusion) at some reference tissue sites of experimental in-vivo
models (e.g. heart muscle vessels). The effect may be cancelled by omission of adenosine, if desirable in special purposes of in-vivo and in-situ experimentation.

d. The basic medium of 91 components contains no antibiotics,
polyamines, hormones or cell-activating agents (except for
serum albumin as a chemokinesin, as discussed below).
However, such variable components, like endogenous or exogenous effectors such as hormones, mediators, lectins, lipo-
polysaccharides, inhibitors, etc., for special purposes may
be alternatively or additionally added for stimulating specific cellular reactions without the loss of the chemically
defined character of the medium. Similarly, this has also
been practised in some cases for component-poorer media (7,
9, 13, 14). The components no.92 to 94 (Table 4) are examples
of such special, variable components added to the basic medium of 91 constituents. On one hand, defined antibiotics for
the suppression of possibly present microbic contaminants are
added in this work in concentrations higher than 1 umol/l as
variable components no.92 and 93 to the basic medium, giving
the reference (REF) medium. It already contains the one necessary, endogenous, humoral positive chemokinesin (serum albumin as component no.24) (2, 34, 81-85, 87, 96, 97,
117-119). On the other hand, the component no.94 (Table 4)
exemplifies an additional constituent of the effector production medium in the form of an exogenous cell-activating substance added in a suitable concentration; e.g. 50.0 nmol/l of
a highly purified, molecularly homogeneous polypeptide lectin

mitogen from Canavalia ensiformis, concanavalin A (CON) (62). Other alternatives to this cell-activating agent used in this work were our own preparations of highly purified endogenous polypeptide chemokinesins, chemotaxins, chemorecruitins, chemotropins and mitogens of humoral and cellular origin, as well as cell surface immune reactions using defined antigens (e.g. bovine serum albumin) to appropriately sensitized cells (1, 2, 34, 47-50, 54-59, 70-74, 81-85, 93-103). Hence, addition of such variable components to the reference or basic medium results in, for example, a cytokine effector production medium. In it, different patterns of effector varieties may be formed upon culture of different cell types, as, in part, will be discussed in the next chapter (Figure 7).

e. The basic medium of 91 components may promote the expression of natural life functions of cultured viable cells in-vitro which may be induced by the variable, additionally provided cell-activating agents, as discussed above. Apart from these essential advantages for the maintenance and stimulation of cells in culture and for effector substance production, the basic medium is characterized by the following additional features:

f. The 91 components of the basic medium are chemically defined. They are mostly balanced in their concentrations according to their physiological concentration ranges in natural blood plasma or serum (3-6, 60, 61, 63, 76, 80) which are a physiological model of "in-vivo culture media". Deviations from this principle in a few cases, such as added serum albumin (component no.24), are dictated by necessity and economic reasons which are further discussed below: topics g) and h).

g. In its basic form, the medium of 91 components contains only one single, defined protein; namely the highly purified, electrophoretically and otherwise molecularly homogenous, natural serum albumin. Its characteristics are given in the footnote of Table 5 and in Figure 2. Normally, preferably, human serum albumin is used. On one hand, human serum albumin at present is the most economic form of a highly purified serum albumin which is commercially available in these qualities required. On the other hand, for the culture of heterologous (animal) cell types, the use of human serum albumin permits analysis of the possible influence of an albumin component of the medium on, and its probable participation in the formation and inactivation of cells and the investigated cell-secreted effector substances. Vice versa, for the culture of normal (non-sensitized) human cells, for such purposes, the same might be achieved by the use of, for example, the more expensive, highly purified bovine or porcine serum albumin; provided it has the qualified purity and is without cytotoxicity for the cells of a distinct species.

418

Fig. 2. Control of molecular homogeneity of commercially available natural human serum albumin (no.24, Tables 4 and 5) used for

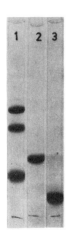

the composition of serum-free, fully synthetic, chemically defined cell culture medium. Electrophoretic pattern under overload (100 ug) and denaturing conditions (0.1% sodium dodecyl sulphate) in 10% polyacrylamide gels, pH 8.8, performed according to Porzio's and Pearson's procedure and conditions (64):

1. Commercially available, natural human serum albumin (Table 5), used for the composition of the medium (molecular weight: 69 000: first band from top as starting point with cathodal to anodal migration) in mixture with two further reference markers for molecular weights, namely ovalbumin (45 000, second band from top) and calmodulin (17 000), third band from top).
2. Reference molecular weight (25 000) marker gel: Chymotrypsinogen a.
3. Reference molecular weight (12 500) marker gel: Cytochrome c.

Except for human serum albumin (Table 5) and calmodulin, the other marker proteins were obtained from Boehringer, Mannheim, Germany. Calmodulin was prepared as a subunit of skeletal muscle phosphorylase kinase (E.C. 2.7.1.38) and kindly supplied by Prof. H.P. Jessissen, Ruhr-University, Bochum Germany (136,137). Contaminating polypeptides (including dimers) in serum albumin, as detectable by this method, are below 1% of the total protein. Other controls and analytical evaluations are presented in Table 5 and Figure 9.

h. The low concentration of serum albumin (7.3 umol/l) is high enough and an optimum concentration to meet economic needs and to confer positive chemokinetic activity to the cells (1, 2, 34, 74, 75, 81-85, 116-119). Essentially, this provides cells, especially the different types of leucocytes, with some necessary further properties which are of paramount importance for cell survival and the expression of cellular life functions such as the motility, the transport of substances from and into the membrane and the regulation of cellular adhesion and aggregation tendencies as well as of cellular secretion and maturation potencies (1, 2, 14, 34, 81-85). Furthermore, this concentration of serum albumin is high enough and optimally balanced for adsorption of all hydrophobic substances present as basic components; or formed and exuded by cells cultured in the medium. To the latter group, in particular, belong cell-derived fatty acid derivatives, like prostaglandins, etc., which represent non-polypeptide cytokine effector substances to be transported from intracellular and interfacial locations to the (serum albumin-containing) aqueous, extracellular spaces, as schematically illustrated in Figure 1. Those reactively formed, and the hydrophobic medium components (e.g., the different free unsaturated fatty acids, no.89-91, Table 4, etc.) which as such are cell-damaging soaps (94), are adsorbed by the serum albumin. For the adsorption of such hydrophobic molecules, one serum albumin molecule has eight binding sites (105). The positive chemokinetic effect of the medium may be cancelled (e.g. for measurement of albumin-independent positive chemokinesis expressed by other substances) (2, 34, 72-74, 81-85, 116-119, 145, 161, 167) by ommission of the serum albumin.

i. For the culture of the mentioned, different cell types so far investigated (2, 74, 75), addition of expensive serum or another biological fluid jeopardizing the fully synthetic character of the medium of 91 components, is not necessary. On the contrary, evidently the addition of other defined variable components for special purposes, for example the defined components no.92-94 (Table 4), however, does not interfere with the fully synthetic, chemically defined nature of the medium.

j. The medium is less expensive in preparation than serum-containing media. It is economic also for large scale serial analytical and biotechnical cultures.

k. The serum-free, fully synthetic, chemically defined nature of the basic medium of 91 components (Table 4) is a prerequisite for permitting a clear distinction, and for avoiding a mixed formation of humoral (serum-derived) and cellular (cytokine) effector substances formed during the maintainance of the cells in it (1, 2, 34, 45, 47-50, 54-59, 70-75, 94, 95, 99, 101, 102).

l. Its composition avoids or minimizes the possibility of the mixed formation of extracellular polypeptide effector substances of different species.

m. It facilitates purification of formed and cell-exuded, extracellular and interfacial trace effector substances from the complex mixture of compounds contained in the culture supernatant solution.

n. The basic medium of 91 components contains no previously added indicator dyes, as do some other media descibed (7). Dyes by hydrophobic or other reactive, irreversible binding may stain cell-secreted trace polypeptides, and, thus, suggest false molecular properties of a (possibly stained) trace effector substance under investigation. However, if required, suitable dyes may be added for distinct purposes separately as additional, variable constituents.

o. The basic medium of 91 components contains no previously added
tensides, as do some other media (7, 143). Tensides in other
media presumably serve to dissolve hydrophobic components.
However, as discussed above, tensides may interfere with, and
be detrimental to the structure, function and purification behaviour of different trace effector substances produced extracellularly by cells. Also, they may not be favourable to the
cultured cells themselves.

p. The basic medium of 91 components contains no previously added
nucleotides, although they are frequently used in some other
media described (7). Nucleotides at higher concentrations are
not normally present extracellularly. However, nucleotides are
synthetized by viable cells intracellularly and interfacially
by vectorial catalysis (138) as components of cellular ener-
getics and of secondary messenger systems. But they are seldom
or never transported as such into or out of cells from or to
the extracellular medium. Therefore, extracellular nucleotides
in media are not normally directly necessary for sustaining
the viability of cells. If occurring extracellularly at higher
concentrations, they are more likely to emerge from
cell-injuring or cell-stimulating reactions. Then, they may
function as effectors carrying information of tissue injury,
for example, for the activation of cellular defense systems.
The role of ADP as a representative of a nucleotide in thrombocyte aggregation exemplifies such a function (126, 139).

q. The basic medium of 91 components contains no previously added
heavy metal ions. By binding to e.g. sulfhydryl groups, such
additives might inhibit or denature heavy metal-sensitive effector substances produced as very trace components in the
proximate environment of cells. Furthermore, at higher concentrations, they may even poison the cells themselves; or exces-
sively promote the growth of possibly present microbial con-
taminations, disturb the redox potential of the medium and
catalyze the degradation of some vitamins (e.g. vitamin C) (4,
31, 60, 120-122, 131-133, 140, 141). The maximally effective
concentrations of so far defined metal and further ions other
than those listed in Tables 4 and 5, as determined by standard
methods (123-125), are presented in Table 6. These are mainly
introduced to the medium as normal contaminants by its
91 components of an analytical or pharmaceutical degree of
purity. The component no.4 (Table 4: NaCl) used in its analytical purity grade for preparation of the medium, mainly con-
tributes to the introduction of these defined contaminants. In
any case, their concentration in the medium is higher than
that of the effector molecules produced by the cells (Table 1)
(1, 2, 34, 45). In part, at such low concentrations (Table 6),
some of the contaminants have also been found necessary for
cell survival and the expression of cellular life functions
(14, 120-122, 132, 140). Thus, trace amounts of metal ions and

selenium are essential in cellular metabolism and in secretory
processes (14, 120-122, 132, 140). However, in culture, the
volume of the medium is kept at least 20 times larger than the
wet cell volume. Therefore, concentrations and total amounts
of such contaminating, essential solutes are high enough and
sufficient (3, 4, 31, 120-122) for the normal promotion and
expression of life functions of eukarions (120-122); in particular, with reference to their natural concentration also in
plasma as a physiological model of a culture medium. Hence,
further addition of some of the metal and other ions in the
range of 10 to 100 nmol/l, as has been suggested to be of advantage for media poorer in components and cellular nutrients
(7-9, 14), is considered not necessary in this component-rich,
basic medium.

Table 6. Maximally effective concentrations of so far defined
metal and further ions other than those listed in Tables 4 and 5
which are introduced to and present in the medium as contaminants
by the 91 components of analytical and pharmaceutical degree of
purity used for its preparation. The determination of these contaminants was carried out according to standard methods (123-125).

```
------------------------------------------------------
Aluminium ions                          </= 200 nmol/l
Arsenate ions                           </=  50 nmol/l
Cadmium ions                            </= 100 nmol/l
Cobalt ions                             </= 100 nmol/l
Copper ions                             </= 200 nmol/l
Iron ions                               </= 300 nmol/l
Lead ions                               </= 100 nmol/l
Manganese ions                          </= 100 nmol/l
Nickel ions                             </= 200 nmol/l
Selenite ions                           </=  50 nmol/l
Thallium ions                           </= 100 nmol/l
Zinc ions                               </= 100 nmol/l
------------------------------------------------------
```

r. During culture, the glucose level, the pH and the oxygen concentration should be measured and kept constant. Then, the
glucose level is constant and remains within the constant physiological plasma concentration range for glucose (3). Therefore, hormone regulation of the glucose level as such is not
necessary. However, at present, a synthetic medium in practice
always is poorer in components than any natural biological
fluid. Therefore, in cultures without biological fluid dynamics and regeneration, crucial to its use is a more frequent
change of the medium for complete removal of formed waste materials and renewal of all components which cannot be kept at
optimum concentration at once in a static culture system.

422

s. The medium has a balanced sulfhydryl group-preserving redox potential which also may maintain sensitive disulfide bridges in polypeptides and in cellular interfaces.

These features of the medium are consistent with the discussed criteria of a useful culture medium (4.0). The following section presents its use for the culture of leucocytes on a large scale for the production and preparation of a variety of cytokine effector substances operating chemical mechanisms for cellular reactions and communication in regenerative tissue morphogenesis by inflammation and healing.

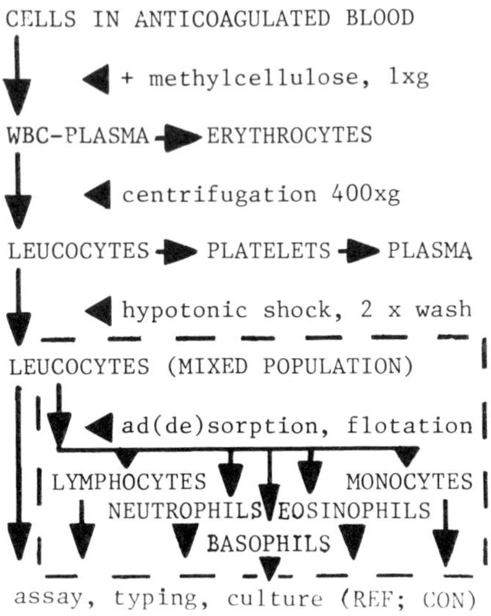

Fig. 3A. Summary of sequence of steps for the biotechnical preparation and purification of blood components in the native, viable state; in particular, leucocytes, thrombocytes, erythrocytes, and blood plasma as natural sources for the production and isolation of cellular and humoral polypeptide effector substances as mediators and hormones of the immune, haematopoietic and cardiovascular systems. They operate chemical mechanisms (1, 2, 34) for cellular reactions and communication in regenerative tissue morphogenesis in inflammation and healing. The methods for performance of the steps are described in Figures 3B, 3C and, together with related references, in the text and elsewhere (74, 144, 145). The physiologically mixed or the homogeneous

CELLS IN ANTICOAGULATED BLOOD

◀ + methylcellulose, 1xg

WBC-PLASMA ▶ ERYTHROCYTES

◀ centrifugation 400xg

LEUCOCYTES ▶ PLATELETS ▶ PLASMA

◀ hypotonic shock, 2 x wash

LEUCOCYTES (MIXED POPULATION)

◀ ad(de)sorption, flotation

LYMPHOCYTES   MONOCYTES
NEUTROPHILS EOSINOPHILS
BASOPHILS

assay, typing, culture (REF; CON)

populations of leucocyte types (granulocytes, monocytes, lymphocytes, Table 7), and platelets isolated, in particular are used as sources for the production and preparation of physical amounts of some of the varieties of cytokine effectors formed and exuded by cells upon their culture and activation. Details of the performance of steps used for the purification of cells (framed by dashed line) are given in Figures 3B and 3C. The plasma obtained served as a source for the production and preparation of humoral (serum-derived) polypeptide effector substances. These are formed upon regulated, limited, bond-specific proteolysis of natural serum proteins as parent molecules of the effector polypeptides (1, 2, 34, 93-103).

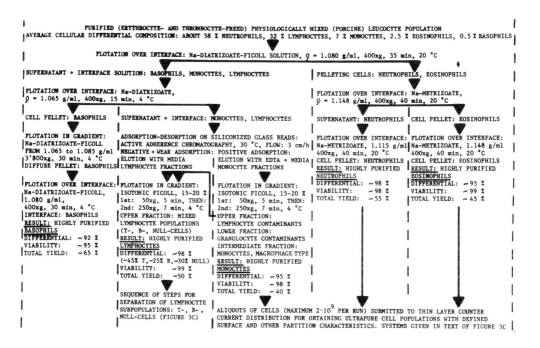

Fig. 3B. Separation and purification of different populations of peripheral leucocyte types: Sequence of steps used for large scale isolation of the cells from peripheral (porcine) blood (continued from Figure 3A). Description of performance of single steps together with related references is given in the text. Density values noted are standardized to rho 20 deg.C/4 deg.C.

424

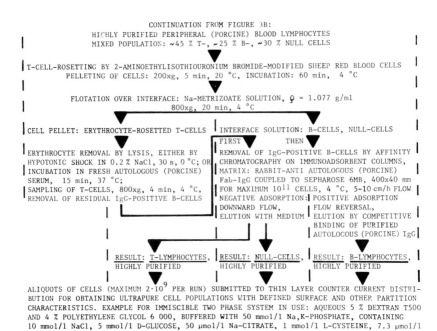

CONTINUATION FROM FIGURE 3B:
HIGHLY PURIFIED PERIPHERAL (PORCINE) BLOOD LYMPHOCYTES
MIXED POPULATION: ~45 % T-, ~25 % B-, ~30 % NULL CELLS

T-CELL-ROSETTING BY 2-AMINOETHYLISOTHIOURONIUM BROMIDE-MODIFIED SHEEP RED BLOOD CELLS
PELLETING OF CELLS: 200xg, 5 min, 20 °C, INCUBATION: 60 min, 4 °C

FLOTATION OVER INTERFACE: Na-METRIZOATE SOLUTION, ρ = 1.077 g/ml
800xg, 20 min, 4 °C

CELL PELLET: ERYTHROCYTE-ROSETTED T-CELLS | INTERFACE SOLUTION: B-CELLS, NULL-CELLS

ERYTHROCYTE REMOVAL BY LYSIS, EITHER BY   FIRST   THEN
HYPOTONIC SHOCK IN 0.2 % NaCl, 30 s, 0 °C; OR REMOVAL OF IgG-POSITIVE B-CELLS BY AFFINITY
INCUBATION IN FRESH AUTOLOGOUS (PORCINE)   CHROMATOGRAPHY ON IMMUNOADSORBENT COLUMNS,
SERUM, 15 min, 37 °C;   MATRIX: RABBIT-ANTI AUTOLOGOUS (PORCINE)
SAMPLING OF T-CELLS, 800xg, 4 min, 4 °C,   Fab-IgG COUPLED TO SEPHAROSE 6MB, 400x40 mm
REMOVAL OF RESIDUAL IgG-POSITIVE B-CELLS   FOR MAXIMUM 10^{11} CELLS, 4 °C, 5-10 cm/h FLOW
                                            NEGATIVE ADSORPTION: POSITIVE ADSORPTION
                                            DOWNWARD FLOW,   FLOW REVERSAL,
                                            ELUTION WITH MEDIUM   ELUTION BY COMPETITIVE
                                                                  BINDING OF PURIFIED
                                                                  AUTOLOGOUS (PORCINE) IgG

RESULT: T-LYMPHOCYTES, | RESULT: NULL-CELLS, | RESULT: B-LYMPHOCYTES,
HIGHLY PURIFIED   HIGHLY PURIFIED   HIGHLY PURIFIED

ALIQUOTS OF CELLS (MAXIMUM $2 \cdot 10^{9}$ PER RUN) SUBMITTED TO THIN LAYER COUNTER CURRENT DISTRI-
BUTION FOR OBTAINING ULTRAPURE CELL POPULATIONS WITH DEFINED SURFACE AND OTHER PARTITION
CHARACTERISTICS. EXAMPLE FOR IMMISCIBLE TWO PHASE SYSTEM IN USE: AQUEOUS 5 % DEXTRAN T500
AND 4 % POLYETHYLENE GLYCOL 6 000, BUFFERED WITH 50 mmol/l Na,K-PHOSPHATE, CONTAINING
10 mmol/l NaCl, 5 mmol/l D-GLUCOSE, 50 µmol/l Na-CITRATE, 1 mmol/l L-CYSTEINE, 7.3 µmol/l
($\triangleq$ 0.5 mg/ml) HIGHLY PURIFIED, MOLECULARLY HOMOGENEOUS, NATURAL SERUM ALBUMIN AND RENDERED
ISOTONICALLY (290 mOsm/kg) WITH 150 mmol/l SUCROSE, pH 7.10, WITH 100 TRANSFERS AT 10 °C

Fig. 3C. Sequence of steps for large scale separation and isolation of lymphocyte subpopulations from highly purified lymphocytes
from peripheral (porcine) blood (Figures 3A,B). Description of
performance of single steps together with related references is
given in the text. Density values noted are standardized to rho 20
deg.C/4 deg.C.

6.0 APPLIED LARGE SCALE AND SERIAL ANALYTICAL BIOTECHNIQUES

This section describes the use of compositions of the
serum-free, fully synthetic, chemically defined medium
for serial analytical and large scale cultures of white
blood cells and for the production, preparation and
characterization of exuded cytokine effector substances
of regenerative tissue m-orphogenesis.

6.1 Isolation and culture of white blood cells

For an approach to basic requirements presented in Table 1
concerning the production and isolation of physical quantities of
cellular trace effector substances which operate chemical mechanisms for cellular reactions and communication in regenerative tissue morphogenesis (1, 2, 34, 45), from cellular homogenates and
culture supernatant solutions, we devised methods for the isolation of defined, viable leucocyte and thrombocyte populations in
biochemical (up to kilogram) amounts for sterile culture techniques. By their culture in the serum-free, fully synthetic, chemically defined medium, the different cell types may be activated to
exude a variety of effector substances, including those of polypeptide nature, with activities basic to functional expressions of
the immune, haematopoietic and cardiovascular systems in inflammation and healing reactions (1, 2, 34, 45, 47-50, 54-59, 70-74,
145-147, 167, 190-194). Such an approach cannot be done at once,
but must be performed batchwise. For the preparation of about 1 kg
(about 2 x 10E12) of leucocytes composed of a physiologically
mixed population as present normally in blood, about 200 l of
fresh, aseptically drawn and anticoagulated blood is necessary
(Table 1). Due to the relatively short life span and functional
sensitivity of white blood cells, such amounts of fresh blood must
be obtained and processed for leucocytes and thrombocytes within a
few hours. Following further the estimates of Table 1, this procedure part must be repeated at least 50 times on a total of 10 tons
of blood, for obtaining the required amount of (about 10E14) cells
for the production and isolation of physical (mg) quantities of
trace (polypeptide) effector substances exuded by cells upon their
culture.
As a result of this investigation (1, 2, 34, 45, 74, 144), a
sequence of steps has been worked out which allows fast isolation
of all the components of fresh blood in the native, viable state.
The isolation strategy is summarized in Figure 3. As a first step
for sequential preparation of all blood components as starting material for the production of humoral and cellular effectors, a
one-phase-batch process has been established to which fresh,
aseptically drawn, anticoagulated blood is submitted. This step
yields all formed elements of blood within a few hours at once,
i.e. plasma, erythrocytes, thrombocytes and a mixture of the vari-

426

ous types of the leucocyte population in the native, viable, sterile form on a technical scale and at a reasonable cost-effect relationship (145). Figures 4, 5, and 6 illustrate some steps in this processing of blood for the isolation of leucocytes, as performed in this laboratory. Then, in a sequence of further steps, namely biotechnical options of adsorption-desorption and flotation processes, we may separate such kilogram quantities of mixed populations of purified leucocytes on the same day into homogeneous cell populations (granulocytes, monocytes, lymphocytes), on a scale euqivalent to the physiological cell differential of the mixed population of leucocytes (Table 7) obtained from blood. Details of the performance of the sequences of the steps and the purification strategy for the isolation of the homogeneous populations of the different types of peripheral leucocytes are presented in Figures 3B and 3C. In essence, technical modifications of established methods are used for this further fractionation of subpopulations and comparable results concerning cell homogeneity, viability and yield are obtained. Firstly, the bulk of mononuclear leucocytes and basophil cells were separated from the bulk of neutrophil and eosinophil granulocytes by flotation of the cells at the interface of lymphoprep (hypaque) – aqueous two phase systems according to methods devised by Boeyum (176), Day (177) and others (189). Then, the basophils were separated from the mononuclear cells and further purified by a modification of Day's procedure (177). The bulk of lymphocytes was separated from adherent mononuclear cells by active adherence chromatography on siliconized glass beads and desorption of a monocyte fraction with EDTA solutions (178, 179). Monocytes (macrophage type) with phagocytic capabilities and lymphocytes were separately further purified by a technical modification of Noble and Cutts' method (180). Elutriation of these cells at 900 x g, 22-42 ml/min and at 10 deg.C in the serum-free, fully synthetic, chemically defined medium may be used as alternative technique (198, 199) for their purification at this step. Similarly, eosinophils and neutrophils were separated and then further purified by modifications of Day's (181) and Gleich and Loegering's methods (182). Lymphocyte subpopulations (Figure 3C) may be obtained from the highly purified peripheral lymphocytes by sequences of technical modifications of Pellegrino et al. (183), Albrechtsen et al. (184) and Chess et al. (185) methods. Finally, the highly purified cell phenotypes were ultrapurified into cell populations with defined surface and other partition characteristics by thin layer counter current distribution (186-188), when special analytical problems required this homogeneity (e.g. cellular source of an effector substance). A suitable separation system is noted in Figure 3C.

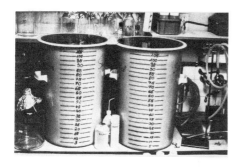

Fig. 4. First step of the biotechnical preparation of at least
1 kg (about 2 trillions) of functionally and morphologically viable leucocytes of a mixed physiological differential composition
(Table 7); or homogeneous cell
populations (granulocytes, monocytes, lymphocytes) thereof, for
sterile culture techniques. They
are sources for the preparation of
(polypeptide) cytokine effectors
which operate the chemical mechan-
isms for cellular reactions and communication in regenerative tissue morphogenesis with activities basic on functional expressions
of the immune, haematopoietic and cardiovascular systems in inflammation and wound healing. Preparation of at least 200 l aseptically drawn, anticoagulated porcine blood per day and investigator. The processing itself is achieved accoording to the scheme in
Figure 3 and, furthermore, as illustrated in Figures 5-8. It is
performed according to the methods described elsewhere (1, 2, 74,
144, 145). A 50-fold repetition of this presented example of blood
preparation corresponds to a processed amount of blood of 10 tons
and yields about 50 kg (about 100 trillions) viable leucocytes of
the mentioned physiological compositions; as a requisite which
follows from the estimates presented in Table 1. Or, an equivalent
thereof of a homogeneous cell population (granulocytes, monocytes,
lymphocytes), as follows from the cell differential of the physiologically mixed population from Table 7; i.e., about 3.5 kg (about
7 trillions) monocytes (macrophage type), appr.16 kg (about
32 trillions) lymphocytes, appr.29 kg (about 58 trillions) neutrophil granulocytes, etc. on an average, when separated by biotechnical modifications of sequences of established adsorption-
desorption and flotation processes (74, 144, 145). Their culture
in the serum-free, fully synthetic, chemically defined medium
(Tables 4 and 5), and the processing of their serum-free culture
supernatant solutions (Figures 5-8), provides the physical (mg)
amounts of some of the varieties of (polypeptide) cytokines formed
and exuded by the cells upon their culture in the medium; for example, mediators for blood vessel sprouting and wound hormones for
the chemorecruitment of leucocytes from the bone marrow into the
blood circulation (Figures 10-13) (1, 2, 34-46, 45, 47-50, 54-59,
70-74, 144, 145, 167).

428

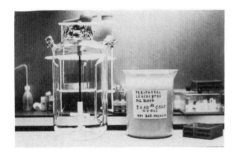

Fig. 5. Processing of freshly prepared, viable leucocytes for the production and preparation of (polypeptide) cytokine effector substances operating chemical mechanisms for cellular reactions and communication in regenerative tissue morphogenesis by inflammation and healing (1, 2, 34): 1 kg (about 2 trillions) of a physiologically mixed population (Table 7) of viable leucocytes which have been obtained within a few hours from about 200 l of aseptically drawn, anticoagulated porcine blood (Figure 4), finally are suspended in about 4 l of the serum-free, fully synthetic, chemically defined reference culture medium (mixture of components no. 1-93, Table 4). Then, they are assayed, typed and cultured; either as this mixed cell population after further dilution with this medium to a maximum density of 10E07 - 10E08 cells/ml and activation of cells (e.g. by addition of component no.94, Table 4, or another activating substance as referenced in the text) in bioreactors shown in Figure 6 for the production of cytokines (145, 167). Or, this suspension of the mixture of isolated leucocyte types serves as starting material for the preparation of technical amounts of homogeneous populations of viable peripheral leucocyte types within the short term of their natural functional viability by a sequence of adsorption-desorption and flotation steps, as described in Figure 3 (74, 145). These isolated different, homogeneous leucocyte populations, then, may be handled for the production of cytokines in the same manner as for the mixed population, or serve another purpose.

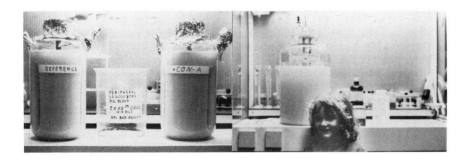

Fig. 6. Sterile culture in bioreactors of the technical (kg) amounts of the (trillions) viable peripheral leucocytes isolated (Figures 3-5) in the serum-free, synthetic, defined medium

(Table 4). It serves in the production and preparation of (poly-peptide) cytokines operating the chemical mechanisms for cellular reactions and communication in regenerative tissue morphogenesis with activities basic to the function expressions of the immune, haematopoietic and cardiovascular systems in inflammation and wound healing. Larger (30 l) (right) (45) and smaller (15 l) types (left) of bioreactors are presented. Others are shown elsewhere (145); e.g. for the culture of homogeneous lymphocyte populations isolated in daily amounts of up to about 6.0 x 10E11 (300 g) cells in one operation from the obtained physiological mixture of iso-lated leucocyte types (Figures 4 and 5). The culture itself is performed in the serum-free, fully synthetic, chemically defined medium (Table 4) at a maximum cell density of 10E07 to 10E08/ml. The reference culture (REF) (left) contains the medium with the components no.1-93 (Table 4). The cytokine production culture con-tains this medium complemented with an additional cell activator component (no.94, Table 4). In the example given in the left fig-ure, a polyvalent polypeptide lectin mitogen from Canavalia ensi-formis, concanavalin A, CON, as native protein (molecular weight 104 000) (62) is used as a cell activator. Under such and other similar conditions, the different leucocyte types may exude or se-crete a variety of newly synthetized or intracellularly preformed, physico-chemically and biologically distinguishable polypeptide and other, simpler structured, non-polypeptide cytokines. They specifically may operate chemical mechanisms for cellular reac-tions and communication (chemopoiesis, chemorecruitment, chemo-kinesis, chemotaxis, chemotropism, chemostasis) (1, 2, 34) in re-generative tissue morphogenesis by inflammation and healing through autocrine, paracrine (mediator) and endocrine (hormonal) information transmission mechanisms (1, 2, 34, 45, 145). For thrombocytes that also may exude similar effector activities on their activation or aggregation, a reference medium for cell sus-pension poorer in components is used than given in Table 4. This exemplifies the advantage of the preparation of the medium from distinct groups of stock solutions (Table 5). For this special purpose, particularly the components no.21 and 22 (calcium and magnesium ions) are omitted from the reference suspension of non-aggregated thrombocytes obtained in the process shown in Figure 3. For activation of thrombocytes, however, adenosine di-phosphate together with calcium and magnesium ions are used as ad-ditional components (alternative to no.94) in the medium for the production of platelet-derived cytokines. The processing of the obtained culture supernatant solutions for isolation of the active cytokines is shown in Figures 7 and 8. Culture methods are des-cribed in section 5.1 and (54, 74, 145, 167).

6.2 Production of cytokines by cells in culture

Leucocytes cultured or subcultured in the serum-free, fully synthetic, chemically defined medium (Table 4) on a technical scale (Figure 6), and activated by appropriate means, exude or secrete a complex mixture of endogenous effector substances. They operate chemical mechanisms for cellular reactions and communication in regenerative tissue morphogenesis with activities basic to the functional expressions of the immune, haematopoietic and cardiovascular systems in inflammation and wound healing through autocrine, paracrine (mediator) and endocrine (hormonal) information transmission mechanisms (1, 2, 34, 45, 145). Appropriate means for culturing and activation of the different cell type populations isolated are met, for example, by exposing the cells in the synthetic medium (components no.1-93, Table 4) to a polyvalent polypeptide lectin mitogen in the form of the additionally added component no.94 (Table 4, Figure 6) for 40 hrs; or, dependent on the life span or proliferation cycle of a distinct cell type, for a longer period at a maximum density of 10E07 to 10E08 cells/ml. Representatives of effector molecule types with biological activities for operation of each of the basic categories of chemical mechanisms known so far (1, 2) for cellular reactions and communication in regenerative tissue morphogenesis, have been found to exist as defined entities. A major portion of the existing variety of effectors are of polypeptide nature having hydrodynamic equivalents of molecular weights in the range of about 500 to 30 000. Nevertheless, under the same in-vitro culture conditions, cells do exude or secrete effector substances of non-polypeptide nature, too, e.g. fatty acid derivatives in the form of prostaglandins, etc. (2).

6.3 Purification and characterization of various leucokines

Our work has been concerned with the evaluation of the nature and variety of formed polypeptide effector substances which until now are the least investigated structural class that may be elucidated by their purification to high molecular homogeneity. As a result of the biotechnically produced polypeptide cytokine effectors (Figures 3-6), a small variety of reaction- and cell-specific or selective cellular effectors could be obtained by a sequence of separation and purification steps from the batchwise produced (cubic metre volumes of) supernatant solutions of serum-free cultures of technical (kg) amounts of (100 trillions) of white blood cells. The strategy of purification and the parts of the technical instrumentation developed for this purpose, are described in Figures 7 and 8.

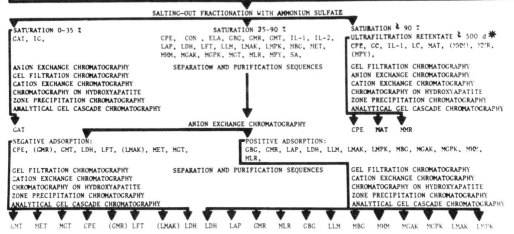

Fig. 7. Cytokines of white blood cells - effector molecules operating chemical mechanisms or cellular reactions and communication in regenerative tissue morphogenesis with activities basic on functional expressions of the immune, haematopoietic and cardiovascular systems in inflammation and wound healing through autocrine, paracrine (mediator) and endocrine (hormonal) information transmission mechanisms. Survey of separation and purification strategy of effector substances for chemopoiesis, chemorecruitment, chemokinesis, chemotaxis, chemotropism and chemostasis of cells as major categories of chemical mechanisms intrinsic to regenerative tissue morphogenesis (1, 2, 34, 45, 145). The consecutive and concomitant isolation of some of a variety of polypeptide cytokines present in supernatant solutions of isolated cells in culture (left, as in-vitro model) and homogenates of inflamed tissue sites or wounds (right, as in-vivo model, in the form of ischaemically injured, infarcted heart muscle sites) is presented as the composition of different separation sequences. The methods of performance of their single steps are described elsewhere (1, 47-50, 54-59, 70-74, 145) and exemplified by the purification of effector substances of the chemotropism reaction of blood vessels produced by different leucocyte types (granulocyto- and monocyto-"angiotropins", GAT and MAT, respectively) in (1, 2, 145). Further abbreviations for effector substances obtainable as by-products of MAT purification of one crude starting supernatant solution of cell culture or tissue homogenate are: For the chemopoiesis reaction: GBG and MBG, LLM and MHM, IL-2, GC and LC, granulocyto- and monocyto-blastogen, lymphocyto-lympho and monocyto-histiomitogen, interleukin-2 (T-cell growth factor), granulocyto- and lympho-

cyto-chalone, respectively, as stimulators (mitogens) and inhibitors (chalones) of granulocyte stem cell (blast), macrophage ("histiocyte") and lymphocyte proliferation and colony formation. For signal substances of the chemorecruitment reaction: GMR, MMR and MLR, granulo- and monocyto-metamyelo- and leucorecruitin, respectively. For signal substances of the chemokinesis reaction: LMAK, MGAK, LMPK and MGPK, lymphocyto-mono- and monocyto-granulo-apokinesin, respectively, as migration-inhibitory factors, and lymphocyto-mono- and monocyto-granulo-proskinesin, respectively, as migration-stimulatory factors. For signal substances of the chemotaxis reaction: GMT, MET and MGT, granulocyto-mono-, monocyto-eosino- and monocyto-granulotaxin, respectively. For signal substances of the chemostasis reaction: IL-1, interleukin-1; MPY, monocyto-pyrogen; LFT, lymphocyto-fibroblasto-toxin; CPE, capillary permeability-enhancing factor. Other abbreviations are: ELA, elastase (E.C. 3.4.21.11); IG, immunoglobulins; LDH, L-lactate: NAD oxidoreductases (E.C. 1.1.1.27); LAP, alpha-aminoacyl-peptide hydrolases (L-leucine aminopeptidases, E.C.3.4.11.1); SA and CON, serum albumin and concanavalin A (from the culture medium given in Table 4). The scheme does not give a full account of all activities present in culture supernatant solutions or tissue homogenates. Moreover, the patterns of activities are different in culture supernatant solutions from the various isolated cell types or mixed cell populations and different inflamed tissue sites. Thus, for example, in lymphocyte-devoid culture, lymphocyte-derived mediators are not detectable, etc. Furthermore, dependent on the culture conditions, the patterns of cytokine substances formed may vary. Thus, for example, the patterns in reference cultures and normal tissues differ from cultures of activated cells and from inflamed tissues. The patterns of activated cells may vary dependent on the activation conditions and agents used. The nomenclature, other definitions, biological assays and further necessary techniques are described in the text, (2) and Figures 8-13.

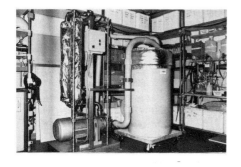

Fig. 8. Technical recycling ultra-filtration apparatus developed for quantitative processing, concentration, desalting and recovery of biologically active, saltsoluble macromolecules with a hydrodynamic equivalent (greater than or equal) 500 dalton. The instrument contains two ultrafiltration membranes mounted in parallel in cartridges with a total surface of about 3 square metres and an exclusion limit of about 500 dalton (Amicon UM 05, Bedford, Mass.). The membrane has a retentate capacity for molecules smaller than the size of bradykinin and larger than those composed of three and more amino acids. Its filtration capacity is about 60-80 l of 1.8 mol/l (45% saturated) ammonium sulphate solution per day at 10 deg.C or about the sixfold volume of salt-free water. Thereby, biologically active molecules are retained, concentrated and desalted. Heat (about 10 KJ/s) developed by the circulation power system must be dissipated by strong cooling effects achieved by some special technical arrangements to prevent heating of circulating solution and destruction of heat-labile, dissolved macromolecules; e.g. by auto-levelling cooling spirals which adjust themselves continuously to volume changes of the circulating solution. The instrument is particularly used for processing of the biologically active, salt-soluble macromolecule fraction (*) (right purification sequence in Figure 7); i.e. the fraction containing macromolecules which cannot be precipitated and concentrated by salting-out with ammonium sulphate at a saturation of 90% (3.6 mol/l). Following Figure 7, this fraction of salt-soluble macromolecules is obtained in a first step for the quantitative isolation of a variety of cytokines from a crude supernatant solution. For the step, salting-out precipitation of salt-insoluble macromolecules with ammonium sulphate is preferably used. This step solves several problems initially intrinsic to the technical preparation of protein cytokines. For the protein precipitate fractions obtained by the salting-out step, the large initial volumes of crude supernatant solutions are largely reduced to laboratory scales (to about 1/50 to 1/200 of original volume), concomitant to an almost quantitative recovery of the different activities originally present. The appr. 1 000 l crude culture supernatant solutions which were obtained batchwise by culture of about 50 kg of leucocytes isolated from about 10 000 l of porcine blood, are reduced to volumes of about 5-20 l of concentrated protein solutions obtained from the different protein precipitate fractions. Such (three) concentrated fractions of salt-insoluble polypeptides may be easily stored frozen over at least 5 years without loss of the investigated biological activities of cytokines, if they are not further processed immediately on normal laboratory scales. Amongst the salt-soluble macro-

molecules contained in the last (greater than or equal 90% ammonium sulphate-saturated) fraction (Figure 7, right panel), are some
interesting, novel, biologically active cytokines; especially
monokines, e.g., monocyto-angiotropin, monocyto-metamyelorecruitin
and also leucocyte chalones, etc. (1, 2, 34, 45, 47-50, 54-57, 70,
71). Together with the fractionation of salt-insoluble polypeptide
cytokines contained in the serum-free cell culture supernatant solution (Figure 6), addition of this method in the given technical
form (*) to the purification sequences (Figure 7), finally alows
the recovery of all more complexly structured, endogenous polypeptide cytokines. Hence, the macromolecule (polypeptide, RNA, polysaccharide, etc.) -containing solution (*) diluted to 45%
(1.8 mol/l) ammonium sulphate saturation, and freed from
salt-insoluble polypeptide cytokines, had a volume of about
2 800 l when prepared from 1 000 l supernatant solutions of cultures of about 50 kg leucocytes obtained from about 10 000 l of
blood. It may be concentrated effectively and quantitatively within about seven weeks to a salt-free, cytokine-containing retentate
solution of about 10-20 l. From this comparatively small volume of
concentrated cytokine solution, all biologically active macromolecules larger in size than 500 dalton can be further purified on
normal laboratory scales (Figure 7).

The same procedures may similarly be applied for the purification of biologically and physico-chemically equivalent effector
substances from their in-vivo production sources, i.e. inflamed
tissue sites. This was practised so far with homogenates of
ischaemically damaged, infarcted heart muscle sites as in-vivo
model and crude starting material (1, 2, 45, 48, 50, 57, 58, 73,
146, 147). From the few polypeptide effectors obtained by these
techniques (Figures 3-8) in physical amounts in a reaction- and
cell-specifically acting, highly purified form, at least one representative with biological activity directed for operation of
each of the basic categories of chemical mechanisms for cellular
reactions and communication in regenerative tissue morphogenesis
(chemopoiesis, chemorecruitment, chemokinesis, chemotaxis, chemotropism and chemostasis of cells), has been described (1, 2, 45).
Among those are leucocytic polypeptide effectors whose properties
conform to the definition of hormones (1, 2, 148). As novel monokines, thus, they are the first evaluated, typical representatives
of wound hormones (1, 2, 34, 45, 47-50, 145, 146). Figure 9 presents some electrophoretic patterns for analyzing the purification
efficiency of the methods devised (Figures 7 and 8) and of the molecular homogeneity obtained for some effector polypeptides investigated (Figures 10-13 and references 1, 2).

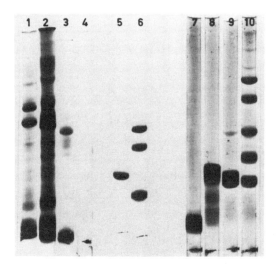

Fig. 9. Evaluation of purification efficiency and molecular homogeneity of some of the biotechnically and serum-free, so far prepared, highly purified, novel polypeptide cytokine substances. They are mediators and hormones of leucocytes operating chemical mechanisms for cellular reactions and communication in regenerative morphogenesis with functional expressions basic to the immune, haematopoietic and cardiovascular systems in inflammation and wound healing: Electrophoretic patterns under overload (100 ug polypeptide applied) and denaturing conditions (as given in Figure 2) (64) in 10% (no.1-6) and 15% (no.7-10) polyacrylamide gels of

1. Supernatant solution of serum-free cultured, isolated, concanavalin A-activated peripheral leucocytes of a mixed, physiological population differential (Figures 3-6, Tables 4-7). Obviously, one of the main components visualized as band stained with Coomassie Brilliant Blue R250 (64), represents serum albumin (reference gel No.6). It was used in its highly purified form as the only polypeptide component of the basic medium of 91 constituents (Table 4, Figure 2) for culture of the cells. The cellular activator component no.94 (Table 4: concanavalin A) used as a variable, additional constituent in the medium at less than 1% of the serum albumin concentration, is hardly visible at its subunit molecular weight position of 25 000 with reference to the molecular weight marker in gel no.5. All other visible bands in this gel originate from macromolecules exuded by the leucocytes in the serum-free culture: This solution serves as crude starting material for the isolation of the polypeptide effectors under investigation (Figures 7, 10-13, gels no.7-9); but none of the polypeptide bands visualized by staining corresponds to any of the biologically active effectors shown, since contained therein on an average of less than 0.001% of the total polypeptide content.
2. Solution of polypeptide fraction obtained from crude starting material (gel no.1) by salting-out fractionation with ammonium sulphate at 45-90% saturation (Figure 7).

Obviously, many of the salt-insoluble polypeptides visible as only faintly stained bands in gel no.1, were concentrated in this fraction together with serum albumin (gel no.6). This solution serves as a crude starting fraction for the purification of the polypeptide effector analyzed in gel no.9. At this stage, it is still not visible as a discrete, stained band, since present at only to about 0.002% of the total polypeptide content. Thus, none of the apparent bands yet correspond to the polypeptide effector entities investigated (Figures 10-13) (1, 2, 34, 45, 54, 145).

3. Retentate solution from the supernatant solution of the salting-out fractionation of the crude cell culture supernatant solution (gel no.1) at (greater than) 90% (3.6 mol/l) ammonium sulphate saturation, obtained by ultrafiltration at membranes with a nominal exclusion limit for hydrodynamic equivalents of a molecular weight of greater than 500 (Figures 7, 8). This solution quantitatively contains all salt-soluble macromolecules with molecular weights greater than 500 of the crude cell culture supernatant solution. It serves as a crude starting fraction for the purification of the polypeptide effectors analyzed in gels no.7 and 8. However, at this stage, they are still not visible as discrete stained bands, since present at a concentration less than 0.1%. Thus, none of the apparent bands correspond yet to the active polypeptide effector entities investigated.

4. Filtrate solution of fraction obtained by ultrafiltration as analyzed in gel no.3 which is freed of all salt-soluble macromolecules. It contains all substances with molecular weights smaller than 500 which also comprise the low molecular weight components of the serum-free, fully synthetic cell culture medium (Table 4). The negative staining of the macromolecule-void gel demonstrates the efficiency of the technical ultrafiltration apparatus shown in Figure 8.

5. Reference molecular weight marker (25 000) for the 10% gel series: Chymotrypsinogen.

6. Reference molecular weight markers (69 000, 45 000, 17 000) for the 10% gel series (no.1-6): Human serum albumin, ovalbumin, calmodulin, respectively.

7. Isolated, biologically active monocyto-angiotropin, MAT: Definition, properties and biological activity are described in Figures 7 and 13.

8. Isolated, biologically active monocyto-metamyelo-recruitin, MMR: Definition, properties and biological activity are described in Figures 7 and 10.

9. Isolated, biologically active monocyto-leuco-recruitin, MLR: Definition, properties and biological activity are described in Figure 7 and reference (2).

10. Reference molecular weight markers (69 000, 45 000, 25 000, 17 000, 12 500) for the 15% gel series (no.7-10): Human serum albumin, ovalbumin, chymotrypsinogen, calmodulin, cytochrome c, respectively.

Further properties, preparation modes and sources of molecular weight markers are described in Figure 2. Band positions are not corrected for different length of gels due to some shrinkage during preparation. Start (cathode) at the top with anodal migration direction (bottom), where the buffer front is indicated by black line (copper needle introduced). All gels intentionally are not extensively destained for good visualization of minor trace contaminants possibly present in preparations which may be easily lost and disappear upon complete destaining (especially low molecular weight macromolecules). Contaminants (or oligomers?) apparent by visual inspection in the overloaded gel patterns of the isolated polypeptide effectors (no.7-9) according to this criterion amount to less than 2% of the total polypeptide applied. At least, the analysis demonstrates the high degree of purity obtained by the purification methods devised (Figures 7 and 8) for some of the investigated polypeptide effector substances.

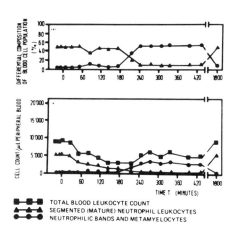

TOTAL BLOOD LEUKOCYTE COUNT
SEGMENTED (MATURE) NEUTROPHIL LEUKOCYTES
NEUTROPHILIC BANDS AND METAMYELOCYTES

Fig. 10. Biological action of isolated monocyto-metamyelo-recruitin (MMR) (Figures 7 and 9) as one of several existing, so far identified representatives of endogenous CHEMORECRUITMENT polypeptide signals of leucocytes (monocytes) (1, 2, 34, 45, 47-50, 54, 145, 146) for their endocrine cellular communication with distinct biological units and functional areas (barriers between poietic, primary storage pools of leucocytes in the bone marrows, and of marginal, secondary stores of leucocytes, and the blood circulation, respectively) (1, 2, 34), remote from the effector production (leucocyte accumulation) site (e.g. reaction site of inflammation in tissue). Endogenously induced, long lasting, transient LEFTWARD SHIFT REACTION (defined as reactive change of the normally constant population differential of circulating blood leucocytes in favour of immature, juvenile cells) (149-151) WITHOUT a general LEUCOCYTOSIS REACTION (defined as a reactive increase in the number above the normally constant level of circulating blood leucocytes) (149-151) by mobilization of immature, juvenile leucocyte phenotypes (neutrophilic bands and metamyelocytes) (30, 151-157) from the bone marrow storage pools into the circulation,

and concomitant sequestration of mature (segmented) neutrophil
leucocytes from the circulation into marginal stores (1, 2, 34).
The figure shows the peripheral blood cell patterns and the kinetics of their changes prior, during (T = 0) and following intravenous application (into Vena saphena dextra) of 25 pmol MMR/kg
guinea pig. These patterns and their kinetics were evaluated by
periodical counting and differentiation of circulating cell types
in the peripheral blood (from Vena saphena sinistra) with classical haematological methods and given nomenclature (30, 149-157).
For transparency, only granulocyte phenotypes are shown in the
differential pattern of cell composition (upper panel). The preparation and isolation in mg-amounts of the highly purified, biologically specific and active MMR polypeptide (molecular weight
given as hydrodynamic equivalent when derived from porcine monocytes: 6 500) was achieved after more than 100 000-fold purification from about 1 000 litres serum-free supernatant solutions of
about 50 kg (100 trillions) biotechnically cultured,
concanavalin A-activated leucocytes (monocytes) with a physiologically mixed cell composition (Table 7); or of 3.5 kg (7 trillions)
monocytes (macrophage type) (54, 145) which may be processed
batchwise by the methods devised (Figures 3-8) from about 10 000
litres porcine blood. Physico-chemically and biologically equivalent MMR-active polypeptide solutes may also be obtained from inflamed tissue sites (Figure 7) as ischaemically injured, infarcted
heart muscle. Phase shifts and reaction amplitudes of leftward
shift reactions induced by MMR solutes are dependent on the applied MMR amount. Endogenous substances for the induction of specific leftward shift reactions, and polypeptide cytokines (chemorecruitins) for the induction of specific leucocytosis reactiones
combined or not with leftward shift reactions as classical phenomena in pathology (3, 30, 149-153, 156, 157), have not been
known, so far. MMR and the other described chemorecruitin cytokines are the first evaluated polypeptides with these biological
properties (1, 2, 34, 45, 47-50, 145, 146). They are distinguishable from humoral (serum-derived) leucorecruitin polypeptide
(101-103). They act highly specifically on target cells and biological units (e.g. bone marrow barrier) remote from their production (leucocyte accumulation) site by endocrine mechanisms of information transmission (Figure 1) and conform in this action to
the definition of hormones (1, 2, 148). Therefore, MMR and the
other chemorecruitins are considered as true leucocytic "WOUND
HORMONES". Hence, for the first time, they provide a chemical
basis and biological function for this historic name (1, 34, 148)
and prove leucocytes as true unicellular, mobile endocrine glands
("SECRETORY LEUCOCYTIC TISSUE") (1, 2). These may convey information by all known transmission mechanisms (Figure 1) (1, 2). For
definitions of nomenclature, see text. For comparison, activity
patterns displayed by other chemorecruitins for leucocytes, so far
isolated, in animals and humans, are shown elsewhere (2, 34, 35,
50, 102, 145, 190-193). Electrophoretic patterns of chemorecruitins as criteria of purification are given in Figure 9.

439

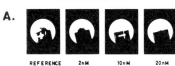

NEGATIVE CHEMOKINETIC ACTIVITY
FOR NEUTROPHIL LEUCOCYTES

A.

REFERENCE   2nM   10nM   20nM

3-5mg OF ACTIVE PROTEIN CAN BE OBTAINED (10% YIELD)
IN MOLECULARLY HOMOGENEOUS FORM FROM ~30-50kg
(60-100·10^{12} CELLS) OF MITOGENICALLY STIMULATED
LEUCOCYTES ISOLATED FROM ABOUT 5'000-10'000 LITERS OF
PORCINE BLOOD AND CULTURED UNDER STERILE CONDITIONS

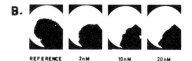

NEGATIVE CHEMOKINETIC ACTIVITY
FOR MONONUCLEAR LEUCOCYTES

B.

REFERENCE   2nM   10nM   20nM

2-3mg OF ACTIVE PROTEIN CAN BE OBTAINED (10% YIELD
IN MOLECULARLY HOMOGENEOUS FORM FROM ~30-50kg
(60-100·10^{12} CELLS) OF MITOGENICALLY STIMULATED
LEUCOCYTES ISOLATED FROM ABOUT 5'000-10'000 LITERS OF
PORCINE BLOOD AND CULTURED UNDER STERILE CONDITIONS

Fig. 11. Paracrine intercellular communication between the different types of leucocytes for the regulation of active random locomotion and displacement (CHEMOKINESIS) of neutrophil granulocytes and monocytes by monocyte- and lymphocyte-derived polypeptide mediators. Biological actions of different concentrations (in nmol/l) of purified (Figure 7)
a. Monocyto-granulo-apokinesin (MGAK) polypeptide (molecular weight given as hydrodynamic equivalent when derived from porcine monocytes: 9 000);
b. Lymphocyto-mono-apokinesin (LMAK) polypeptide (molecular weight given as hydrodynamic equivalent when derived from porcine lymphocytes: (14 000) (2);
in terms of negative (apo-) chemokinesis (159) of porcine granulocytes (A) and monocytes (macrophage type) (B), respectively. Together with some other identified, in part counteracting polypeptide mediators (2, 34, 54, 73, 74, 145, 167), the monocyte- and lymphocyte-derived polypeptides are representatives of regulatory effectors operating mechanisms of CHEMOKINESIS in leucocytes (granulocytes and monocytes, respectively): They reversibly inhibit (non-cytotoxically) the migration and displacement of granulocytes and monocytes, respectively, migrating by active locomotion at random on surfaces. Their preparation was achieved as for MMR (Figure 10) from biotechnically, serum-free and batchwise cultured, concanavalin A-activated porcine leucocytes (about 7 trillions monocytes and about 30 trillions lymphocytes, respectively) (Table 7) according to the described methods (Figure 3-9). The assay shown was performed according to the classical method of Rich and Lewis (2, 99, 145, 160) as inhibition of the emigration of freshly isolated porcine granulocytes and monocytes, respectively, from glass capillaries (Sahli type, 20 ul). In them, the cells had been densely packed. For reference assays, the serum-free, fully synthetic, chemically defined reference medium comprising the components no.1-93 (Table 4) was used only. In the other assays, the cytokine polypeptides were added as variable components no.94 at the given concentrations to this medium. The migration areas of granulocytes and monocytes were measured after incubation of the assembly at 37 deg.C (99% humidity, 3% carbon-

440

dioxide) for either 10 h or 20 h, respectively. Polystyrol well-type incubation chambers (total volume: 500 ul) in which the capillaries are mounted with sterile silicone grease at the closed end, were covered with a gas-permeable membrane during the incubation period. Smaller migration areas with respect to controls (in reference medium, 100% migration) indicate negative chemokinetic activity of the leucocyte-derived polypeptides under investigation; when possible cytotoxicity effects on cellular migration could be ruled out by proving viability of the cells after the assay by morphological (negative vital staining by the trypan blue dye exclusion test) (95, 145) and functional criteria (capability of chemotactic migration of cells in response to our own preparations of endogenous polypeptide leucotaxins, described in Figure 12 and elsewhere) (2, 34, 54, 85, 87, 93-100, 116-119, 145, 161). The assay system shows the usefulness of the newly designed, serum-free, fully synthetic, chemically defined medium (Table 4) and its composition of groups of stock solutions also in serial analytical test performance. Definitions of nomenclature are described in the text.

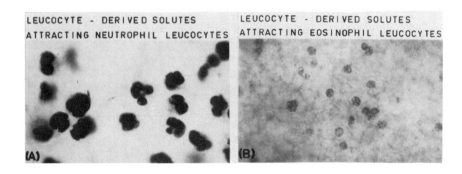

Fig. 12. Paracrine intercellular communication between the different types of leucocytes for the regulation of directional locomotion and displacement (CHEMOTAXIS) of neutrophil and eosinophil granulocytes by monocyte-derived polypeptide mediators: Biological actions of purified (Figure 7)
      a. Monocyto-granulo-taxin (MGT) polypeptide (having a hydrodynamic equivalent of molecular weight of 11 000, when derived from porcine monocytes);
      b. Monocyto-eosino-taxin (MET) polypeptide (having a hydrodynamic equivalent of molecular weight of 5 000, when derived from porcine monocytes);
on freshly isolated porcine neutrophil (A) and eosinophil (B) granulocytes, respectively (2, 34, 96-99, 145, 167), in terms of directional locomotion through a filter membrane (3 um and 8 um pore size for neutrophils and eosinophils, respectively). A modified Boyden chamber assay system was used for this purpose as des-

cribed and schematically drawn elsewhere (96, 97). It had been adapted to the double filter technique (catching filter: 0.45 um pore size) (161) and miniaturized (200 ul test volume in the lower compartment and 200 ul cell suspension with 10E06 cells/ml in the upper compartment). Figures show (A) neutrophils and (B) eosinophils which migrated through, and are adhering to the lowermost surface of the upper (cell migration) filter after having responded chemotactically to 10 nmol/l MGT and MET, respectively, during incubation at 37 deg.C (99% humidity, 3% carbondioxide for 3 hrs (neutrophils) and 4 hrs (eosinophils); and after having been stained by described histological techniques (96, 145) with Weigert's iron-haematotoxylin (A) and phosphate-buffered (0.15 mol/l, pH 7.0) Giemsa's solution (B), respectively. Together with other identified representatives of leucocyte-derived polypeptide mediators operating chemotaxis mechanisms in distinct leucocyte types (2, 54, 72-74, 145), the preparation of MGT and MET was achieved as for other isolated polypeptide effectors (Figures 10 and 11), from biotechnically, serum-free and batchwise cultured, concanavalin A-activated porcine leucocytes (about 7 trillions monocytes) (Table 7) according to the described methods (Figures 3-9) (54, 73, 74, 145, 167). Reference assays were performed in a component-poorer medium as given in Table 3; namely, in a medium composed of the components no.1-24, 45-47, 92 and 93 (Table 4). For the chemotactic stimulation of the cells, the taxin probes were added as additional, variable components to this medium. It contains already a positively acting chemokinesin (proschemokinesin) (159) for leucocytes in the form of serum albumin (2, 34, 81-85, 87, 116-119). It allows control and correction of chemotactic values for possible stimulatory or inhibitory (chemokinetic) effects on intrinsic motility of cells migrating at random by the added taxin probes, when assayed under diffusion equilibrium and non-equilibrium conditions in the chamber (161). This assay shows the usefulness of the serum-free, fully synthetic medium and its composition of groups of stock solutions for building up the appropriate fluid system in serial analytical test performance. Definitions of nomenclature are given in the text. For comparison, activity display of another isolated leucocyte-derived chemotaxin (granulocyto-mono-taxin, GMT) (Figure 7) is shown elsewhere (2, 73).

Figure 10 presents the biological action and molecular properties of one of the evaluated and isolated wound hormones (monocyto-metamyelo-recruitin, MMR). Figures 11-13 illustrate the biological and other molecular properties of a few other, highly purified leucocytic mediators obtained: Monocyto-granulo-apokinesin (MGAK), lymphocyto-mono-apokinesin (LMAK), monocyto-granulo-taxin (MGT), monocyto-eosino-taxin (MET) and monocyto-angiotropin (MAT) (Figures 7 and 9). Table 7 summarizes this part of the investigation of polypeptide effectors exuded by leucocytes in serum-free cultures as a trigger of chemical mechanisms for cellular reactions and communication in regenerative tissue morphogenesis with

activities basic to functional expressions of the immune, haematopoietic and cardiovascular systems in inflammation and wound healing through autocrine, paracrine (mediator) and endocrine (hormonal) information transmission mechanisms.

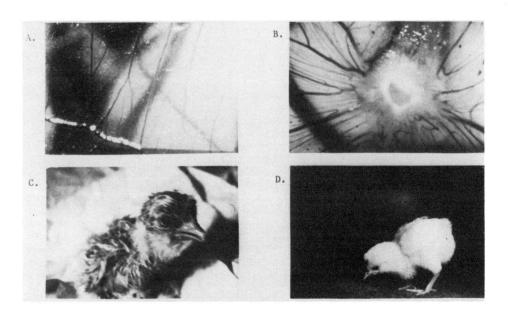

Fig. 13. Paracrine intercellular communication of leucocytes (monocytes) with blood vessel (endothelial) cells for the operation
of cellular CHEMOTROPISM (directional hyperplastic growth) mechanisms by leucocyte (monocyte)-derived polypeptide mediators. Neovascularization of embryonic tissue (chorio-allantois membrane,
CAM, of a chick embryo) by the biological action of a focally applied, highly purified (Figures 7 and 9), porcine monocyte-derived
polypeptide effector ("monocyto-angiotropin", MAT, hydrodynamic
equivalent of molecular weight: 4 500) (1, 2, 36, 45, 54-57, 145,
147) for chemotropism (directional sprouting) of endothelial
cells. Figure A shows a reference tissue. It represents a normal
CAM of an eight day old chick embryo having a life-experienced original (conservative) physiological blood vessel pattern, as expressed in ontogeny (1, 2). Figure B shows an experimentally vascularized CAM of a 7 day old chick embryo to which on the fifth
day of its life 5 fmol MAT was applied by implantation of a
MAT-soaked filter paper (cellulose acetate) (visible in centre of
shell window). The directional growth of vessels to the MAT-soaked
filter paper and the modification of the conservative, physiological blood vessel pattern is obvious: The resulting abnormal ("pathological"), star-like blood vessel pattern shown deviates signi-

ficantly from the reference, conservative pattern (A), as expressed in undisturbed ontogeny of the embryo. The filter paper alone (only soaked with a medium containing the components no.1-91, Table 4) does not lead to such significant changes. Are such artificially induced, non-conservative (blood vessel) tissue patterns induced by the focal application of the endogenous effector molecules of leucocytes in a normally differently vascularized tissue compatible with development and life? Figures C and D answer this question: They show (C) the normal birth of a chick baby and (D) well-being of the growing-up chick which CAM had been neovascularized and modified in their blood vessel patterns by MAT, as shown in Figure B. Apparently, the endogenous effectors of leucocytes for chemotropism of blood vessels are not noxious agents. The experimentally altered morphogenic patterns of the CAM tissue do not significantly disturb the biological functions in development, birth and later life. CAM is considered as an embryonal "lung" for gas exchange (168, 169). At birth, the CAM tissue is partially rejected and incorporated in the body. No disturbance of this function, too, could be observed in artificially vascularized tissues. Further experimental sets on MAT-induced neovascularization of tissues, the structure, (haemodynamic) function and turnover of MAT-mediated vessel patterns are presented elsewhere (1, 2, 36, 45, 54-57, 145, 194). The preparation of MAT in a highly purified form (Figure 9) and mg-amounts was achieved concomitantly and as given for MMR (Figures 7-10) from biotechnically, serum-free and batchwise cultured (Figures 3-6), concanavalin A-activated porcine leucocytes (about 7 trillions monocytes) (Table 7). Physico-chemically and biologically equivalent MAT-active polypeptide solutes may also be obtained from inflamed tissue sites (Figure 7) in the form of ischaemically injured, infarcted heart muscle as an in-vivo model source. An electrophoretic pattern of this MAT preparation as a criterion of purification is given in Figure 9. Definitions of nomenclature are given in the text.

Table 7. Summary of investigations and results on the biotechnical preparation and characterization of humoral and cellular polypeptide effectors of white blood cells, operating chemical mechanisms for cellular reactions and communication in regenerative tissue morphogenesis with activities basic to functional expressions of the immune, haematopoietic and cardiovascular systems in inflammation and wound healing through autocrine, paracrine (mediator) and endocrine (hormonal) information transmission mechanisms. For the nomenclature, other definitions, biological assays and further necessary techniques see text, Figures 3-13, and references (1, 2, 34, 47, 50, 55-59, 74, 85, 93-99, 101, 102, 144, 145, 167, 190-194).

a. Preparation of at least 1 kilogram (about 2.0 x 10E12) viable leucocytes of a physiologically composed population mixture from a minimum volume of about 200 litres of aseptically drawn, anticoagulated, fresh blood, preferably porcine blood, per day and investigator by a new biotechnical process. Its first step is a one-phase-batch process providing kilogram amounts of peripheral white blood cells in yields of (greater than or equal) 50% within a few hours. Concomitant preparation by the same process of all other blood components in their native state, especially thrombocytes, erythrocytes, and blood plasma in kilogram amounts and at hectolitre scales, respectively, per day and per investigator.

b. Separation of the prepared kilogram amounts of mixed leucocyte population into homogenous cell populations, especially neutrophil, eosinophil and basophil granulocytes, monocytes and lymphocytes by a sequence of further (adsorption-desorption and flotation) steps of the biotechnical process within a few hours.

c. Sterile culture of the kilogram quantities of isolated leucocytes and thrombocytes in bioreactors of ten to fifty litre culture volumes in a new, fully synthetic, serumfree, chemically defined cell culture medium for the production of cellular effectors (cytokines) operating basic chemical mechanisms of cellular reactions and communication in regenerative tissue morphogenesis processes, with activities basic to functional expressions of the haematopoietic and immune system.

d. Twenty- to fifty-fold repetition of processes a) to c) provide from 10 000 litres of blood about fifty kilograms (one hundred trillion) of peripheral leucocytes of a physiological cell population mixture, or, correspondingly, about 29 kilograms (58%) neutrophil, 1.25 kilograms (2.5%) eosinophil and 0.25 kilograms (0.5%) basophil granulocytes, 3.5 kilograms (7%) monocytes (macrophages) and 16 kilograms (32%) lymphocytes.

e. Production, isolation, crystallization and characterization of biologically active, humoral polypeptide effectors of inflammation from the isolated native blood plasma.

f. Production, physical isolation and characterization of biologically active polypeptide cytokine effectors for autocrine, paracrine (mediator) and endocrine (hormonal) information transmission in cellular communication systems: The kilogram amounts of isolated leucocytes and thrombocytes obtained from about 10 000 litres of blood result in appr. 1 000 litres of culture supernatant solution. Then, on average, 1-10 milligram quantities of highly purified, biologically active, reaction- and cell-specific inflammatory polypeptide mediators and wound hormones can be obtained with yields of about 10% by sequences of multiple purification steps. These polypeptide cytokine effectors display their reaction- and cell-specific biological activity above thresholds of picomolar concentrations or femtomol amounts.

g. For the first time, physical (milligram) quantities of at least one representative effector for the specific operation of each of the known basic categories of chemical mechanisms for cellular reactions and communication in regenerative tissue morphogenesis processes can be obtained separately by the biotechnical methods devised. These basic categories of chemical mechanisms are chemopoiesis, chemorecruitment, chemokinesis, chemotaxis, chemotropism and chemostasis of cells and biological units. Biological specificity of action of isolated leucocytic effector polypeptides implies specific mechanisms in signal reception, discrimination and transmission into cellular reactions within the cell and its membrane with which effectors interact.

446

h. "Wound hormones" as a new class of leucocytic effector polypeptides have been shown to exist for the first time. Hence, they substantiate this classical term by chemical objects and biological activities which were missing, so far. In contrast to leucocytic mediators, wound hormones specifically act by endocrine mechanisms of information transmission and conform to hormone definitions. Their existence proves leucocytes as truly unicellular, mobile endocrine glands ("secretory leucocytic tissue"). By their mediators, however, leucocytes may convey information also by autocrine and paracrine mechanisms of transmission for the operation of certain chemical mechanisms of cellular reactions and communication in regenerative tissue morphogenesis processes.

i. Wound hormones comprise novel cytokine entities for classical reactions in pathophysiology, e.g. the leucocytosis and, especially, "leftward shift reactions", i.e., the reactive increase in the number and the band/segmented ratio of circulating leucocyte phenotypes.

j. Molecular properties of mediators (angiotropins) for directional blood vessel sprouting (chemotropism of endothelial cells) suggest a novel mechanism operating the atherogenetic reaction: An endogenous "lesion" in the endothelium of the vessel ("intravascular leaky tip") is formed as a normal biological response in terms of a cellular reaction, i.e. impaired, intravascular sprouting, induced by angiotropins derived from intravascular monocytes. Such a "lesion" ("intravascular leaky tip") is not the response to intrinsic or extrinsic injury of endothelial cells itself, but a physiological, cellular reaction operated by wrong transmission mechanisms of information of the effector system to which cellular reactions and communication in the regenerative morphogenesis of tissues are subjected. Impaired (increased) permeability and perfusion disorders are brought about spot-wise in the asymmetrical endothelium of the vessel by this mechanism as a first step promoting the atherogenetic reaction. The directionally wrong hyperplastic growth of cells intrinsic to this mediator-disordered cellular reaction may be of monoclonal or of polyclonal origin.

k. Highly purified mediators of inflammation and wound hormones are potential models of natural pharmaceuticals whose specificity of action has been selected in evolution.

6.4 Applied nomenclature for effector substances

The nomenclature in use for cells, enzymes and effectors investigated follows existing and agreed nomenclature proposals (1,
2, 34, 148-159, 162-164). In this context, if no agreed nomenclature proposals are in existence, or available nomenclature (163,
164) is not applicable on novel, biologically active effector substances, newly identified mediators and wound hormones are tenta-
tively termed in names composed basically of three syllables. The
fist is derived from the cell producing the effector molecule, as
far as identified. The second is derived from the target cell or
biological unit on which the effector obviously acts, as determined by the biological assay system and the biological specificity of the effector substance. The third syllable qualifies the activity elicited by the effector molecule according to the chemical
mechanism for cellular reactions and communication (1, 2, 34)
which is triggered by the effector. The pre-syllables "apo-" and
"pros-" (Figures 7 and 11) are used according to Rothert (159) to
briefly qualify "negative" and "positive" chemokinetic effects expressed by some of the mediators on cells in terms of their random
locomotion (2, 34, 54, 73, 74, 145, 163). The distinction between
mediators and hormones as used in this context for the effector
substances, is described in (1, 2). It follows proposals on hormone nomenclature (148). Essentially, it considers the different
transmission mechanisms of the information residing in the effector molecules (Figure 1: autocrine, paracrine and endocrine mechanisms).

6.5 Cellular exudation mechanisms of produced cytokines

The exudation or secretion of some of the so far investigated
effector substances into the extracellular medium is obviously induced by a cellular activation reaction, when they are in a steady
state equilibrium in the medium in a measurable amount or concentration. However, as we found (34, 165), in principle, such an activation (e.g. by a polyvalent polypeptide lectin mitogen in the
form of concanavalin A, CON, as the variable, additional component
no.94 to the basic medium, Table 4) is not an absolutely necessary
requirement for cellular formation, exudation or secretion of at
least some of the evaluated effector substances. As far as determined for monocytes and lymphocytes, these leucocyte types secrete
or exude also without activation by a lectin mitogen or a surface
immune reaction some effector entities (monocyto-angiotropin,
monocyto-metamyelo-recruitin, monocyto-leuco-recruitin, monocyto-
granulo-apokinesin, lymphocyto-mono-apokinesin) (Figures 7 and
9-13) (1, 2, 34, 45, 145). However, in contrast to activated leucocytes, resting leucocytes in a reference medium composed of the
first 93 components (Table 4), exude or secrete such effector polypeptides only at a very low rate. The resulting low steady-state

concentration of the biologically active effectors in reference culture solutions and crude fractions thereof, is below the active threshold detectable by normal biological assay systems. The activation reaction at the cell surface potentiates the exudation or secretion rate of the effector molecules. Dependent on the type of the effector polypeptide, its turnover rate and the cell activation process, it results in approximately a 50- to 1 000-fold higher steady-state concentration of these effectors in the extracellular fluid around activated cells with reference to controls (non-activated cells). By this increase, the activities of these effector polypeptides become measurable in crude fractions of the culture supernatant solutions of activated cells and form the basis for the estimates presented in Table 1. Therefore, by analytical variants of, or by the shown biotechnical procedures themselves, in principle, thus, these polypeptide effectors may also be detected by the presented assay systems (Figures 10-13) (1, 2, 145) in reference cultures of non-activated cells, but only after concentration by about 50- to 1 000-fold purification. Therefore, their isolation from activated cell cultures is much more efficient than from non-activated, reference cultures. This phenomenon is independent of whether cells had been isolated from blood of a single animal, or mixed from a number of the same species which might be supposed to induce a low level activation of leucocytes cultured under reference conditions.

My interpretation of these results is (34, 165) that exudation of at least some leucocytic effector entities operating chemical mechanisms for cellular reactions and communication in regenerative tissue morphogenesis, follows mechanisms which correspond, or are similar to mechanisms of quantal neurotransmitter release (166). Hence, exudation or secretion of effector molecules as chemical signals for the organization of the inflammatory and healing processes, multiplies and amplifies the intrinsic cellular activation trigger (mitogenic or immune activation) (2, 34). Preliminary turnover studies with monocyto-angiotropin (Figure 13) and leucotaxin polypeptide cytokines (Figure 12) show (1, 34, 165, 167) that approximately 10E04 to 10E05 activated and secreting cells may already be sufficient to augment the steady-state sub-threshold effector concentration derived from non-activated, biologically "quiescent" cells to high steady-state effector concentrations as they are usually found with activated cells (about 5 000 active molecules per mitotic cell). Such levels may be detected by current assay systems in crude culture fluids. The high steady-state concentration corresponds to about the 2- to 30-fold of the biologically active threshold of an effector substance. This "noise-response" limit in transmission of the information of effector molecules represents about the apparent picomolar concentration or femtomol amount range in which a leucocytic mediator (e.g. monocyto-angiotropin, Figure 13) or wound hormone (e.g. monocyto-metamyelo-recruitin, Figure 10) displays its specific biological activity. However, as far as determined for the turnover of angiotropin, only about 1 of 1 000 of these molecules ex-

uded by the cells into the extracellular fluid into a steady-state
equilibrium actively come to interaction with a target cell. Taken
this relation into consideration, then, a total of about 10E06 molecules monocyto-angiotropin derived from a maximum of 10 to 100
activated (secreting) cells (monocytes) are sufficient to achieve
full expression of the apparent biological activity investigated.
In this case, it is full vascularization of about 0.5 cu.cm tissue
(e.g. cornea surface) (1, 45, 55).

Furthermore, there are humoral serum-derived effectors with
biological activity triggering similar or comparable chemical mechanisms for cellular reactions and communication, as do some
(leucocytic) polypeptide cytokines (e.g. for chemorecruitment and
chemotaxis) (1, 2, 34, 35, 45, 47-50, 54, 73, 74, 93-103). In all
cases, however, polypeptide cytokines have been found different
and distinguishable in their physico-chemical nature from corresponding humoral polypeptide effectors. In addition, different
cell types (e.g. monocytes and granulocytes) may form and exude
different effector polypeptides with biological activity directed
at the operation of comparable mechanisms (Figures 11 and 12) (1,
2, 34, 45, 47-50, 54-59, 70-74, 145-147). This distinguishable nature of effectors originating from the various sources, may allow
leucocytes (or other target cells), when stimulated by them to a
specific (e.g. chemotactic or chemorecruitment) function, to discriminate signals emitted from different sources. Thus, for example, leucocytes may discriminate between finding the direction to
the site of tissue injury through a chemotaxin formed by interaction of intruded foreign matter with plasma components (humoral
chemotaxin), or through a chemotaxin exuded by cellular "colle-
gues" (2, 34, 54, 74, 165, 167).

6.6 Species specificity and clinical usefulness of effectors

As shown in Table 2, highly purified, endogenous effectors of
regenerative tissue morphogenesis may be considered as models of
future natural pharmaceuticals the structure and specificity of
action of which has been selected by evolution. The presently intensified clinical investigations of the treatment of several diseases by available endogenous non-polypeptide and polypeptide effectors of inflammatory and healing processes, such as prostaglandins and interferons, by enzymes and by hormones of endocrine
glands, exemplify natural substances as potential pharmaceuticals
of choice and presumably superior to conventional drugs (35-37,
39-44, 51-53, 90-92, 134, 148, 150, 190-194).

In general, several basic aspects are associated with the
clinical use of a biologically active, natural chemical. Firstly,
specific treatment is a matter of the specificity of action and
the toxicity of a pharmaceutical in use. Secondly, basic to any
clinical application of a specifically acting endogenous substance
is its availability in physical amounts and versatile pharmaceuti-

cal compositions, rather than just as biological activity. For
human use, efficient and economic technical processes are necessary to prepare natural substances of homologous (human) or heterologous structure by one of the technical procedures compiled in
Table 3. Thirdly, in the case of heterologous origin of a biologically active substance, its species specificity and immunological
compatibility in humans has to be evaluated. Fourthly, clinical
application forms and techniques for the natural substance have to
be evaluated.

Concerning the specificity of polypeptide effectors of regenerative tissue morphogenesis, they mostly are reaction and/or cell
specific, and non-toxic natural chemicals. Mostly they are not,
and, if so, only to a limited extent, species-specific in their
action. This becomes quite evident from the biotechniques shown in
Figures 10-13, and in other papers (1, 2, 35, 36, 57, 93-102). In
general, species specificity may depend (at least) on two terms:
namely the maximum magnitude of the effect itself expressed by a
biological reaction, one one hand, and/or the threshold concentration of the activity displayed by an effector substance, on the
other hand.

Comparison of biological effects in homologous and heterologous assay systems in some cases may show differences. If at
all, they mostly are obvious rather in terms of a varying threshold concentration than in terms of a strong variation of the
maximum magnitude of the effect itself (59, 96, 98, 99, 101). Exceptions from this rule have also been suggested, e.g. for interferons (43, 44). So far, in this respect, in general, inflammatory
mediators and wound hormones of polypeptide structure share properties with respect to species-non-specificity in common with effector substances of non-polypeptide nature and with hormones of
different structural classes produced by known endocrine glands.
Thus, e.g. insulin as a polypeptide hormone, when isolated from
porcine or bovine pancreas, or other synthetic derivatives, having
a primary structure different from human insulin (195), also are
biologically active in humans with similar or even the same magnitude of effect. However, their threshold concentrations of activity significantly vary by several orders of magnitudes (195). If
thresholds for an effector activity expressed in homologous and
heterologous systems are not too different, a comparable magnitude
of the effect may be apparent in heterologous and homologous systems as well with crude extracts and fractions thereof. For highly
purified effectors with a threshold for activity in the picomolar
concentration range, therefore, small species differences may be
balanced even over a range of two orders of magnitude of their
concentration, since augmenting the concentration mostly does not
provoke side effects as is the case for crude extract. Thus, until
recently, insulin of heterologous origin exclusively served for
medical treatment of diabetes in humans.

Similar considerations hold for the potential use of polypeptide effectors of regenerative tissue morphogenesis of heterologous and homologous origin for diagnostic and therapeutic pur-

poses in medical care of humans. As for insulin of heterologous origin, the application fields and potential clinical usefulness of some of the highly purified effectors of regenerative tissue morphogenesis (pesented in this and other papers: 1, 2, 34, 47-50, 54-59, 70-74, 85, 93-103, 145-147) have been demonstrated (35, 190-193). A number of further potential applications of the presently known effector substances of heterologous origin have been suggested (50, 57, 58, 73, 97, 100, 102); in particular from experimental investigations of neovascularization of muscles (1, 36), embryonic tissue (1, 2,) (Figure 13) and skin (194). Since the homologous (human) effectors are not available, the porcine effectors derived from the large scale techniques and biotechniques (as described in this paper) offer the possibility of initiating such investigations.

6.7 Efficiency of the applied biotechniques

The development of new alternative biotechnical procedures (Table 3) might, in the future, additionally provide an economic production mode for sufficient amounts of some effector substances preferably of human origin. Presently practized classical biotechnical method is indispensable: Firstly, novel, so far unknown natural compounds may be elaborated only by means of the classical procedure applied either to animal or human cells or tissue. Secondly, only this method provides an approach to the elaboration of the structure and mode of action of human polypeptide cytokines as it also allows the comparison of their differences to equivalents of animal sources. Nevertheless, worth of consideration is also the favourable cost-effect relationship of the presented classical biotechnical procedure devised for the preparation of physical amounts of higly purified, biologically active effector substances of the inflammatory and healing process: in Table 8, such a cost-effect relationship of the method is compiled, as far as the procedure is practized in a scientific-technical laboratory under normal working conditions. The calculated example may be met by a highly purified polypeptide mediator like monocyto-angiotropin: With one application unit of less than 100 fmol, about 0.5 - 1.0 cu.cm of tissue may be fully neovascularized, as shown for different tissues (1, 2, 36, 194).

About 8-10 mg of this cytokine can be obtained in highly purified form from about 1.000 l supernatant solutions of cultures of about 50 kg (10E14) leucocytes composed of a physiologically mixed population (Table 7) or, correspondingly, of about 3.5 kg (about 7.0 x 10E12) isolated monocytes. Therefore, about 10E5 to 10E7 of such application units may be obtained, including the inevitable loss of material during its handling. Each of these application units can be prepared by the presently practized biotechnical procedure for a value in the range of a cent, when derived from animal cells, or of a dollar, when derived from human cells.

ECONOMY OF PRODUCTION OF EFFECTOR MOLECULES
BY THE CLASSICAL BIOTECHNICAL PROCEDURE

A. EFFECTOR MOLECULE ($\sim$5'000 DALTON) WITH
   OPTIMUM EFFECT AT $\sim^{\leq}$ 100 FMOL.

B. $\sim$10 MG SUBSTANCE YIELDS $\sim 10^5$ - $2 \cdot 10^7$
   ACTIVE APPLICATION UNITS.

C. $\sim$10 MG SUBSTANCE ARE OBTAINED FROM 10 TONS
   OF BLOOD (ABOUT 100 TRILLIONS OR 50 KG
   LEUKOCYTES).

D. 4 INVESTIGATORS MAY PRODUCE 1 SUBSTANCE,
   10 INVESTIGATORS MAY PRODUCE 8 SUBSTANCES
   WITHIN 2 YEARS.

E. 1 INVESTIGATOR, ENERGY AND MATERIALS
   COST 200'000,-- DM PER YEAR.

F. ONE APPLICATION UNIT OF 1 SUBSTANCE
   (8 SUBSTANCES) DERIVED FROM PORCINE BLOOD
   COSTS 0.08 - 16,-- DM (0.025 - 5,-- DM).

Table 8. Economy and efficiency of production and preparation of a set of endogenous polypeptide cytokine effector substances of regenerative tissue morphogenesis by the applied large scale and biotechnical procedures as they are practiced under conditions of a scientific-technical laboratory.

This calculation shows that the devised classical biotechnical process as practiced presently for the preparation of clinically useful amounts of natural substances, has also unsurpassing premises for the future. It is at least competitive to any alternative process yet to consider realizable (Table 3). In addition, it is one of its outstanding features that its costs do not linearly increase with the number of perceivable, natural effector substances of the inflammatory and healing process to be prepared consecutively or concurrently in the future: The process becomes the more economic, the larger the number of effector substances is which are isolated from the same starting lot of blood, or of cultured cells.

453

7.0   CONCLUSIONS: EFFECTOR VARIETY AND INFORMATION NETWORK

Evaluation of the possibly existing variety of   effector
substances   triggering   chemical mechanisms for cellular
reactions   and   communication   in   regenerative   tissue
morphogenesis by inflammation and wound healing:

The first evaluation of several   leucocytic   wound   hormones,
and of at least one representative of a leucocytic polypeptide effector substance as specific trigger for each basic category of so
far   known chemical mechanisms for cellular reactions and communication in regenerative tissue morphogenesis   through   inflammation
and   healing   processes, prompts the question as to the variety of
effector substances which possibly exist for the operation of   the
biological   (effector)   information   network   of the various cells
within interactive tissues of the body (1, 2, 34, 54). An estimate
as   to how many effectors might exist to achieve an organized formation of the different types of morphogenic patterns   (1,   2)   in
regenerative   growth,   is not available so far. From my viewpoint,
however, an estimate of this possibly existing variety may be made
by the following approach:
In a higher (mammalian) organism, about 100   types   of   cells
can be distinguished. (168, 169). For their cellular reactions and
communication in the organization   of   the   different   morphogenic
patterns   (1,   2),   they provide themselves with specific instructions within the control circuits of the information networks discussed   elsewhere   (1,   2,   34, 99) for the effector system. These
chemical instructions concern the six basic categories of chemical
mechanisms, with about 20 first subgroups taken into consideration
(1, 2), for the organization of the cellular reactions and communication   in   regenerative morphogenesis processes. Supposedly only
4 effector types with specific information   should   be   minimally
sufficient   in   a simple control circuit, consisting of activation
and (negative) feedback regulation (inhibition); and all are   suggested   to be equally likely. Then, roughly about 10E04 (cell- and
reaction-specific) different necessary signals, for example, types
of the effector molecules, result from this estimate on an average
under the constraints given. According to the   basic   theorems   of
the   information   theory   (170-172) which apply to the function of
signalling devices and information networks, a maximum information
I = log(2)10E04   (2) and about 13.3 bits per specific response can
be calculated. This probably too low estimate has been made   under
the   constraints   that cross-reactivity does not reduce the amount
of information transmitted   in   the   effector   network   system   to
achieve   organization   of regenerative tissue morphogenesis by inflammation and wound healing. If,   further,   intensity   parameters
(gradients,   boundaries,   etc.)   and   other information increments
(compartmentation, etc.) (2)   are   included   in   this   estimate   to
which the variety of effectors are constrained in the transmission
of their information (Figure 1), a maximum   information   of   25-30
bits per specific response may be appreciated (1, 54).

Accordingly, following one of the basic theorems of the information theory (170), the reliable conveyance of information in a signalling device (2) requires that the entropy of the signal source or the channel input of the device, cannot exceed the entropy of the transmission channel itself (1,2). In addition, for the effective control of a given system, the "law of requisite variety" (173) was derived for neuronal control mechanisms from the fundamental theorems of information theory (170). It says that a controller has to generate at least as much variety, as the controlled system does itself. This means for regenerative tissue morphogenesis by inflammation and healing processes, and for the chemical mechanisms to which their intrinsic cellular reactions and communication processes are subjected, that adequate control is obtained only, when the variety generated by the effector system meets at least the variety inherent in the pattern formation processes in regenerative morphogenesis. It means, too, that variety is not obtained by cross-reactivity, since information is lost by this reaction. Cross reactive effectors cannot replace the needs for a variety of biologically highly specific types of the effector molecule. From this rough estimate of the probably existing, but not yet elucidated variety of effector molecules, I may draw at least several conclusions:

Firstly, the effector information network of the immune, haematopoietic and other tissue systems which triggers chemical mechanisms for cellular reactions and communication for the organized regenerative tissue morphogenesis through inflammation and healing, should be as similarly complex, as the information network of the immune system itself. The "information network" of the immune system has been estimated to have an information - entropy in the range of 30 bits per response (174). Comparably, my estimate resulted in 25-30 bits per response for information - entropy of the effector network system, when maximum information is to be reliably transmitted. Hence the effector system is similarly complex, as the catalyst (enzyme) system of biological metabolism. About 10 000 enzymes are known to exist, so far (162).

Secondly, polypeptide structures may be considered superior in having intrinsic properties for the generation of the variety of specific chemical signals (effectors) necessary to trigger the chemical mechanisms for cellular reactions and communication to which organized pattern formation and changes in regenerative tissue morphogenesis are confined. Therefore, probably a larger portion of effector substances of the inflammatory and healing processes with specific activity are more likely to be of a polypeptide nature than of any other structure. Furthermore, for intrinsic biological specificity of action, polypeptide effectors should have more than three normal amino acids in sequence. The roughly estimated number (about 10E04) of specific chemical signals necessary under the given constraints, was made for a simply controlled cellular signalling device. A peptide composed of at least 4 amino acids, and, thus having an average molecular weight of about 500, should represent the minimum size for a highly specific chemical signal. The maximum variability possible for such a peptide is 20E04, or approximately 160 000 different tetrapeptides. Thus, it exceeds the estimated variety of necessary chemical signals (effectors) as a specific trigger of chemical mechanisms for cellular reactions and communication in the organization of regenerative tissue morphogenesis. In contrast, such variability for a tripeptide (20E03) would be somewhat lower than the estimated necessary variety. Therefore, tripeptides operative as effectors should be expected to have less biological specificity of action. These facts also influence the choice of performance of ultrafiltration on membranes with nominal exclusion limits for molecular weights of about 500 for quantitative processing and evaluation of effector types produced by leucocytes (Figure 8) upon culture in a serum-free, fully synthetic, chemically defined medium (Tables 4 and 5, Figures 3-7).

Thirdly, the estimate of about 10 000 different effector molecules is probably too low. The uncertainty concerning this present estimate is not surprising. Thus, for example, knowledge of the chemistry and biophysics of the control of cellular cooperation in the macrophage-lymphocyte system, in leucocyte differentiation and maturation in the bone marrow, or in situations which lead to changes in vascular patterns in their interaction with the host muscle tissue, is still very fragmentary. The total number and properties are yet uncertain. The number which was evaluated from the same basic viewpoints as the number of possibly existing immunoglobulin molecules has been realised (174), and nature has evolved them by the generation of variety. Thus, for comparison, 43 hormone structures were already isolated in 1960 from the cortex of the adrenal gland. Only seven of them were active hormones (46). Finally, it is of basic interest whether or not entities like iso-effectors produced by one and the same types of cells exist, comparable to isoenzymes with a low activity; or whether or not genetic variants of effectors may be evaluated. So long as the majority of mediator and wound hormone entities are unknown and the mechanisms by which the variety of existing types of cells intercommunicate is unknown, the scientific basis for the regenerative morphogenesis processes will remain obscure.

Fourthly, from the estimate of effector variety, it is conceivable that, additionally to the already (about 100) known ones, a large number of further effector entities exist which have not been considered yet. Hence, essential to an aproach to the full understanding of the formation or change of tissue patterns in regenerative (and, thus, also degenerative) morphogenesis by inflammation with (or without) a consecutive healing process (or for the understanding why sometimes such reactions may fail to occur), is the identification and characterization of novel effector entities with specific biological activity triggering chemical mechanisms of cellular reactions and communication. For this purpose, various techniques for the production and preparation of effector molecule types are needed as a prerequisite to this approach. It is a necessity to learn what nature - or the white blood cells as the

456

basic part of the body's system of defense and regenerative morphogenesis (1, 2, 34, 168, 169, 175) - already know: That is, how to achieve the formation of new life-compatible tissue patterns at sites of damaged tissue.

Acknowledgements

The author thanks Prof. Dr. H.P. Jennissen for his cooperation and hospitality in his laboratories at the Institutes of Physiological Chemistry of the Universities of Bochum and Munich, in particular in performing electrophoresis experiments (Figures 2 and 9), after a flood affected the town of Bad Nauheim in August 1981, and destroyed large parts of our laboratories and transiently abrogated our experimental work. I owe special appreciation to Mr. Helmut Renner who put all his efforts in helping the reconstructing of the laboratories, and for his expert assistance in the performance of the experimental work. I am very grateful to Dr. E. Logeman, University of Freiburg, Germany, for his numerous discussions, recommendations, and general assistance concerning trace analytics with which he contributed to this work.

SUMMARY

Some principles in the culturing of cells and criteria of useful media are evaluated. The preparation and properties of a novel serum-free, fully synthetic, component-rich medium are described. Its chemical definition has been approached. In addition to usual components of cell culture media, in its basic composition of 91 constituents, it contains also three unsaturated fatty acids bound to serum albumin, a flavanoid, one ubiquinone, vitamin U, mevalolactone, carnosine and carnitine, and some otherwise unusual combinations of further basic substances. The medium contains no serum or any other undefined biological fluid. However, its composition comprises one defined protein which is highly purified, molecularly homogenous, natural serum albumin. Most of the components are equilibrated in their concentration ratios according to their normal plasma or serum content as an in-vivo model of a physiological fluid. Primarily, this basic medium has been designed for maintenance of cells, not for cellular activation. However, for purposes of stimulating cells, it may be supplemented by further chemically defined, variable additional or alternative constituents for directing cells to express distinct functions. The cell culture medium has been proven suitable for culturing some eukariontic cells, in particular such of the immune, haematopoietic and cardiovascular systems (leucocytes, fibroblasts, endothelial and heart muscle cells). Its usefulness will be shown in serial analytical assay and large scale work inherent to biotechnical preparation and culturing (of up to kilogram or trillion quantities) of peripheral leucocytes; and isolation of their secretory products in the form of some polypeptide effector substances (cytokine mediators and hormones) as minute trace components present in (milligram amounts in cubic metres of) culture supernatant solutions. In special consideration are leucocytic polypeptide cytokines with activities basic to functional expressions of the immune, haematopoietic and cardiovascular systems in inflammation and wound healing. These effectors specifically operate chemical mechanisms for cellular reactions and communication for organized renewal of tissue patterns in regenerative morphogenesis through autocrine, paracrine (mediator) and endocrine (hormonal) information transmission mechanisms. The possibly existing secretion or exudation mode and variety of these effector substances upon cellular activation, and basic problems intrinsic to their preparation in terms of presently available technical procedures and culture conditions, are evaluated. Isolated effectors for intercellular communication are exemplified in the form of monocytic mediators for chemotaxis and chemokinesis of leucocytes, chemotropism of blood vessel (endothelial) cells; and of monocytic (wound) hormones for the chemorecruitment of specific phenotypes of leucocytes, providing first a chemical basis for leftward shift with or without leucocytosis reactions in the regulation of blood cell patterns.

REFERENCES

1. Wissler J.H.: Inflammatory mediators and wound hormones: Chemical signals for differentiation and morphogenesis in tissue regeneration and healing. In: Proc. 33th Mosbach Colloquium 1982: Biochemistry of Differentiation and Morphogenesis, edited by L. Jaenicke, pp.257-274. Springer Verlag, Heidelberg, 1982.
2. Wissler J.H.: Inflammatory effectors and mechanisms of information processing for cellular reactions and communication in regenerative tissue morphogenesis by leucocytes: Chemical signalling in poiesis, recruitment, kinesis, taxis, tropism and stasis of cells. Chapter 4, this book, pp.41-102.
3. Diem K. and C. Lentner (Eds.): Documenta Geigy. Wissenschaftliche Tabellen, 7th Ed. J.R. Geigy SA, Basel, 1968.
4. Fox C.H. and K.K. Sanford: Chemical analysis of mammalian sera commonly used as supplements for tissue culture media. In: Tissue Culture Association Manual, Vol.1, edited by Tissue Culture Association, pp.233-237. Rockville Maryland, 1975.
5. Paul J. (Ed.): Cell and Tissue Culture, 5th Ed. Churchill Livingstone, Edinburgh, 1975.
6. Kruse jr. P.F. and M.K. Patterson jr. (Eds.): Tissue Culture. Methods and Applications. Academic Press, New York, 1973.
7. Morton H.J.: A survey of commercially available tissue culture media. In Vitro 6:89-108, 1970.
8. Rechcigl jr., M. (Ed.): Culture Media for Cells, Organs and Embryos. CRC Press, Boca Raton, Florida, 1977.
9. Rizzino A., H. Rizzino and G. Sato: Defined media and the determination of nutritional and hormonal requirements of mammalian cells in culture. Nutr. Rev. 37:369-378, 1979.
10. Higuchi K.: Cultivation of animal cells in chemically defined media, a review. Adv. Appl. Microbiol. 16:111-136, 1973.
11. Sato G. and L. Reid: Replacement of serum in cell culture by hormones. In: Biochemistry and Mode of Action of Hormones, Part.II, Int. Rev. Biochem., Vol.20, edited by H.V. Rickenberg, University Park Press, Baltimore, pp.219-251, 1978.
12. Barnes D. and G. Sato: Growth of a human mammary tumor cell line in a serum-free medium. Nature 281:388-389, 1979.
13. Hayashi I. and G.H. Sato: Replacement of serum by hormones permits growth of cells in a defined medium. Nature 259:132-134, 1976.
14. Iscove N.N. and F. Melchers: Complete replacement of serum by albumin, transferrin, and soybean lipid in cultures of lipopolysaccharide-reactive B lymphocytes. J. Exp. Med. 147:923-933, 1978.
15. Maciag T., B. Kelley, J. Cerundolo, S. Ilsley, P.R. Kelley, J. Gaudreau and R. Forand: Hormonal requirements of baby hamster kidney cells in culture. Cell Biol. Int. Rep. 4:43-50, 1980.

16. Allegra J.C. and M.E. Lippman: Growth of a human breast cancer cell line in serum-free hormone-supplemented medium. Cancer Res. 38:3823-3829, 1978.
17. Stanley E.R., R.E. Palmer and U. Sohn: Development of methods for the quantitative in vitro analysis of androgen-dependent and autonomous Shionogi carcinoma 115 cells. Cell 10:35-44, 1977.
18. Takaoka T. and H. Katsuta: Long-term cultivation of mammalian cell strains in protein- and lipid-free chemically defined synthetic media. Exp. Cell Res. 67:295-304, 1971.
19. Donta S.T.: The growth of functional rat glial cells in a serumless medium. Exp. Cell Res. 82:119-124, 1973.
20. Florini J.R. and S.B. Roberts: A serum-free medium for the growth of muscle cells in culture. In Vitro 15:983-992, 1979.
21. Holmes R., G. Mercer and N. Mohamed: Studies of alpha-protein in human cell cultures. In Vitro 15:522-530, 1979.
22. McKeehan W.L., K.A. McKeehan, S.L. Hammond and R.G. Ham: Improved medium for clonal growth of human diploid fibroblasts at low concentrations of serum protein. In Vitro 13:399-416, 1977.
23. Hamilton W.G. and R.G. Ham: Clonal growth of chinese hamster cell lines in protein-free media. In Vitro 13:537-547, 1977.
24. Golde D.W. and M.J. Cline: Cultivation of normal and neoplastic human bone marrow leucocytes in liquid suspension. In: Proc. 7th Leucocyte Culture Conf. Manoir Richelieu 1972, edited by F. Daguillard, Academic Press, New York, pp.3-13, 1973.
25. Chen J.M.: The cultivation in fluid medium of organised liver, pancreas and other tissues of foetal rats. Exp. Cell Res. 7:518-529, 1954.
26. Morgan J.F., H.J. Morton and R.C. Parker: Nutrition of animal cells in tissue culture. I. Initial studies on a synthetic medium. Proc. Soc. Exp. Biol. Med. 73:1-8, 1950.
27. Waymouth C.: Rapid proliferation of sublines of NCTC clone 929 (strain L) mouse cells in a simple chemically defined medium (MB 752/1). J. Natl. Cancer Inst. 22:1003-1017, 1959.
28. Gey G.O. and M.K. Gey: The maintenance of human normal cells and tumor cells in continuous culture. I. Preliminary report: Cultivation of mesoblastic tumors and normal tissue and notes on methods of cultivation. Am. J. Cancer 27: 45-76, 1936.
29. Lembeck F. and D. Winne (Eds.): Pharmakologisches Praktikum. Georg Thieme Verlag, Stuttgart, 1965.
30. Hallmann L. (Ed.): Klinische Chemie und Mikroskopie, 11th ed. Georg Thieme Verlag Stuttgart, 1980.
31. Glassman A.B., R.S. Rydzewski and C.E. Bennet: Trace metal levels in commercially prepared tissue culture media. Tissue and Cell 12: 613-617, 1980.
32. Monod J., J. Wyman and J.-P. Changeux: On the nature of allosteric transitions: A plausible model J. Mol. Biol. 12:88-118, 1965.

460

33. Monod J., J.-P. Changeux and F. Jacob: Allosteric proteins and cellular control systems. J. Mol. Biol. 6:306-329, 1963.

34. Wissler J.H.: Entzuendungsmediatoren: Chemische Anlockung, Motilitaetsbeeinflussung und molekulare Mechanismen biologischer Nachrichtenuebertragung bei der Ansammlung von Leukozyten. Forschungsberichte aus Technik und Naturwissenschaften 3: 10, pp.1-36. Technische Informationsbibliothek Hannover 06A 2154, Physik Verlag, Weinheim, 1982.

35. Burdach St.E.G., K.G. Evers and J.H. Wissler: Infantile genetische Agranulozytose (IGA). Leukorecrutin im diagnostisch-therapeutischen Versuch (Diagnostic-therapeutic trial in infantile genetic agranulocytosis with leucorecruitin). Monatsschr. Kinderheilkd. 130:789-791, 1982.

36. Gottwik M., H. Renner and J.H. Wissler: Biochemical neovascularization of muscles by leukocyte-derived polypeptide effectors: Morphogenesis and turnover of blood vessel patterns with active hemodynamics in vivo. Z. Physiol. Chem. 363:938-939, 1982.

37. Feder J. and W.R. Tolbert: The large-scale cultivation of mammalian cells. Scientific American 248:36-43, 1983.

38. Jakoby W.B. and I.H. Pastan (Eds.): Cell culture. Meth. Enzymol. 58:3-590, 1979.

39. Praeve P., U. Faust, W. Sittig and D.A. Sukatsch (Eds.): Handbuch der Biotechnologie. Akademische Verlagsgesellschaft, Wiesbaden, 1982.

40. Haemmerling G.J., U. Haemmerling and J.F. Kearney (Eds.): Research Monographs in Immunology, Vol.3: Monoclonal Antibodies and T-Cell Hybridomas. Elsevier - North Holland, Amsterdam, 1981.

41. Chakrabarty A.M. (Ed.): Genetic Engineering. CRC Press, Boca Raton, Florida, 1978.

42. Beers jr., R.F., and E.G. Bassett (Eds.): Miles Int. Symp., Series 12: Polypeptide Hormones. Raven Press, New York, 1980.

43. Stewart II, W.E. (Ed.): The Interferon System. Springer Verlag, Wien, 1979.

44. Friedman R.M. (Ed.): Interferons. A Primer. Academic Press, New York, 1981.

45. Wissler J.H.: Biotechnik der Gewinnung leukozytaerer Entzuendungsmediatoren und Wundhormone. In: BMFT-Statusseminar: T-ierische Zellkulturen, Juelich 1981, edited by Bundesministerium fuer Forschung und Technologie (BMFT), pp.293-303. Projekttraeger Biotechnologie Kernforschungsanlage, Juelich, 1982.

46. Fieser L. and M. Fieser (Eds.): Lehrbuch der organischen Chemie, 3rd. Ed., Verlag Chemie, Weinheim, pp.1145-1160, 1960.

47. Wissler J.H., H. Renner, U. Gerlach and A.M. Wissler: Inflammation, cell mitosis and differentiation signals: Novel hormones in homeostatic regulatory mechanisms of hematopoiesis and left shift recruitment of leucocytes. Z. Physiol. Chem. 362:244-245, 1981.

48. Wissler J.H., H. Renner, U. Gerlach, M. Gottwik and A.M. Wissler: Cell division, differentiation signals and chemo-recruitment of leucocytes: Isolation of novel monokine and leucocyte-derived hormones ("leuco- and metamyelorecruitins") regulating homeostasis of hematopoiesis and left shift of white blood cells in circulation and at tissue repair sites. Immunbiology 159:121-122, 1981.
49. Wissler J.H., H. Renner, F. Bodzian, U. Gerlach and A.M. Wissler: Chemorecruitment of leukocytes (leucocytosis and leftward shift reactions): A novel class of leukocyte-derived leukopoietin hormones and their biotechnical preparation and purification. Exp. Hematol. 9, Suppl. 9:35, 1981.
50. Wissler J.H.: Chemorecruitins of leukocytes and inflamed tissues: A new class of natural leukopoietin proteins for chemo-recruitment of specific leukocyte types from the bone marrow into blood circulation (leukocytosis and leftward shift reactions), process for their biotechnical preparation and pharmaceutical compositions. Eur. Pat. Publ. EP 0 061 140 A2 Bull. 82/39, DOS DE 31 10 561 Al, pp.1-72. Max-Planck-Gesellschaft zur Foerderung der Wissenschaften, Muenchen, 1982.
51. Wuensch E., L. Moroder, M. Gemeiner, E. Jaeger, A. Ribet, L. Pradayrol and N. Vaysse: Totalsynthese von Somatostatin-28 (Big-Somatostatin). Z. Naturforsch. 35b:911-919, 1980.
52. Wuensch E.: Synthese von Peptid-Naturstoffen: Problematik des heutigen Forschungsstandes. Angew. Chem. 83:773-782, 1971.
53. Gattner, H.G., G. Krail, W. Dahno, R. Knorr, H.J. Wieneke, E.E. Buellesbach, B. Schartmann, D. Brandenburg and H. Zahn: Eine verbesserte Methode der Kombination von Insulinketten zur Darstellung von Insulinanalogen. Z. Physiol. Chem. 362:1043-1049, 1981.
54. Wissler J.H. and H. Renner: Specific polypeptide mediators and wound hormones of monocytes: Leukopoiesis, leukocytosis, leukopenia, leftward shift reactions, leukokinesis, leukotaxis, angiogenesis, and fever. Immunobiology 162:438. Abstr. Commun. 5th Eur. Immunol. Meeting, Istanbul 1982, p.45, 1982.
55. Wissler J.H. and H. Renner: Inflammation, chemotropism and morphogenesis: Novel leucocyte-derived mediators for directional growth of blood vessels and regulation of tissue neovascularization. Z. Physiol. Chem. 362:244, 1981.
56. Wissler J.H.: A novel, biologically specific chemotropic blood vessel growth factor ("monocyto-angiotropin") derived from monocytes. Immunobiology 160:131-132, 1981.
57. Wissler J.H. and W. Schaper: Angiotropins of leukocytes and inflamed tissue: A new class of natural chemotropic protein mitogens for specific induction of directional growth of blood vessels, neovascularization of tissues and morphogenesis of blood vessel patterns, process for their biotechnical preparation and pharmaceutical compositions. Eur. Pat. Publ. EP 0 061 138 A2 Bull. 82/39, DOS DE 31 10 560 Al, pp.1-64. Max-Planck-Gesellschaft zur Foerderung der Wissenschaften, Muenchen, 1982.

462

58. Wissler J.H.: Mitogens of leukocytes and inflamed tissue: Natural leukopoietin proteins for specific induction of proliferation and differentiation of leukocytes, process for their biotechnical preparation and pharmaceutical compositions. Eur. Pat. Publ. EP 0 061 139 A2 Bull. 82/39, DOS DE 31 10 611 Al, pp.1-64. Max-Planck-Gesellschaft zur Foerderung der Wissenschaften, Muenchen, 1982.

59. Neumeier R., H.R. Maurer, M. Arnold, U. Gerlach, K. Glendinning, H. Renner and J.H. Wissler: Identification of two granulocyte/macrophage colony-stimulating factors from porcine leukocyte cultures. Z. Physiol. Chem. 363:193-195, 1982.

60. Sebrell jr., W.H. and R.S. Harris (Eds.): The Vitamins. Chemistry, Physiology, Pathology, Vol.1-3. Academic Press, New York, 1954.

61. Rauen H.M. (Ed.): Biochemisches Taschenbuch, Part 1 and 2. Springer Verlag, Heidelberg, 1964.

62. Edelman G.M. (Ed.): Cellular Selection and Regulation in the Immune Response. Soc. Gen. Physiol. Ser., Vol.29. Raven Press, New York, 1974.

63. Sober H.A. (Ed.): Handbook of Biochemistry. Selected Data for Molecular Biology. CRC The Chemical Rubber Co., Cleveland, Ohio, 1970.

64. Porzio M.A. and A.M. Pearson: Improved resolution of myofibrillar proteins with sodium dodecyl sulfate - polyacrylamide gel electrophoresis. Biochem. Biophys. Acta 490:27-34, 1977.

65. LKB (Ed.): Ultrogel. Vorgequollenes Polyamid-Agarose Gel fuer die hochaufloesende Gelfiltration. LKB 2204-T01, Uppsala, 1977.

66. Merck E. (Ed.): Diagnostica Merck: Extrelut. Neues Verfahren zur Extraktion lipophiler Stoffe. E. Merck 24/825/10/677D, Darmstadt, 1977.

67. Donike M., W. Hollmann and D. Stratmann: Qquantitative gaschromatographische Bestimmung von gesaettigten und ungesaettigten Fettsaeuren als Trimethylsilyester. J. Chromatog. 43:490-492, 1969.

68. Melcher F. and E. Renner: Untersuchungen ueber Minorfettsaeuren des Milchfettes: 1. Zur gaschromatographischen Analyse von Minorfettsaeuren. Milchwissenschaft 31:70-76; 2. Minorfettsaeuren in Humanmilch. Milchwissenschaft 31:193-199, 1976.

69. Kannan R., A. Rajiah, M.R. Subbaram and K.T. Achaya: Analysis of some hydroxy fatty compounds as their trimethylsilyl ethers by gas-liquid chromatography. J. Chromatog. 55:402-404, 1971.

70. Maurer H.R., M. Kastner, R. Maschler, R. Neumeier, M. Arnold, U. Gerlach, K. Glendinning, B. Pfefferkorn and J.H. Wissler: Biotechnologische Isolierung und Charakterisierung von Poetinen und Chalonen der Granulopoese. Z. Physiol. Chem. 362:221, 1981.

71. Maurer H.R., M. Kastner, R. Maschler and J.H. Wissler: Isolation and some properties of a specific granulopoiesis inhibitor (chalone) from bovine and porcine leukocytes. Exp. Hematol. 9, Suppl. 9: 34, 1981.
72. Wissler J.H., H.R. Maurer, M. Kastner, R. Maschler, R. Neumeier, M. Arnold, U. Gerlach, B. Pfefferkorn, H. Tschesche and W. Schaper: Lymphokines, monokines, leucokines: Large scale production, isolation and properties of porcine leucocyte-derived cytotaxins, cytokinesins, cytotoxins, mitogens, stimulators (CSF) and inhibitors (chalones) of colony formation. Eur. J. Cell Biol. 22:387, 1980.
73. Wissler J.H.: Chemokinesins and chemotaxins of leukocytes and inflamed tissues: Natural mediator proteins for reversible promotion of random and directional locomotion (chemokinesis and chemotaxis) for accumulation of specific leukocyte types, process of their biotechnical preparation and pharmaceutical compositions. Eur. Pat. Publ. EP 0 061 141 A2 Bull. 82/39, DOS DE 31 10 610 Al, pp.1-82. Max-Planck-Gesellschaft zur Foerderung der Wissenschaften, Muenchen, 1982.
74. Wissler J.H., M. Arnold, U. Gerlach and W. Schaper: Leukocyte-derived protein hormones for tissue repair (lympho-, mono- and leucokines): Large scale production, isolation and properties of cell-derived cytotaxins, cytokinesins, cytotoxins and mitogens. Z. Physiol. Chem. 361:351-352, 1980.
75. Wissler J.H.: Fully synthetic cell culture medium. Eur. Pat. Publ. EP 0 060 565 A2 Bull. 82/38, DOS DE 31 10 559 Al, pp.1-27. Max-Planck-Gesellschaft zur Foerderung der Wissenschaften, Muenchen, 1982.
76. Allison A.C. (Ed.): Structure and Function of Plasma Proteins. Plenum Press, New York, 1975.
77. Bradshaw R.A. and J.S. Rubin: Polypeptide growth factors: Some structural and mechanistic considerations. J. Supramol. Struct. 14: 183-199, 1980.
78. Bottenstein J., I. Hayashi, S. Hutchings, H. Masui, J.Mather, D.B. McClure, S. Ohasa, A. Rizzino, G. Sato, G. Serrero, R. Wolfe and R. Wu: The growth of cells in serum-free hormone-supplemented media. Meth. Enzymol. 58:94-109, 1979.
79. Ham R.G. and W.L. McKeehan: Media and growth requirements. Meth. Enzymol. 58:44-93, 1979.
80. Jamieson G.A. and T.J. Greenwalt (Eds.): Trace Components of Plasma: Isolation and Clinical Significance. Progr. Clin. Biol. Res., Vol.5. Alan R. Liss, New York, 1976.
81. Wissler J.H.: Fluidity (microviscosity) of surface lipid hydrocarbon layers of membranes of chemokinetically and chemotactically stimulated neutrophil polymorphonuclear leucocytes. Z. Physiol. Chem. 359:339-340, 1978.
82. Wissler J.H.: Mode of action of chemotactic and chemokinetic solutes and physical properties of membranes of neutrophil leukocytes in relation to cellular recognition in chemotaxis and locomotion in chemokinesis. Z. Physiol. Chem. 359:1167-1168, 1978.

464

83. Wissler J.H. and E. Logemann: Biological memory and meta-
    stable membrane states associated with recognition and infor-
    mation processing in directional locomotion (chemotaxis) of
    leukocytes. Z. Physiol. Chem. 360:1204-1205, 1979.
84. Wissler J.H., H.P. Jennissen and H.U. Keller: Regulation of
    cellular transport of lipid-hydrocarbon molecules and of cel-
    lular contact phenomena of viable adherent leucocytes by
    serum albumin. Z. Physiol. Chem. 359:1462, 1978.
85. Keller H.U., J.H. Wissler, M.W. Hess and H. Cottier: Distinct
    chemokinetic and chemotactic responses in neutrophil granulo-
    cytes. Eur. J. Immunol. 8:1-7, 1978.
86. Warburg O. and F. Kubowitz: Stoffwechsel wachsender Zellen
    (Fibroblasten, Herz, Chorion). Biochem. Z. 189:242-250, 1927.
87. Keller H.U., G. Gerisch and J.H. Wissler: A transient rise in
    cyclic AMP levels following chemotactic stimulation of neu-
    trophil granulocytes. Cell Biol. Int. Rep. 3:759-765, 1979.
88. Wissler J.H., V.J. Stecher and E. Sorkin: Cyclic AMP and che-
    motaxis of leukocytes. In: Proc. Conf. Cyclic AMP, Cell
    Growth and the Immune Response, Marco Islands Florida 1973,
    edited by W. Braun, L.M. Lichtenstein and C.W. Parker,
    pp.270-283. Springer Verlag, New York, 1974.
89. Meissl H., C.S. Donley and J.H. Wissler: Free amino acids and
    amines in the pineal organ of the rainbow trout (Salmo gaird-
    neri): Influence of light and dark. Comp. Biochem. Physiol.
    61C:401-405, 1978.
90. Belz G.G., K.O. Vollmer and J.H. Wissler: Zur Hemmwirkung von
    Herzglykosiden auf die 86-Rb-Aufnahme der Erythrozyten:
    I. Methodische Untersuchungen zur Konzentrationsbestimmung
    von Cymarin und Digitoxin. Eur. J. Clin. Pharmacol. 4:92-98,
    1972.
91. Vollmer K.O., J.H. Wissler and G.G. Belz: Zur Hemmwirkung von
    Herzglykosiden auf die 86-Rb-Aufname der Erythrozyten:
    II. Spezifitaet der Hemmwirkung unter besonderer Beruueck-
    sichtigung der Cymarin-Reihe. Eur. J. Clin. Pharmacol.
    4:99-103, 1972.
92. Wissler J.H., Belz G.G. and K.O. Vollmer: Zur Hemmwirkung von
    Herzglykosiden auf die 86-Rb-Aufnahme der Erythrozyten:
    III. Ueber die Beeinflussbarkeit der durch Cymarin bewirkten
    86-Rb-Aufnahmehemmung der Erythrozyten. Eur. J. Clin. Pharma-
    col. 4:104-106, 1972.
93. Wissler J.H.: A new biologically active peptide system relat-
    ed to classical anaphylatoxin. Experientia 27:1447-1448,
    1971.
94. Wissler J.H.: Chemistry and biology of the anaphylatoxin-
    related serum peptide system. I. Purification, crystalliza-
    tion, and properties of classical anaphylatoxin from rat
    serum. Eur. J. Immunol. 2:73-83, 1972.
95. Wissler J.H.: Chemistry and biology of the anaphylatoxin-
    related serum peptide system. II. Purification, crystalliza-
    tion, and properties of a new basic peptide, cocytotaxin,
    from rat serum. Eur. J. Immunol. 2:84-89, 1972.

465

96. Wissler J.H., V.J. Stecher and E. Sorkin: Chemistry and biology of the anaphylatoxin-related serum peptide system. III. Evaluation of leukotactic activity as a property of a new peptide system with classical anaphylatoxin and cocytotaxin as components. Eur. J. Immunol. 2:90-96, 1972.
97. Wissler J.H., V.J. Stecher and E. Sorkin: Biochemistry and biology of a leucotactic binary serum peptide system related to anaphylatoxin. Int. Arch. Allergy 42:722-747, 1972.
98. Wissler J.H., V.J. Stecher and E. Sorkin: Regulation of chemotaxis of leucocytes by the anaphylatoxin-related peptide system. In: Proc. 20th Coll. Protides of the Biological Fluids, Brugge 1972, edited by H. Peeters, pp.411-416. Pergamon Press, Oxford, 1973.
99. Wissler J.H.: Evaluation and action of biological mediators generated from normal serum by interaction with foreign macromolecules. In: Proc. Immunosymp. Wien 1973: Gram-negative Bacterial Infections and Mode of Endotoxin Actions; Pathophysiological, Immunological and Clinical Aspects, edited by B. Urbaschek, R. Urbaschek and E. Neter, pp.91-105. Springer Verlag, Wien, 1975.
100. Wissler J.H.: A process for producing and obtaining anaphylatoxin- and cocytotaxin-containing leukotaxin preparations and anaphylatoxin and cocytotaxin proteins in molecularly homogeneous, biologically active form. Eur. Pat. Publ. EP 0 042 560 A2 Bull. 81/52, DOS DE 30 22 914 A1, pp.1-53. Max-Planck-Gesellschaft zur Foerderung der Wissenschaften, Muenchen, 1981.
101. Wissler J.H., B. Pfefferkorn, K. Rother, U. Rother, L. Schramm, H. Renner, H. Renker, A.M. Wissler and W. Schaper: Inflammation and the leukocytosis reaction: Purification, crystallization and properties of a serum-derived protein mediator with bone marrow leukocyte-mobilizing activity. Z. Physiol. Chem. 361:1358, 1980.
102. Wissler J.H.: Serum-derived "Leukorecruitin": A protein mediator of inflammation from mammalian serum for specific induction of a leukocytosis reaction, a process for its biotechnical production and isolation in molecularly homogeneous, crystallizable, biologically specific, active form, and leukorecruitin-containing pharmaceutical compositions. Eur. Pat. Spec. EP 0 047 979 B1 Bull. 82/12, Courier Press, Leamington, Spa, pp.1-48; German Patent DE 30 34 529 C2. Max Planck Gesellschaft zur Foerderung der Wissenschaften, Muenchen, pp.1-44, 1982.
103. Logemann E. and J.H. Wissler: Humoral polypeptide mediators of inflammation (leukorecruitin, anaphylatoxin, cocytotaxin): Homogeneity criteria and separation of identified nutrition pollutants as companion products present in blood. Z. Physiol. Chem. 363:939-940, 1982.
104. Tanford C. (Ed.): The Hydrophobic Effect. Formation of Micelles and Biological Membranes, 2nd Ed. Wiley-Interscience, New York, 1980.

466

105. Rosenoer V.M., M. Oratz and M.A. Rothschild (Eds.): Albumin Structure, Function and Uses. Pergamon Press, Oxford, 1977.
106. ASTM (Ed.): Standard Specification for Reagent Water D-1193-70. Annual Book of ASTM Standards 1970. ASTM, Easton Maryland, 1970.
107. Kenyon R.L. (Ed.): Reagent Chemicals. Suppl.1, 4th Ed. American Chemical Society Publications, Washington D.C., 1969.
108. Stier A.P., L.K. Miller and R.J. Smith (Eds.): Reagent Water, Specifications and Methods of Quality Control. College of American Pathologists (CAP) Comission on Laboratory Inspection and Accreditation, Skokie, Illinois, 1971.
109. Millipore Corporation Bedford Massachusetts (Ed.): Milli-Q-Systems for High Purity Water. Bull. MB 414. Millipore Corporation, Bedford, 1973.
110. Millipore Corporation Bedford Massachusetts (Ed.): Super-Q-System. Bull. MB 403. Millipore Corporation, Bedford, 1972.
111. Millipore Corporation Bedford Massachusetts (Ed.): Pellicon Membrane Casette Systems for Molecular Filtration. Bull. PB 802/DM 130. Millipore Corporation, Bedford, 1975.
112. Organikum: Organisch-chemisches Grundpraktikum, 13th Ed. VEB Verlag der Wissenschaften, Berlin, 1974.
113. Kratky O., H. Leopold and H. Stabinger: Dichtemessungen an Fluessigkeiten und Gasen auf 10E-06 g/cu.cm bei 0.6 cu.cm Praeparatvolumen. Z. Angew. Physik 4:273-277, 1969.
114. Bauer N., K. Fajans and S.Z. Lewin: Refractometry. In: Techniques of Organic Chemistry, Vol.1, Part 2: Physical Methods of Chemistry, edited by A. Weissberger. Wiley-Interscience, New York, 1960.
115. Amicon (Ed.): Concentrating, Desalting, Separating Solutions and Suspensions. Application Manual Publication no.427. Amicon Technical Library, Oosterhout Holland, 1977.
116. Keller H.U., J.H. Wissler and B. Damerau: Diverging effects of chemotactic serum peptides and synthetic f-Met-Leu-Phe on neutrophil locomotion and adhesion. Immunology 42:379-383, 1981.
117. Keller H.U., J.H. Wissler, M.W. Hess and H. Cottier: Relation between stimulus intensity and chemotactic response. Experientia 33:534-536, 1977.
118. Keller H.U., J.H. Wissler and J. Ploem: Chemotaxis is not a special case of haptotaxis. Experientia 35:1669-1671, 1979.
119. Keller H.U., J.H. Wissler, M.W. Hess and H. Cottier: Chemokinesis and chemotaxis of phagocytes. In: Proc. 1st. Eur. Conf. Biochemistry of Phagocytes, Trieste 1976: Movement, Metabolism, and Bactericidal Mechanisms of Phagocytes, edited by F. Rossi, P.L. Patriarca and D. Romeo, pp. 15-20. Piccin Medical Books, Padova, 1977.
120. Gawthorne J.M., J.McC. Howell and C.L. White: Trace Element Metabolism in Man and Animals. Springer Verlag, Berlin, 1982.

121. Kevander O.A. and L. Cheng (Eds.): Micronutrient Interactions. Vitamins, Minerals and Hazardous Elements. Ann. N.Y. Acad. Sci. 355:1-372, 1980.
122. Sarkar B. (Ed.): Biological Aspects of Metals and Metal-Related Diseases. Raven Press, New York, 1983.
123. Merck E. (Ed.): Merck Standards. E. Merck, Darmstadt, 1971.
124. Jander G. and E. Blasius (Eds.): Lehrbuch der analytischen und praeparativen anorganischen Chemie. S. Hirzel Verlag, Stuttgart, 1966.
125. Mueller G.O. (Ed.): Praktikum der quantitativen chemischen Analyse, 6th Ed. S. Hirzel Verlag, Stuttgart, 1962.
126. Holmsen H.: Secretable storage pools in platelets. Annu. Rev. Med. 30:119-134, 1979.
127. Good N.E. and S. Izawa: Hydrogen ion buffers. Meth. Enzymol. 24:53-68, 1972.
128. Papper S (Ed.): Sodium: Its Biological Significance. CRC Press, Boca Raton, Florida, 1982.
129. Aikawa J.K. (Ed.): Magnesium: Its Biological Significance. CRC Press, Boca Raton, Florida, 1981.
130. Anghileri L.J. and A.M. Tuffet-Anghileri (Eds.): The Role of Calcium in Biological Systems, Vol.1-3. CRC Press, Boca Raton, Florida, 1982.
131. Briggs M.H. (Ed.): Vitamins in Human Biology and Medicine. CRC Press, Boca Raton, Florida, 1981.
132. Rechcigl jr. M. (Ed.): Nutritional Disorders, Vol.1-3. CRC Press, Boca Raton, Florida, 1978.
133. Rechcigl jr. M. (Ed.): Nutritional Requirements, Vol.1: Comparative and Qualitative Requirements. CRC Press, Boca Raton, Florida, 1977.
134. Voelter W. and G. Jung (Eds.): 0-(beta-Hydroxyethyl)-rutoside - Experimentelle und klinische Ergebnisse. Springer Verlag, Berlin, 1978.
135. Middleton jr. E., G. Drzewiecki and D. Krishnarao: Quercetin: An inhibitor of antigen-induced human basophil histamine release. J. Immunol. 127:546-550, 1981.
136. Jenissen H.P.: The binding and regulation of biologically active proteins on cellular interfaces: Model studies of enzyme adsorption on hydrophobic binding site lattices and biomembranes. Adv. Enzyme Regulation 19:377-406, 1981.
137. Jennissen H.P., J.H. Wissler, G. Botzet and W. Schaper: Phosphorylase kinase from dog skeletal muscle. Z. Physiol. Chem. 361:275-276, 1980.
138. McLaren A.D. and L. Packer: Some aspects of enzyme reactions in heterogeneous systems. Adv. Enzymol. 33:245-308, 1970.
139. Mustard J.F. and M.A. Packham: Factors influencing platelet function: Adhesion, release, and aggregation. Pharmacol. Rev. 22:97-187, 1970.
140. Prasad A.S. (Ed.): Zinc in Human Nutrition. CRC Press, Boca Raton, Florida, 1979.
141. Burrows D. (Ed.): Chromium: Metabolism and Toxicity. CRC Press, Boca Raton, Florida, 1983.

142. Ozawa H., K. Momose and Y. Koseki: Effect of ubiquinone on respiration of cultured cells. Yakugaku Zasshi 89:1604-1612, 1969.

143. Cartaya O.A.: Serum-free cell culture medium, pp.1-10. United States Patent 4,205,126, Washington, 1978.

144. Wissler J.H.: Process for obtaining intact and viable leucocytes and thrombocytes from blood. United States Patent 4,343,793, pp.1-10. Max-Planck-Gesellschaft zur Foerderung der Wissenschaften, Washington, 1981.

145. Wissler J.H.: Cellular Communication in tissue morphogenesis by leukocytes: Methods for biotechnical preparation of cultures, mediators and wound hormones of leukocytes for chemopoiesis, chemorecruitment, chemokinesis, chemotaxis, chemotropism and chemostasis of cells. Proc. 1st World Conf. on Inflammation, Venezia 1984, Bioscience Ediprint, Geneva, in press.

146. Wissler J.H., H. Renner, B. Pfefferkorn, M. Gottwik and A.M. Wissler: Inflammation, cell division and differentiation: Infarct-associated mediators for cardiac tissue repair and description of a novel monokine. Biochem. Soc. Trans. 9:257P, 1981.

147. Wissler J.H., M. Gottwik, H. Renner, H.H. Klein, U. Gerlach, A.M. Wissler, R. Schuurmans and W. Schaper: Inflammation, chemotropisms and morphogenesis: Isolation of novel monokine and leukocyte-derived protein mediators ("angiotropins") for a directional angiogenesis reaction from cell cultures and infarcted heart muscle sites. Fed. Proc. 40:1638, 1981.

148. Karlson P.: Was sind Hormone? Der Hormonbegriff in Geschichte und Gegenwart. Naturwissenschaften 69:3-14, 1982.

149. Boggs D.R.: Homeostatic regulatory mechanisms of hematopoiesis. Annu. Rev. Physiol. 28:39-56, 1966.

150. Whipple H.E., M.I. Spitzer and H.R. Bierman (Eds.): Leukopoiesis in Health and Disease. Ann. N.Y. Acad. Sci. 113:511-1092, 1964.

151. Schilling V. (Ed.): Das Blutbild und seine klinische Verwertung (mit Einschluss der Tropenkrankheiten). Gustav Fischer Verlag, Jena, 1929.

152. Mathy K.A. and J.A. Koepke: The clinical usefulness of segmented vs. stab neutrophil criteria for differential leukocyte counts. Amer. J. Clin. Pathol. 61:947-958, 1974.

153. Peirson E.L.: Hematology problem of the month: Band or seg? Amer. J. Med. Technol. 42:288-296, 1976.

154. Committee for Clarification of the Nomenclature of Cells and Diseases of the Blood and Blood Forming Organs (Ed.): First Report. Amer. J. Clin. Pathol. 18:443-450, 1948.

155. College of American Pathologists (Ed.): Quality Evaluation Program (1970-1978). College of American Pathologists, Skokie, Illinois, 1978.

156. Begeman H. and J. Rastetter (Eds.): Atlas of Clinical Hematology, 3rd. Ed. Springer Verlag, Berlin, 1979.

157. Schulten H. (Ed.): Lehrbuch der klinischen Haematologie. Georg Thieme Verlag, Stuttgart, 1948.
158. Eur. Vortragsreihe (Europarat) no.50: Pruefung auf Pyrogene. Eur. Arzneibuch (Eur. Pharmacopoeia), Vol.2, pp.56-59. Deutscher Apotheker-Verlag, Stuttgart, 1975.
Medicine Commission, Medicine Act: I. Test for Pyrogens. Brit. Pharmacopoeia, Appendix XIV I, p.A115. Her Majesty's Stationery Office, London, 1973.
The United States Pharmacopeia,19th revision: Pyrogen Test. United States Pharmacopeial Convention USP, p.613. Rockville, Maryland, 1975.
159. Rothert W.: Beobachtungen und Betrachtungen ueber taktische Reizerscheinungen. Flora 88:371-421, 1901.
160. Rich A.R. and M.R. Lewis: The nature of allergy in tuberculosis as revealed by tissue culture studies. Bull. Johns Hopkins Hosp. 50:115-131, 1932.
161. Keller H.U., J.H. Wissler, B. Damerau, M.W. Hess and H. Cottier: The filter technique for measuring leucocyte locomotion in vitro. Comparison of three modifications. J. Immunol. Meth. 36:41-53, 1980.
162. Nomenclature Committee of the International Union of Biochemistry (Ed.): Enzyme Nomenclature 1978. Recommendations of the Nomenclature Committee of the IUB on the Nomenclature and Classification of Enzymes. Academic Press, New York, 1979.
163. Letter to the Editor: A proposal for the definition of terms related to locomotion of leukocytes and other cells. J. Immunol. 121:2122-2124, 1978.
164. Letter to the Editor: Revised nomenclature for antigen-non-specific T cell proliferation and helper factors. J. Immunol. 123:2928-2929, 1979.
165. Wissler J.H.: Cellular communication between leucocytes: Production from large scale cultures, isolation and properties of leucocyte-derived cytotaxins, cytokinesins, cytotoxins and mitogens. Abstr. Commun. 2nd Eur. Conf. Biochemistry of Phagocytes, p.5. Trieste, 1980.
166. Katz B.: Quantal mechanism of neural transmitter release. Science 173:123-126, 1971.
167. Wissler J.H. and M. Arnold: Large scale production, isolation and characterization of pig leucocyte-derived activities (lymphokines) affecting random migration (chemokinesis) and directional locomotion (chemotaxis) of neutrophil, eosinophil and mononuclear leucocytes. Z. Immun.-Forsch.-Immunobiology 157:301-302, 1979.
168. Bloom W. and D.W. Fawcett: Textbook of Histology, 10th Ed. W.B. Saunders Company, Philadelphia, 1975.
169. Stark D. (Ed.): Embryologie. Ein Lehrbuch auf allgemein biologischer Grundlage, 3rd. Ed. Georg Thieme Verlag, Stuttgart, 1975.
170. Shannon C.E. and V. Weaver (Eds.): The Mathematical Theory of Communication. University of Illinois Press, Chicago, 1949.

470

171. Brillouin L. (Ed.): Science and Information Theory. Academic Press, New York. 1962.
172. Khinchin A.I. (Ed.): Mathematical Foundations of Information Theory. Dover Publications, New York, 1957.
173. Ross Ashby W. (Ed.): An Introduction to Cybernetics. Chapman and Hall, London, 1956.
174. Ebringer A.: Information theory and limitations in antibody diversity. J. Theoret. Biol. 51:293-302, 1975.
175. Cline M.J. (Ed.): The White Cell. Harvard University Press, Cambridge, Massachusetts, 1975.
176. Boeyum A.: Separation of leucocytes from blood and bone marrow. Scand. J. Clin. Lab. Invest. 21, Suppl.97:1-109, 1968.
177. Day R.P.: Basophil leucocyte separation from human peripheral blood: a technique for their isolation in high purity and high yield. Clin. Allergy 2:205-212, 1972.
178. Shortman K., N. Williams, H. Jackson, P. Russel, P. Byrt and E. Diener: The separation of different cell classes from lymphoid organs. IV. The separation of lymphocytes from phagocytes on glass bead columns, and its effect on subpopulations of lymphocytes and antibody-forming cells. J. Cell. Biol. 48:566-579, 1971.
179. Rabinowitz Y.: Separation of lymphocytes, polymorphonuclear leukocytes and monocytes on glass columns, including tissue culture observations. Blood 23:811-828, 1964.
180. Noble P.B. and J.H. Cutts: Isolation of individual leukocyte types from peripheral blood. J. Lab. Clin. Med. 72:533-538, 1968.
181. Day R.P.: Eosinophil cell separation from human peripheral blood. Immunology 18:955-959, 1970.
182. Gleich G.J. and D. Loegering: Selective stimulation and purification of eosinophils and neutrophils from guinea pig peritoneal fluids. J. Lab. Clin. Med. 82:522-528, 1973.
183. Pellegrino M.A., S. Ferrone and A.N. Theofilopoulos: Isolation of human T and B lymphocytes by rosette formation with 2-aminoethylisothiouronium bromide (AET)-treated sheep red blood cells and with monkey red blood cells. J. Immunol. Meth. 11:273-279, 1976.
184. Albrechtsen D., B.G. Solheim and E. Thorsby: Serological identification of five HLA-D associated (Ia-like) determinants. Tissue Antigens 9:153-162, 1977.
185. Chess L., R.P. MacDermott and S.F. Schlossman: Immunologic functions of isolated human lymphocyte subpopulations. I. Quantitative isolation of human T ad B cells and response to mitogens. J. Immunol. 113:1113-1121, 1974.
186. Albertsson P.-A.: Partition of cell particles and macromolecules in polymer two-phase systems. Adv. Protein Chem. 24:309-341, 1970.
187. Albertsson P.-A., B. Andersson, C. Larsson and H.-E. Akerlund: Phase partition - A metod for purification and analysis of cell organelles and membrane vesicles. Meth. Biochem. Analysis 28:115-150, 1982.

188. Walter H., E.J. Krob and G.S. Ascher: Separation of lympho-
     cytes and polymorphonuclear leukocytes by countercurrent dis-
     tribution in aqueous two-polymer phase systems. Exp. Cell
     Res. 55:279-283, 1969.
189. Thorsby E. and A. Bratlie: A rapid method for preparation of
     pure lymphocyte suspensions. In: Histocompatibility Testing,
     edited by P.I. Terasaki, pp.655-656. Munksgaard, Copenhagen,
     1970.
190. Burdach St.E.G., K.G. Evers and J.H. Wissler: Specific induc-
     tion of leukocytosis reactions in humans by highly purified,
     serum-derived leukorecruitin and their diagnostic value. Im-
     munobiology 160:13-14, 1981.
191. Burdach St.E.G., J.H. Wissler and K.G. Evers: Evaluation of
     neutropenia with maturation stage-specific chemorecruitins.
     Abstr. Commun. 4th Eur. Meeting Plasma Proteins in Clinical
     Diagnosis, p.24, Milano 1983.
192. Burdach St.E.G., J.H. Wissler, K.G. Evers and E. Godehardt:
     Evaluation of neutropenia with a maturation stage-specific
     chemorecruitin. Res. Clin. Lab. 1984 (in press).
193. Burdach St.E.G., K.G. Evers and J.H. Wissler: Recruitment of
     different maturation stages of polymorphonuclear granulocytes
     from human bone marrow by specific polypeptide effectors for
     leukocytosis and leftward shift reactions. In: Proc. Int.
     Symp.: Peptide Hormones as Mediators in Immunology and Oncol-
     ogy, Celle 1983, edited by R.-D. Hesch. Academic Press, New
     York, 1984 (in press).
194. Hoeckel M., W. Wagner, H. Renner and J.H. Wissler: Chemotro-
     pic morphogenesis of new blood vessel patterns with active
     hemodynamics in rabbit by monocyto-angiotropin: Evidence for
     resulting tissue hyperfunctions (hair growth). Z. Physiol.
     Chem. 364:1146-1147, 1983.
195. Maerki F., M. De Gasparo, K. Eisler, B. Kamber, B. Riniker,
     W. Rittel and P. Sieber: Synthesis and biological activity of
     seventeen analogues of human insulin. Z. Physiol. Chem.
     360:1619-1632, 1979.
196. Berne R.M.: Cardiac nucleotides in hypoxia. Possible role in
     regulation of coronary blood flow. Amer. J. Physiol.
     204:317-322, 1963.
197. Drury A.N. and A. Szent-Gyoergyi: The physiological activity
     of adenine compounds with special reference to their action
     upon mammalian heart. J. Physiol. (London) 68:213-226, 1929.
198. Beckman-Spinco (Ed.): J-21 Elutriator Rotor for Separation of
     Cells and Large Particles in an Isotonic Medium. Technical
     Bulletin DS-125, 4SP64802-472-4P. Beckman Instruments, Palo
     Alto, 1972.
199. McEwen C.R., E.Th. Juhos, R.W. Stallard, J.V. Schnell, W.A.
     Siddiqui and Q.M. Geiman: Centrifugal elutriation for the re-
     moval of leukocytes from malaria-infected monkey blood.
     J. Parasitol. 57:887-890, 1971.

INDEX